Anal Fistula

Herand Abcarian

Editor

Anal Fistula

Principles and Management

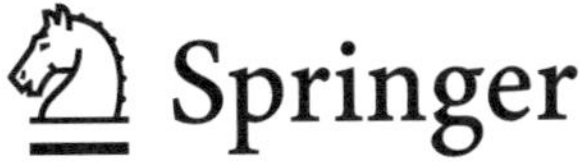 Springer

Editor
Herand Abcarian, M.D., F.A.C.S.
Professor of Surgery
The University of Illinois at Chicago
Chairman, Division of Colon and Rectal Surgery
John Stroger Hospital of Cook Country
Chicago, IL, USA

ISBN 978-1-4939-5362-2   ISBN 978-1-4614-9014-2 (eBook)
DOI 10.1007/978-1-4614-9014-2
Springer New York Heidelberg Dordrecht London

Printed on acid-free paper

Springer is part of Springer Science+Business Media (www.springer.com)

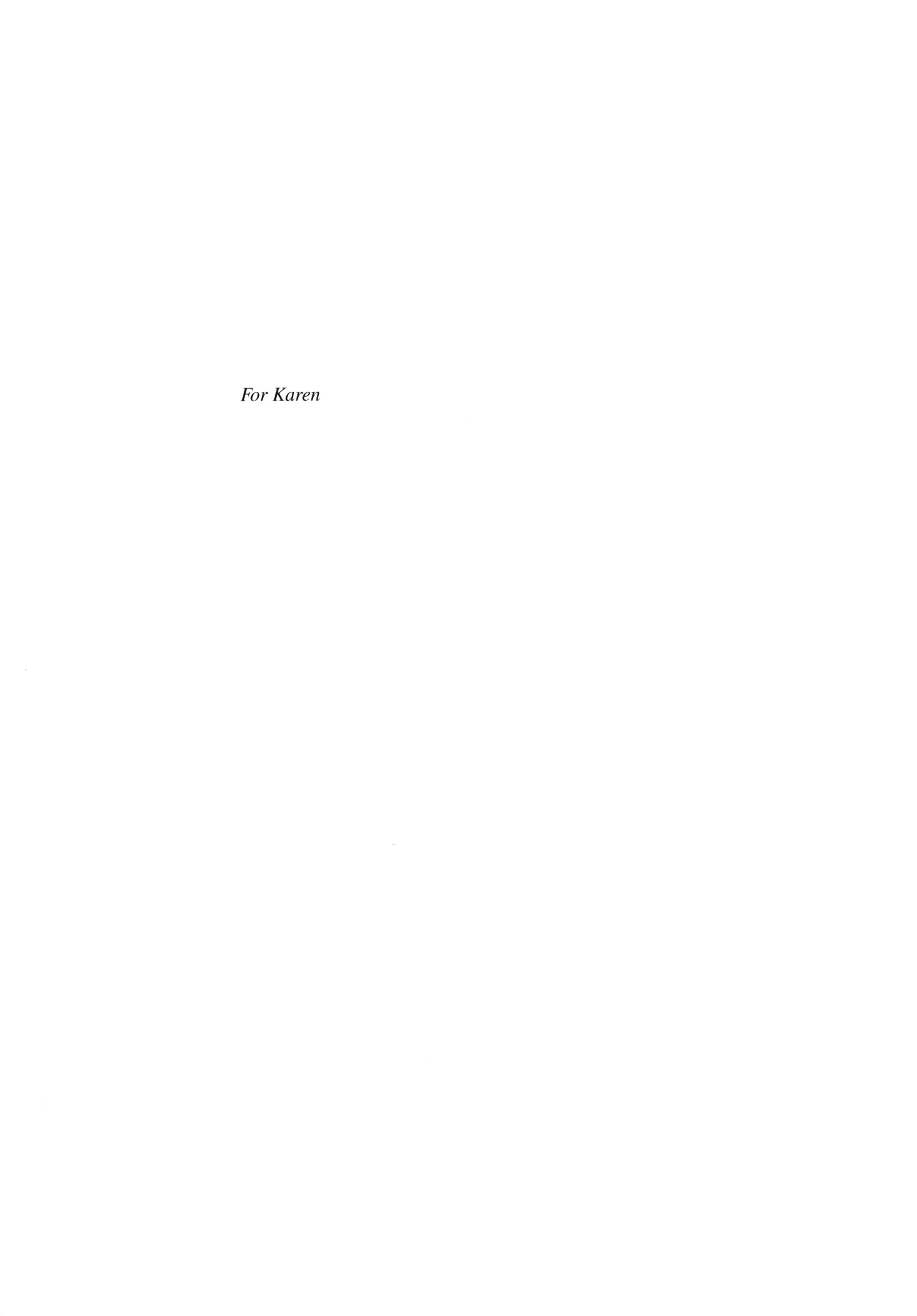

For Karen

Foreword

Anal abscess and fistula have been a scourge of civilization for centuries. Hippocrates offered a treatise on fistula in ancient Greece. In the 1300s John of Arderne, considered by many to be the father of modern British surgery, was notorious for his successful treatment of fistulas in Knights of the Round Table. King Louis XIV of France suffered from a famous chronic fistula that gave rise to the use of a cutting seton in the1600s. Frederick Salmon in 1854 opened in downtown London the St. Mark's Hospital for Fistula and other Diseases of the Rectum. This institution is considered to be the birthplace of modern colon and rectal surgery. To this institution Dr. Joseph Mathews traveled to study anal surgery and returned to Louisville, Kentucky, to establish the first Department of Proctology in the United States, applying the knowledge gained at St. Mark's. Dr. Mathews was the first American surgeon to limit his practice to anorectal surgery and went on to become a founder of the American Proctologic Association (the precursor of the American Society of Colon and Rectal Surgeons) and its first president. Consistent among these historical developments is the clinicopathologic entity of anal fistula.

Despite the relatively high frequency of this disease, treatment remains controversial primarily because of the risk of incontinence after surgery. As a result, alternate operative procedures and other palliative adjuncts that control infection without sacrificing muscle continue to evolve. Increasingly sophisticated diagnostic evaluation and imaging studies have resulted in an increasing array of possible treatments, including in some instances a return to more basic fistula operations.

This volume on anal fistula is, to my knowledge, the most recent and comprehensive reference for this disease, including even a discussion of the use of stem cells. The contributors are all experienced clinicians; this lends immeasurable credibility to each of their chapters. Of equal or greater importance is the experience and expertise of the editor. As a result, we are presented with an invaluable resource to assist in the diagnosis and treatment of a historically challenging problem.

Boston, MA, USA   David J. Schoetz Jr., M.D.

Preface

It is almost 2 decades since the publication of the last book dedicated solely to fistula in ano by Phillips and Lunniss [1]. Since then the readers interested in management of fistula in ano have had to search the textbooks of Surgery and Colon and Rectal Surgery for relevant information. The need for a more recent book dedicated to fistula in ano arises from the proliferation of sphincter sparing procedures which have dominated the colon and rectal surgery literature since the mid 1990s.

This volume represents a compilation of many chapters dealing with alternatives in sphincter sparing surgery as well as traditional fistulotomy. In addition, basic topics such as applied anatomy, relationship of anorectal abscess and fistulas, clinical assessment, and current imaging modalities have been covered. The most recent developments include the use of adipose-derived stem cells in the treatment of anal fistula, video-assisted anal fistula treatment (VAAFT), and ligation of intersphincteric fistula tract (LIFT).

In addition to incidence and prevalence, causes of operative failures, fistula surgery in the era of evidence-based medicine, as well as alternative approaches to fistulas which recur despite all therapeutic measures are also addressed in this volume.

It is impossible to have a multi-author book and not have any redundancy among chapters. However, the repetition if any, within the context of the covered topics, in my opinion, is a plus rather than a distraction.

It is my hope that this volume will be a useful companion for the interested surgeon and will be a source of reference for many alternative treatments of this frustrating disease.

Chicago, IL, USA   Herand Abcarian, M.D., F.A.C.S.

Reference

Phillips RK, Lunniss PJ, editors. Anal fistula: surgical evaluation and management. London: Hodder Education; 1995.

Contents

Contributors

Herand Abcarian, M.D., F.A.C.S. The University of Illinois at Chicago, Division of Colon and Rectal Surgery, John Stroger Hospital of Cook Country, IL, USA

Maher Aref Abbass, M.D., F.A.C.S., F.A.S.C.R.S. Department of Surgery, Kaiser Permanente, Los Angeles, CA, USA
Center for Minimally Invasive Surgery, Los Angeles Medical Center, Los Angeles, CA, USA

Mohammad Ali Abbas, M.D. Department of Surgery, Kaiser Permanente, Los Angeles Medical Center, Los Angeles, CA, USA

Ariane M. Abcarian, M.D. Department of Surgery, University of Minnesota, Chicago, MN, USA

José R. Cintron, M.D., F.A.C.S., F.A.S.C.R.S. Division of Colon and Rectal Surgery, John H. Stroger Jr. Hospital of Cook County, Chicago, IL, USA

Kyle G. Cologne, M.D. Clinic Tower, Los Angeles, CA, USA

Samuel Eisenstein, M.D. Department of Surgery, Mount Sinai School of Medicine, New York, NY, USA

James Fleshman, M.D., F.A.C.S., F.A.S.C.R.S. Department of Surgery, Baylor University Medical Center, Dallas, TX, USA

Ross Fraser, C.I.S.S.P., I.S.S.A.P. Sextant Corporation, Toronto, ON, Canada

Damian Garcia-Olmo, M.D., Ph.D. Colorectal Surgery Unit, La Paz University Hospital, Universidad Autonoma de Madrid, Madrid, Spain

Hector Guadalajara-Labajo, M.D. Colorectal Surgery Unit, La Paz University Hospital, Universidad Autonoma de Madrid, Madrid, Spain

Alexander Herold, M.D., Ph.D. Deutches End-und Dickdarm-Zentrum Mannheim, Mannheim, Germany

Pravin Jaiprakash Gupta, MS, F.I.C.A., F.I.C.S., F.A.I.S., F.A.S.C.R.S. Fine Morning Hospital and Research Center, Nagpur, India

Christine C. Jensen, M.D., M.P.H. Department of Surgery, University of Minnesota, St. Paul, MN, USA

Alex Jenny Ky, B.A., M.D. Department of Surgery, Mount Sinai School of Medicine, New York, NY, USA

Piercarlo Meinero, M.D. Department of General Surgery, Sestri Levante Hospital, ASL 4 Chiavarese, Sestri Levante, Genova, Italy

Enrique Montaño-Torres, M.D. Clinica Especializada en Colon, Recto y Ano (CECRA) and Hospital General Regional de Iztapalapa, Mexico DF, Mexico

Lorenzo Mori, M.D. Department of General Surgery, Sestri Levante Hospital, ASL 4 Chiavarese, Sestri Levante, Genova, Italy

Alero T. Nanna, B.S., M.D. Department of Surgery, Mount Sinai School of Medicine, New York, NY, USA

Richard L. Nelson, M.D., F.A.C.S. Northern General Hospital, Herr Road Sheffield, South Yorkshire, UK

Adrian E. Ortega, M.D. Clinic Tower, Los Angeles, CA, USA

Russell K. Pearl, M.D., M.S. (Surg.) Division of Colon and Rectal Surgery, University of Illinois at Chicago, Chicago, IL, USA

Robin K.S. Phillips, M.B.B.S., M.S., F.R.C.S. St. Mark's Hospital, London, UK

Michael Polcino, M.D. Department of Surgery, Mount Sinai Hospital, New York, NY, USA

Rachel Tay, M.D. Department of Surgery, Baylor University Medical Center, Dallas, TX, USA

Philip Tozer, M.B.B.S., M.D. (Res.), M.R.C.S., M.C.E.M. St. Mark's Fistula Research Unit, St. Mark's Hospital, London, UK

Vamsi R. Velchuru, M.B.B.S., F.R.C.S. (Edin.), F.R.C.S. (Gen. Surg.) Department of General Surgery, James Paget University Hospitals Foundation Trust, Yarmouth, Norfolk, UK

Juan Antonio Villanueva-Herrero, M.D. Clinica Especializada en Colon Recto y Ano (Cecra) and Hospital General de Mexico, Mexico City, Mexico

Epidemiology, Incidence and Prevalence of Fistula in Ano

Richard L. Nelson and Herand Abcarian

Incidence

Anorectal fistulas have been the subject of medical and lay literature for over 2,500 years. The term fistula is ascribed to John Arderne (1307–1392) whose classic work on anal fistula is still in print. However, it is important to note that in Ayurvedic medicine, Suhruta (b ~800 BC) described both fistulotomy and fistulectomy as well as the chemical seton using Kshara Sutra [1]. Hippocrates (b ~460 BC) described the use of horsehair (seta) in the treatment of anal fistulas. Fistulas have been written about in many languages and geographical locations throughout the years [2–4]. The true incidence of anal fistulas is unknown.

Most publications on anal fistula reflect the authors' experience, some quite large, from a single institution [4–6]. This, however, does not address the incidence of the disease due to the lack of proper denominator. Also it is difficult, if not impossible, to accurately assess the incidence of anorectal abscess because so many drain spontaneously or are incised and drained in a surgeon's office, emergency department or surgicenter. On the other hand, hospital discharges or formal operations in the operation rooms are usually recorded and are available for statistical evaluation. Thus among the 1,000 patients presented to the Surgical Section of the Diagnostic Clinic at the University of Virginia, 150 had anorectal pathology, 4 (0.4 %) had an abscess and 8 (0.8 %) had fistula. This is quite comparable to 532 fistulas treated in a population of 77,372 patients admitted to Brooklyn Hospital between 1930 and 1939 for an incidence of 0.69 % [7]. Also Buie reported an incidence of 5 % anal fistulas in patients with anorectal abscesses seen at the Mayo Clinic [8].

Using operating room data in Helsinki Finland (1969–1978), the incidence of fistulas was calculated to be 8.6 per 100,000 populations (males 12.3 %, females 5.6 %). Nelson in his meta-analysis equated this with 20,000–25,000 fistulas treated annually in the US [9]. Interestingly, the ambulatory case of the National Center for Health Statistics reported 24,000 patients with a primary diagnosis of fistula treated in US Hospitals in 1979. This number has decreased drastically to 3,800 in 1999 possibly due to more and more ambulatory approaches [9].

The incidence of anorectal fistula can be estimated from the number of anorectal abscesses. In a series reported by Ramanujam from a large inner city hospital, the incidence of fistula was 34 % [4]. This is almost identical to another US study [10] and a Canadian study [11] both reporting from single institutions. Calculating backward, this would translate to an estimated annual incidence of 68,000–96,000 cases in the US [9].

Etiology

Fistulas in the overwhelming majority of cases arise from prior abscesses. Other causes such as hemorrhoidectomy, foreign body perforation, and trauma are of less frequency. Inflammatory bowel disease, more commonly Crohn's disease, has been known to be associated with anorectal fistulas. Specific diseases such as tuberculosis and actinomycosis are much less frequent in the Western world. Tubercular fistulas are covered in a separate section. The origin of anal abscess and the relationship of abscesses to fistulas is covered in Chap. 3.

Age and Sex

Data on age and sex can be extracted from single series. Most patients with anal fistula are between the ages of 20 and 60 with mean age of 40 in both genders. In the Sainio report,

R.L. Nelson, M.D., F.A.C.S.
Northern General Hospital, Herr Road Sheffield, South Yorkshire, S5 7AU, UK

H. Abcarian, M.D., F.A.C.S. (✉)
The University of Illinois at Chicago, Division of Colon and Rectal Surgery, John Stroger Hospital of Cook Country, IL 60612, USA
e-mail: abcarian@uic.edu

H. Abcarian (ed.), *Anal Fistula: Principles and Management*, DOI 10.1007/978-1-4614-9014-2_1,
© Springer Science+Business Media New York 2014

men were afflicted twice as frequently as women (12.3 % vs. 5.6 %) [5]. In two large series reported from Cook County Hospital in Chicago, the male to female ratio was also 2:1 [4, 12]. Hill reported treating 636 patients of whom nine were less than 9 years old and were all boys [13]. Similarly, Mazier reported 1,000 cases of fistula treated at the Ferguson Clinic of whom 25 were younger than 10 years of age and nine of the ten were boys [14]. Piazza and Radhakrishnan reported anorectal abscesses in the pediatric population. Of 40 patients, 33 were boys and seven girls. Twenty-one were younger than 2 years old, 20 were less than 9 months of age and all were boys [15].

Rosen and colleagues reported 18 infants who were treated with incision and drainage of abscess and expectant therapy of established fistulas. In 18 of 18 patients (100 %), the fistula resolved without the need for surgery [16]. This might reinforce the concept put forward by Fitzgerald et al. that fistulas in childhood are of congenital etiology [17].

Race

There are few epidemiologic studies regarding racial distribution of fistulas. In the series reported by Read and Abcarian [12], 92 % of the patients were African American which closely corresponded to the racial makeup of that particular inner city hospital population. However, the patients were younger with a peak incidence in ages 20–29 years and 61 % were between the ages of 15–29 [12].

Seasonal Occurrence

No seasonal variation has been found in incidence of abscess fistulas, although the study by Vasilavsky and Gordon reported the higher incidence in June and lowest in the months of August and September in Montreal, Canada [11].

Personal Hygiene and Sedentary Occupation

Although both implicated, personal hygiene and sedentary lifestyle have not been shown to have a statistical significance [12].

Bowel Habits

Vasilavsky and Gordon reported that of 103 patients, diarrhea was the presenting symptom in 7 % [11]. However in most published series in adults, diarrhea or constipation was infrequently seen to be significant risk for fistulas [14].

Risk of Cancer

Long-standing chronic draining wounds predispose to development of cancer. Such is also the case of anal fistulas [18, 19]. Nelson and colleagues reported six cancers in chronic fistulas which on the average were present for 13.8 years [20, 21]. None of the six cancers had an intraluminal component and were not suspected preoperatively. Several case-control and cohort studies have also shown an association between intractable fistulas and development of cancer [22]. In cases where cancers develop in a clinically preexisting fistula, it is easy to blame the fistula as a contributing factor. Adenocarcinoma of the anal canal is an aggressive disease [23]. The pathology of cancer in chronic inflammation has been well documented in diseases such as ulcerative colitis [24]. Because chronic inflammation due to anal fistulas can be easily treated operatively with low morbidity (in contrast to restorative proctocolectomy and ileal pouch anal anastomosis in chronic ulcerative colitis), it stands to reason that anal fistulas should be treated surgically and expeditiously soon after diagnosis.

Conclusion

Although the etiology of abscess fistulas is clear and less controversial, the exact incidence and prevalence of fistulas is not known due to poor data available from outpatient treatment centers. The disease predominates in adults with a male to female ratio of 2:1. The rare but potentially lethal development of cancer in long-standing fistulas mandates early treatment of this disease soon after diagnosis.

References

1. Sankaran PS. Sushruta's contribution to surgery. Varanasi: Ideological Book House; 1976.
2. Akinola DO, Hamed AD. Fistula in ano in Nigerians. Trop Gastroenterol. 1989;10:153–7.
3. Navruzov SN, Dul'tsev IV, Salamov KN. Causes and prevention of rectal fistula recurrences. Vestn Khir Im I I Grek. 1981;27:43–6.
4. Ramanujam PS, Prasad ML, Abcarian H, Tan AB. Perianal abscess and fistulas; a study of 1023 patients. Dis Colon Rectum. 1984;27: 593–7.
5. Sainio P. Fistula in ano in a defined population. Incidence and epidemiologic aspects. Ann Chir Gynaecol. 1984;73:219–24.
6. Shrum RC. Anorectal pathology in 1000 consecutive patients with suspected surgical disorders. Dis Colon Rectum. 1959;2:469–72.
7. Buda AM. General candidates of fistula in ano: the role of foreign bodies as causative factors fistulas. Am J Surg. 1941;54:384–7.
8. Buie SL. Sr practice proctology. 2nd ed. Springfield, IL: Charles C Thomas; 1960.
9. Nelson RL. Anorectal Abscess fistulas. What do we know? Surg Clin North Am. 2002;82:1139–51.

10. Scoma JA, Salvati EP, Rubin RJ. Incidence of fistulas subsequent to anal abscesses. Dis Colon Rectum. 1974;17(3):357–9.
11. Vasilevsky CA, Gordon PH. The incidence of recurrent abscesses or fistula-in-ano following anorectal suppuration. Dis Colon Rectum. 1984;27(2):126–30.
12. Read DR, Abcarian H. A prospective survey of 474 patients with anorectal abscess. Dis Colon Rectum. 1979;22(8):566–8.
13. Hill JR. Fistulas and fistulous abscesses in the anorectal region: personal experience in management. Dis Colon Rectum. 1967;10(6):421–34.
14. Mazier WP. The treatment and care of anal fistulas: a study of 1,000 patients. Dis Colon Rectum. 1971;14(2):134–44.
15. Piazza DJ, Radhakrishnan J. Perianal abscess and fistula-in-ano in children. Dis Colon Rectum. 1990;33(12):1014–6.
16. Rosen NG, Gibbs DL, Soffer SZ, Hong A, Sher M, Pena A. The non-operative treatment of fistula in ano. J Pediatr Surg. 2000;35:938–9.
17. Fitzgerald RJ, Harding B, Ryan W. Fistula in ano in childhood: a congenital etiology. J Pediatr Surg. 1985;20:80–1.
18. Corman BC. All's well that ends well Shakespeare's treatment of anal fistula. Dis Colon Rectum. 1998;41:914–24.
19. Abcarian H. Anorectal infections: abscess-fistula. Clin Colon Rectal Surg. 2011;24:14–21.
20. Nelson RL, Malik A. Anorectal fistula. Sheffield: Northern General Hospital; 2010.
21. Nelson RL, Prasad ML, Abcarian H. Anal carcinoma presenting as a perirectal abscess or fistula. Arch Surg. 1985;120:632–5.
22. Nelson RL, Abcarian H. Do hemorrhoids cure cancer? Sem Colon Rectal Surg. 1996;6:178–81.
23. Tarazi R, Nelson RL. Adenocarcinoma of the anus. Sem Colon Rectal Surg. 1995;6:169–73.
24. Shacter E, Weitzman SA. Chronic inflammation and cancer. Oncology. 2002;16:217–36.

Applied Anatomy

2

Russell K. Pearl

Introduction

A thorough understanding of anorectal anatomy is essential for the surgeon treating a patient with an anorectal fistula. Proper surgical decision-making mandates intimate knowledge of factors such as the architecture of the sphincter muscles, the distribution of anal glands, and the geography of the anorectal spaces. This chapter begins with a brief overview of current concepts of anorectal anatomy with emphasis on structures contributing to the etiology and surgical management of fistulas. It is followed by a discussion of practical guidelines such as operative recommendations as to the amount of sphincter that can be divided safely at one setting, when to use marking or dividing setons, tips to avoid nerve injury, and the anatomic reasons why certain treatment options fail.

Overview of Pelvic Floor and Anorectal Anatomy

The Pelvic Floor

The pelvic floor is formed by overlapping paired musculotendinous sheets of predominantly striated fibers known as the levator ani muscles (Fig. 2.1). The major components of this pelvic diaphragm are the pubococcygeus and the iliococcygeus muscles, although the posteriorly situated coccygeus muscles are sometimes included in this group. Recent evidence suggests that the puborectalis sling, which functions to angulate the anorectal junction anteriorly, is actually an integral part of both the levator ani and external anal sphincter complexes [1]. The levator ani is innervated from branches of the fourth sacral nerves on its pelvic surface and by the perineal branch of the pudendal nerve on its underside. The puborectalis receives additional innervation from below through the inferior rectal nerves.

The pubococcygeus originates from the posterior inferior aspect of the pubis and the inner anterior surface of the obturator fascia, including a portion of the arcus tendineus of the levator ani. Its anterior fibers insert medially into the central tendon of the perineum (hiatal ligament), where they fuse with the musculature of the prostate, vagina, and perineal body to form the levator prostate, pubovaginalis, and pubourethralis muscles. Some of these intermediate fibers also travel caudally along the intersphincteric plane and contribute to the conjoined longitudinal coat of the anal canal. The muscular fibers of the pubococcygeus merge posteriorly into the broad fibrous band that inserts into the anococcygeal ligament, anterior sacrococcygeal ligament, and coccyx.

The iliococcygeus arises from the arcus tendineus of the fascia of the internal obturator muscle posterior and caudal to the origin of the pubococcygeus. The fibers run posteromedially, where they merge and insert into the anococcygeal ligament and the last two segments of sacrum.

The puborectalis is the most caudal and controversial component of the levator ani complex. It arises from the posterior aspects of the body of the pubis, the inferior pubic ramis, the superior fascia of the urogenital diaphragm, and the adjacent obturator internus fascia and loops around the rectum to form a strong U-shaped sling. Medial fibers of the puborectalis fan out and insert into the central tendon of the perineum where they intermingle with fibers from the pubococcygeus and contribute to the conjoined longitudinal muscle of the anal canal. The puborectalis sling, together with the upper borders of the internal and external sphincters, forms the anorectal ring, which delineates the surgical anal canal from the rectum.

R.K. Pearl, M.D., M.S. (Surg.) (✉)
Division of Colon and Rectal Surgery, University of Illinois at Chicago, 840 S. Wood Street, 518E CSB, MC 958, Chicago, IL 60612, USA
e-mail: rkpearlmd@yahoo.com

H. Abcarian (ed.), *Anal Fistula: Principles and Management*, DOI 10.1007/978-1-4614-9014-2_2,
© Springer Science+Business Media New York 2014

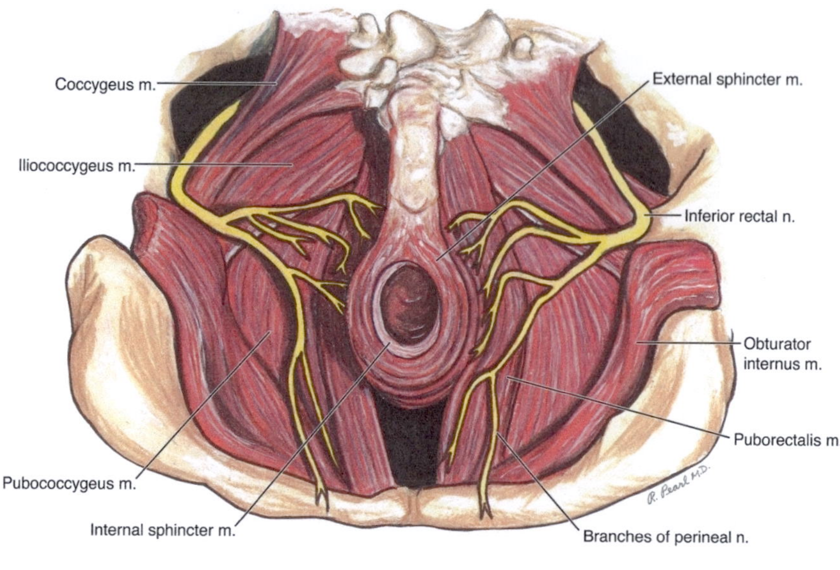

Fig. 2.1 Overview of the pelvic floor muscles and anal sphincters seen from below

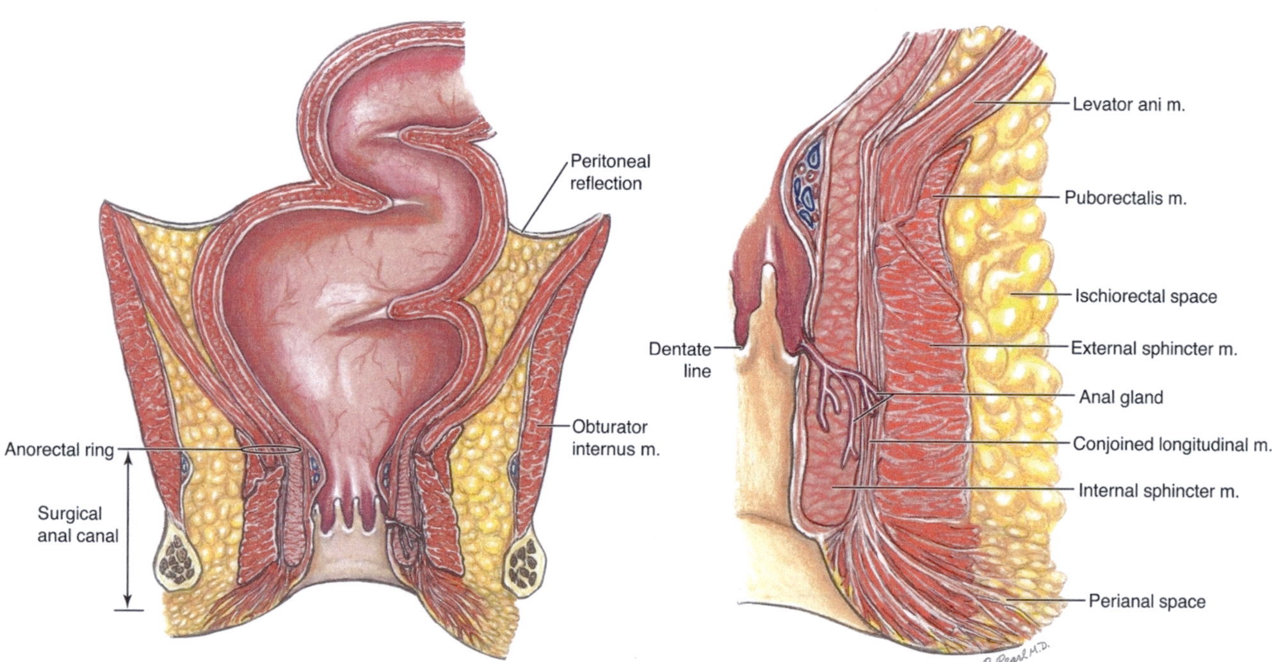

Fig. 2.2 Coronal view of the anal canal, lower rectum, and surrounding spaces. The enlarged view on the right highlights the architecture of the sphincter muscles and anal glands

Rectum and Anal Canal

The rectum begins at the level of the third sacral vertebra and in general follows along the curvature of the sacrum and coccyx for its entire length of 12–15 cm (Fig. 2.2). In addition, it has three lateral curves; the upper and lower ones are convex to the right, the middle one convex to the left. The inner aspects of these three transverse infoldings correspond to the rectal valves of Houston. At the rectosigmoid junction, the fibers of the taenia spread out to form the longitudinal muscle layer of the rectum, which surrounds the inner circular muscle layer. The outer muscle coat is slightly thicker on the anterior and posterior rectal walls than on its lateral surfaces, contributing to the formation of three lateral curves.

The upper surface of the rectum is covered by the peritoneum on its anterior and lateral surfaces. The middle third is covered on its anterior surface only, and the lower third is entirely below the peritoneal reflection. The middle valve of Houston is approximately at the level of the anterior peritoneal reflection.

The posterior wall of the rectum is covered with a thick layer of pelvic fascia (fascia propria). A strong sheet of fascia (Waldeyer's or rectosacral fascia) arises from the fourth sacral segment, tracks forward and downward, and attaches to the fascia propria on the posterior surface of the rectal wall at the anorectal junction. The lower portion of the rectum is supported on each side by reflections of endopelvic fascia known as the lateral stalks of the rectum. The anterior extraperitoneal surface of the rectum is covered by Denonvilliers' visceral pelvic fascia which extends to the urogenital diaphragm running between the rectum and prostate or vagina.

As the rectum passes through the pelvic diaphragm at the level of the anorectal ring, it changes its name, shape, and direction. The anal canal begins at this point and extends for approximately 4 cm to the anal verge (surgical anal canal). The circular lumen of the rectum flattens into an anteroposterior slit because of its attachment to the perineal body and coccyx along with the medial pressure exerted by the ischiorectal fat pads. The puborectalis sling in its normal contracted state angulates the anorectal junction forward to create an 80° bend, the perineal flexure, which may assist the external sphincter mechanism in maintaining fecal continence.

The internal sphincter is a continuation of the involuntary layer of circular smooth muscle of the rectum that begins at the level of the anorectal ring. As it proceeds distally, it becomes appreciably thicker, and its rounded lower margin can usually be palpated about 1–2 cm below the dentate line. The internal sphincter, like the puborectalis, is tonically contracted "at rest".

The conjoined longitudinal muscle coat that surrounds the internal sphincter arises from medial fibers of the pubococcygeus and puborectalis. These striated voluntary fibers course along the intersphincteric plane, fan out through the subcutaneous portion of the external sphincter, and attach to the anoderm and perianal skin, constituting the corrugator cutis ani muscle.

Several versions of the musculature of the external sphincter have been proposed, ranging from the single continuous muscle sheet model of Goligher to the three distinct loop theory of Shafik [2, 3]. The inconsistencies of these various descriptions are most likely based on differences in age, sex, and individual variation among the subjects, as well as on differences in points of orientation among investigators (anatomists, physiologists, radiologists, clinical surgeons). For example, a clinical surgeon repairing a sphincter injury with an overlapping sphincteroplasty generally does not appreciate several subdivisions of the external sphincter. In addition, the external sphincter complex acts as a single functional unit, as demonstrated by electromyography. More recently anal sphincter anatomy has been investigated by high-spatial-resolution endoanal MR imaging [4]. These findings will be discussed in more detail later in this chapter.

Perhaps all that can be stated definitively with respect to structure is that the external anal sphincter is an elliptical cylinder of striated muscle that surrounds the anal canal, and at least the large central portion (superficial component) is firmly tethered to the coccyx, forming the anococcygeal ligament.

Of particular interest is the composition of the fibers of the external sphincter. It is made up of two different types of striated muscle, type I and type II which function independently, even though they are fully integrated with each other. The type I muscle fibers, although voluntary in appearance, behave as involuntary smooth muscle by maintaining a state of tonic contraction in much of the same manner as the internal sphincter. The type II muscle mass is capable of powerful contractions far exceeding the baseline level of the type I fibers. However, these type II fibers can only maintain this maximal level of contraction for a short time before they become fatigued.

The mucosa of the upper portion of the anal canal is lined primarily by columnar epithelium. The lower portion or anatomic anal canal extends from the dentate line to the anal verge and is lined with anoderm, a thin layer of stratified squamous epithelium that lacks sweat glands and hair follicles. Interspersed between the mucosa of the proximal anal canal and the serrated margin of the dentate line is a narrow indistinct band of cuboidal epithelium known as the transitional zone, which represents the embryological remnants of the cloacal membrane.

Several longitudinal mucosal folds, the columns of Morgagni, arise in the proximal anal canal and terminate at the dentate line, where they surround the anal crypts. The majority of the branched tubular anal glands that originate from the depths of these crypts are located in the posterior quadrant of the anal canal, and will be discussed in more detail later. In addition, the normally pink mucosa of the upper anal canal appears purple where it overlies the three vascular anal cushions often referred to as the internal hemorrhoids.

The mucosa proximal to the dentate line lacks somatic innervation. In contrast, the anoderm is richly endowed with cutaneous sensory nerve endings. The blood supply to the rectum and anal canal originates at three levels (Fig. 2.3). The superior rectal artery, the principal blood supply to the upper and middle portion of the rectum, begins as the terminal branch of the inferior mesenteric artery, where it crosses over the left common iliac vessels. As it descends within the sigmoid mesocolon, it bifurcates at the level of the third sacral vertebra into right and left branches that course along and within either side of the rectal wall. Each vessel divides further so that an average of five small mucosal arteries terminate at the level of the anal valves. There appears to be a paucity of anastomoses on the anterior and posterior surfaces of the rectum between the two collateral branches of the superior rectal artery.

The middle rectal arteries usually arise from the internal iliac arteries, travel along the anterolateral surface of the

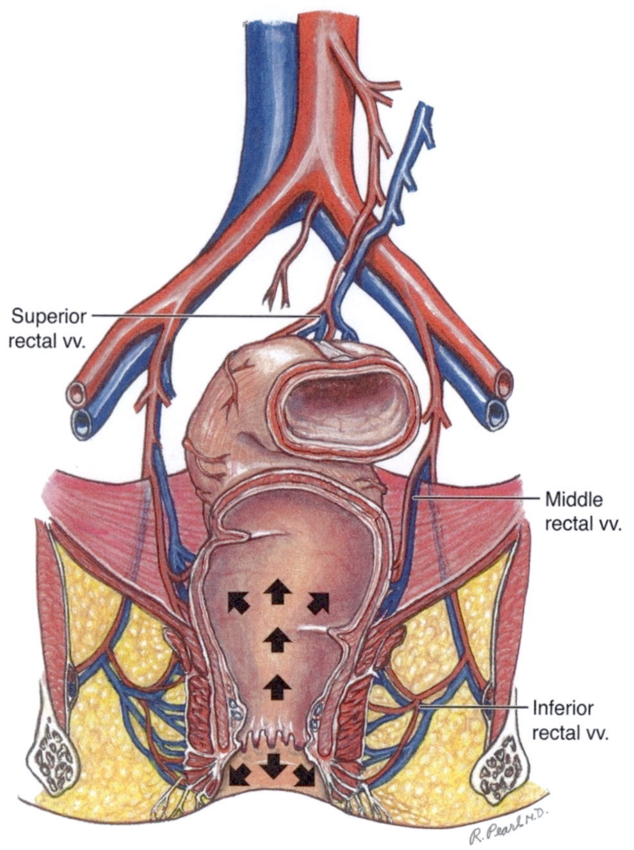

Fig. 2.3 The blood supply and venous drainage of the rectum and anal canal. The *arrows* indicate the direction of lymphatic drainage

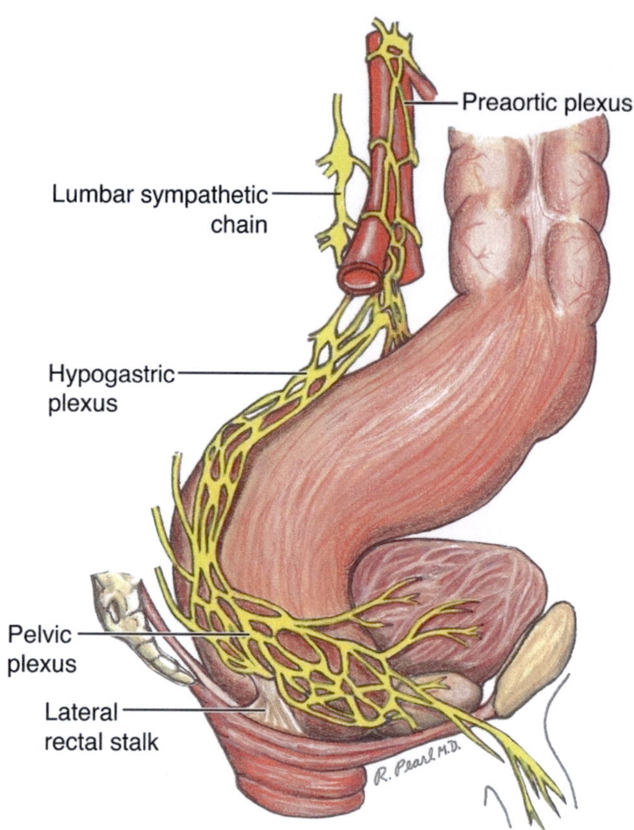

Fig. 2.4 Lateral view of the rectum and anal canal illustrating the course and distribution of the pelvic autonomic nerves. Note the proximity of the pelvic plexus to the lower third of the rectum

lower rectum, traversing Denonvilliers' fascia, and enter the rectal wall at the level of the anorectal ring. Although the middle rectal arteries do not run within the lateral stalks, accessory branches may occasionally be found coursing through these ligaments.

The inferior rectal arteries enter the posterolateral aspects of the isciorectal fossae as offshoots of the internal pudendal arteries, which run in Alcock's canals. Each of these arteries divides further into two to four vessels that supply the external and internal sphincter, as well as the lining of the anal canal.

Although the degree of confluence between the vessels supplying the rectum and anal canal is controversial, it appears that all three vascular systems are interconnected by a rich intramural plexus. The contribution of the middle sacral artery to this network is at best small and variable.

The venous drainage of the rectum and anal canal parallels the arterial supply. Therefore, blood from the rectum and upper part of the anal canal returns through the superior rectal vein into the portal system, whereas the middle and inferior rectal veins empty into the caval circulation. The submucosal veins of the distal anal canal do not have a special connection with the portal circulation. Contrary to earlier beliefs, there is no significant increase in the incidence of symptomatic hemorrhoids in patients with portal hypertension.

The lymphatic system of rectum and anal canal follows the course of the regional blood supply. Lymphatic drainage from the anal canal proximal to the dentate line courses cephalad along the superior rectal vessels and laterally by way of the middle rectal lymphatics to the internal iliac nodes. Lymph from the anal canal below the dentate line usually drains to the inguinal lymph nodes.

The rectum, upper portion of the anal canal, bladder, and genitals are innervated by fibers of the autonomic nervous system (Fig. 2.4). The external sphincter and anoderm are supplied by somatic nerves.

The sympathetic nerves to these pelvic structures originate from the lower thoracic and upper lumbar spinal segments as preganglionic sympathetic fibers that synapse with postganglionic fibers in the preaortic plexus and lumbar sympathetic chains. They then course the pelvis adjacent to the ilicac vessels, ureters, and lateral pelvic wall. The preaortic plexus is adherent to the anterior wall of the aorta and the common iliac arteries. The lumbar sympathetic chains pass underneath the common iliac vessels and join the fibers from the preaortic plexus to form the left and right hypogastric plexuses just distal to the bifurcation of the aorta. These plexuses are covered by pelvic peritoneum and are generally adherent to the posterolateral pelvic walls.

Preganglionic parasympathetic nerves that arise from the second, third, and fourth sacral segments (nervi erigentes) descend into the pelvis and intermingle with the sympathetic fibers from the hypogastric nerves to form the pelvic plexuses [5]. The pelvic plexuses are at the level of the lower third of the rectum just above the levator ani muscles and are situated well lateral to the pararectal reflections of the endopelvic fascia known as the lateral stalks of the rectum. This dense reticulum of sympathetic and parasympathetic nerves continues anterolaterally around the bladder and into the prostate and penis.

Sensation to the perianal region and anal canal distal to the dentate line is conveyed by afferent fibers of the inferior rectal nerves. The mucosa of the rectum and proximal anal canal lacks somatic sensory innervation so that mucosa injury caused by biopsy, cauterization, polypectomy, or rubber bands ligation is not perceived as painful. The dull, aching sensation sometimes experienced in this region during transanal procedures is probably mediated via the pelvic parasympathetic nerves.

Anatomic Considerations Relating to Fistula Surgery: Anal Glands

Situated within the 4–12 pockets or anal crypts found at the dentate line are the openings to a variable number of straight and branched anal glands (Fig. 2.2) [6]. These glands are lined with stratified squamous epithelium and were first described by Chiari in 1878. More than one gland may open into the same crypt, while half the crypts have no communication with the gland. These tubular glands extend into the submucosa in a downward and outward direction with two-thirds of them entering the internal sphincter. In addition, half of them extend out as far as the intersphincteric plane. Parks first addressed their role in the pathogenesis of anorectal abscesses and fistulas [7]. Immunochemical staining methods have confirmed the presence of mucous secreting cells as well as intraluminal secretions within the glands. It is controversial whether these glands have a definite active secretory function such as lubricating stool as it passes through the anal canal, or merely are static outgrowths of the anal crypts that can potentially become blocked with debris. Regardless, it seems logical that an obstructed gland extending into the intershincteric space can develop into an abscess that can track along or through adjacent tissue planes and upon spontaneous or surgical drainage develop into a fistula. This concept is substantiated clinically since most internal fistulous openings are found within the crypts at the dentate line.

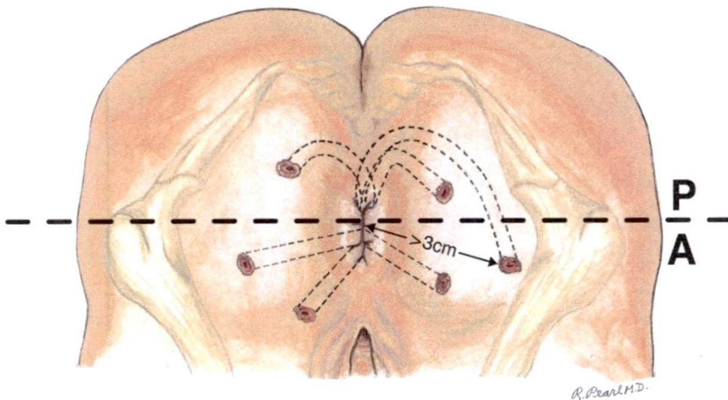

Fig. 2.5 Illustration of Goodsall's rule

The majority of the anal glands are located in the posterior midline, which explains the prevalence of anorectal abscesses in this region. When these posterior midline abcesses erode into the adjacent deep postanal space, the septic process gains access to the left and right ischiorectal spaces to form a horseshoe abscess/fistula. The high concentration of anal glands in this region helps explain Goodsall's rule, which is often useful in identifying the primary opening of a fistula (Fig. 2.5). This guideline states that if the secondary opening is situated around the posterior half of the anus or more than 3 cm away from the anus, the primary opening will usually be located at the posterior midline. Conversely, if the secondary opening is found within the anterior half of the anus, the internal opening will be directly in line (radially located) with the secondary opening at the dentate line. However, there is evidence suggesting that Goodsall's rule is less accurate for identifying fistulas with an anterior external opening [8].

Sphincter Architecture Based on Refined Imaging Techniques

Traditional descriptions of sphincter architecture were based on anatomic dissections and operative observations. With the advent of endoanal ultrasound, in vivo evaluation of anal anatomy and pathology became available. However, the shortcoming of this technique was suboptimal delineation of the external sphincter and levator ani muscles. High-spatial-resolution endoanal MR imaging using a coil affords excellent resolution of all of the sphincter muscles. By utilizing this technique, normal sphincter anatomy in both men and women was definitively presented. Among the major findings in this study were that the anterior part of the external sphincter was about half as long in women compared with men (14.0 mm vs. 27.0 mm). The thickness of each sphincter component was roughly equivalent between the sexes, and that there was a substantial difference in the arrangement of muscle fibers anterior to the sphincter. In men the central perineal tendon is a strong insertion point directly anterior to the external sphincter, whereas in women it is a less well-defined insertion area of woven muscle fibers slightly superior to the external sphincter. The significance of this finding is that during vaginal delivery this tissue becomes markedly attenuated predisposing it to obstetrical tears which can clearly impact fecal continence. This anatomic arrangement in women along with the fact that the puborectalis muscle is absent anteriorly should alert the surgeon to exercise caution when encountering an anterior fistula tract. Unless the fistula is extremely superficial, primary fistulotomy should probably be avoided.

The Geography of the Anorectal Spaces

There are several spaces and potential spaces surrounding the rectum and anal canal that are of surgical significance (Fig. 2.6). The ischiorectal fossa is divided into the perianal space and ischioanal space. The perianal space surrounds the lowest portion of the anal canal and is confined by the radiating elastic septae of the conjoined longitudinal muscle attachments to the anoderm and perianal skin and contains finely lobulated fat, delicate branches of hemorrhoidal vessels, nerves, and lymphatics. When blood or pus accumulates in this closed space the stretching and irritation of the many nerve endings results in the severe anal pain associated with perianal abscesses and thrombosed external hemorrhoids.

The ischioanal fossa surrounds the upper portion of the anal canal to the level of the anorectal ring. The roof of this pyramid-shaped space is composed of the levator ani muscles, and laterally it is bounded by the obturator internus muscle which lines the pelvic sidewalls. It is filled with coarsely lobulated fat and contains the inferior rectal vessels and nerves. It is a relatively large space and can harbor a substantial abscess with only minimal involvement of the overlying gluteal skin. These clinical findings can mislead an

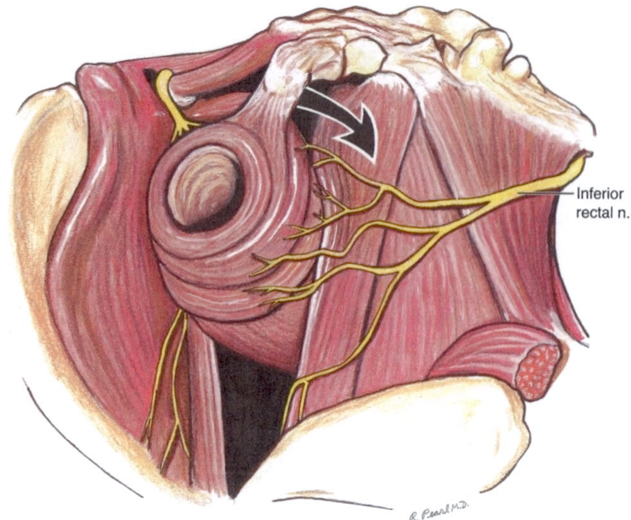

Fig. 2.7 Partial oblique view of the pelvic floor and anal sphincter muscles from below. The *arrow* illustrates how the deep postanal space serves as a window to the left and right ischiorectal spaces, which is how horseshoe abscess/fistula forms. The location and course of the inferior rectal nerves are shown to emphasize how they can be readily avulsed by overaggressive spreading of curved clamps during drainage of ischiorectal abscesses

inexperienced clinician into making the diagnosis of celluitis rather than a drainable abscess with disastrous results especially in the case of a diabetic of immunocompromised patient. The abscess cavity may extend around one-half the circumference of the anus (horseshoe) or extend completely around the anus (floating freestanding anus).

Another pitfall that sometimes occurs when draining a large ischiorectal abscess is inadvertently mistaking the fanned out array of branches of the inferior rectal nerve as "loculations" inhibiting adequate drainage. Tearing these branches by recklessly spreading a large curved clamp can result in significant injury to the nerve supply to the external sphincter. If this procedure is carried out on both sides as in the case of a horseshoe abscess, complete denervation of the sphincter can occur.

The superficial postanal space is located in the posterior midline between the skin and anococcygeal ligament and is frequently involved with anorectal abscesses. The deep postanal space (retrosphincteric space of Courtney) located deep to the anococcygeal ligament and the upper portions of the external sphincter and levator muscles is of special surgical significance first because of the frequency of abscesses occurring in this region, and secondly because the deep postanal space serves as a window to the left and right ischiorectal spaces which can result in horseshoe abscesses or fistulas (Fig. 2.7).

In longstanding horseshoe fistulas, the deep postanal space can become quite indurated and rigid. Attempts to sterilize and completely fill this infected cavity with collagen

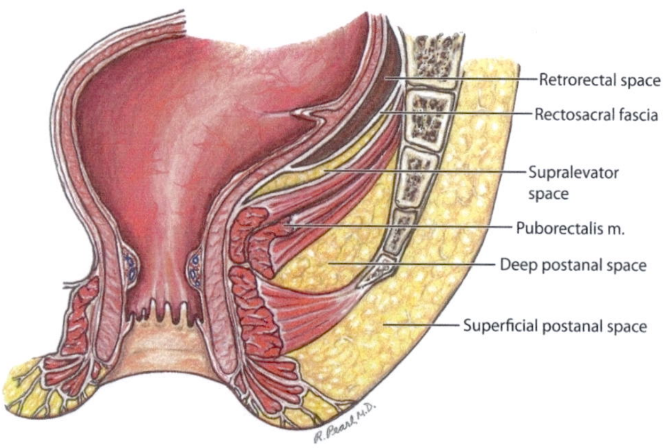

Fig. 2.6 Mid-sagittal view of the lower rectum and anal canal emphasizing the anorectal spaces

plugs or fibrin glue often fail because residual contaminated space is left behind to reactivate the septic process.

The supralevator space is sandwiched between the upper surface of the levators and pelvic peritoneum. Abscess presenting in this location may be difficult to diagnose especially when there are no visible clinical findings around the perineum. Approximately 9 % of large ischiorectal abscesses have an associated supralevator component, which resulted from the septic process eroding through the adjacent levator ani muscle resulting in an hourglass-shaped abscess [9, 10].

When to Avoid Primary Fistulotomy

Anorectal examination under anesthesia is an important step to assess the location and extent of the abscess/fistula process, as well as a means to determine how much sphincter muscle is encircled by the tract. There are several circumstances where these findings can be particularly helpful in preventing overly aggressive fistulotomy which may result in fecal incontinence. In each of the following cases complete primary fistulotomy should be avoided and be replaced by more conservative procedures such as the judicious use of setons, fistula plugs, fibrin glue, or eventually mucosal or cutaneous advancement flap procedures:

1. The presence of a high transsphincteric fistula which can be defined as involving more than 50 % of the external sphincter posteriorly or laterally or 30 % of the external sphincter anteriorly.
2. A transsphincteric fistula in cases of massive anorectal sepsis (floating, freestanding anus) where the normal anatomic landmarks have been severely distorted such that primary fistulotomy may compromise proper wound healing resulting in a large gap or step-off deformity.
3. The existence of an anterior, high transsphincteric fistula in a woman. The external sphincter is quite tenuous and the puborectalis is absent in this region. Primary fistulotomy may result in fecal incontinence.
4. The presence of a high transsphincteric fistula in a patient with poorly controlled acquired immunodeficiency syndrome (AIDS). Healing of anorectal wounds is notoriously poor in these individuals. Moreover, many patients with AIDS have chronic diarrhea, which further exacerbates the problem.
5. The presence of a high fistula in a patient with Crohn's disease. In these instances, it is prudent to mark the fistula tract with a long-term seton such as a silastic vessel loop to promote drainage and deter the development of recurrent abscesses.
6. A marking seton should be placed whenever there is a reasonable clinical suspicion that primary fistulotomy will disrupt fecal continence.

Summary

- Anatomic considerations relating to fistula surgery
- Sphincter architecture based on refined imaging techniques
- Geography of the anal glands and anorectal spaces
- When to avoid primary fistulotomy

References

1. Dalley AF. The riddle of the sphincters, the morphophysiology of the anorectal mechanism reviewed. Am Surg. 1987;53:298–306.
2. Goligher JC. Surgical anatomy and physiology of the colon, rectum, and anus. In: Goligher JC, editor. Surgery of the anus, rectum, and colon. 5th ed. London: Balliere-Tindall; 1984.
3. Shafik A. A new concept of the anatomy of the anal sphincter mechanism and the physiology of defecation. The external anal sphincter: a triple-loop system. Invest Urol. 1975;12:412–9.
4. Rociu E, Stoker J, Eiijkemans MJC, Lameris JS. Normal anal sphincter anatomy and age and sex-related variations at high spatial-resolution endoanal MR imaging. Radiology. 2000; 217:395–401.
5. Pearl RK, Monsen H, Abcarian H. Surgical anatomy of the pelvic autonomic nerves, a practical approach. Am Surg. 1986;52:236–7.
6. Seow-Choen F, Ho JM. Histoanatomy of anal glands. Dis Colon Rectum. 1994;37:1215–8.
7. Parks AG. Pathogenesis and treatment of fistula-in-ano. Br Med J. 1961;1:463–9.
8. Cirocco WC, Reilly JC. Challenging the predictive accuracy of Goodsall's rule for anal fistulas. Dis Colon Rectum. 1992;35: 537–42.
9. Prasad ML, Read DR, Abcarian H. Supralevator abscess: diagnosis and treatment. Dis Colon Rectum. 1981;24:456–61.
10. Pearl RK. Anorectal fistula; role of the seton. In: Cameron JL, editor. Current surgical therapy. 4th ed. St. Louis: Mosby-Year Book; 1992.

Relationship of Abscess to Fistula

Herand Abcarian

Introduction

The true incidence of the anorectal abscess fistula is not known because most reports come from a large colorectal surgery practice or a single institution. In addition many cases of anorectal abscess are drained in the office, outpatient clinic, surgicenters, or emergency departments and as such no formal records, e.g., operating room or hospital discharge data accounts for such treatments.

The incidence of anorectal abscess fistula is covered in a separate chapter. In one large series of anorectal abscesses treated in the operating room, the incidence of fistula was 34 % [1]. In two single-institution series, the incidence of fistula was similar at 26 % [2] and 37 % [3]. If one extrapolates the number of abscesses based on fistula data, the incidence of abscess in the US falls between 68,000 and 96,000 per annum [4].

Etiology

Anorectal abscess is believed to originate from infected anal glands. These were originally described by Hermann and Desfosses in 1880s who demonstrated that the anal glands opened into the anal crypts, and branched within the internal sphincter and ended in the space between the internal and external sphincters. They were also the first to suggest that infection in these glands spread through the intersphincteric space to the perianal skin [5]. In 1933 Tucker and Hellwing published on the histopathology of the anal gland, and demonstrated conclusively that anal sepsis originates in the gland ducts and extends from anal lumen into the walls of the anal canal [6]. Hill and colleagues in 1943 published and stressed

the role of anal glands in the pathogenesis of anorectal infection [7]. Similarly, Kratzer in 1950 stressed the clinical significance of anal glands and ducts [8]. Eisenhammer in 1956 stated that all fistulas originate from intermuscular gland infections [9]. Parks demonstrated typical stratified, mucus-secreting, columnar epithelium of anal glandular type in biopsy material from 21 of 30 patients with fistula in ano. In 13 this formed part of the lining of the internal opening of the fistula tract or an intersphincteric abscess. In his opinion, this conclusively supported the case for regarding anal glands as the essential etiologic function in most anal fistulae. However, in 1967, Goligher and colleagues challenged this etiologic theory. In a series of 29 patients with acute abscess (20 perianal, eight ischiorectal, one perirectal) they carefully inspected the lining of the anal canal and its valves with a bivalve anoscope. Then putting firm presser on the abscess they looked for whether pus could be expressed from any anal crypt [10][1]. The crypts were probed gently in search of an internal opening. In only five out of 29 cases (all perianal) they found communication with the crypt region, supporting the argument that in about two-thirds of the anorectal infections the cryptoglandular etiology does not apply [11].

The infection, originally an intersphincteric abscess, finds a path of least resistance to spread. If it extends caudad between the internal and external sphincter to reach the anal verge, it produces a *perianal abscess*. If it ruptures through the external sphincter to reach the ischiorectal fossa, it is called *ischiorectal abscess*. If the abscess extended in a cephalad direction between the layer of the rectal smooth muscle it will produce a *high intermuscular abscess* which on occasion is labeled a *submucosal abscess*. Rarely, infection may spread above the levator space producing a *supralevator abscess* (Fig. 3.1). A deep postanal abscess may spread to one or both ischiorectal fossae and results in a *horseshoe abscess*.

Aside from cryptoglandular origin, the other causes of anorectal suppuration may result from the downward spread of *pelvic infection* from appendicitis, diverticulitis, and gynecologic sepsis resulting in *supralevator abscess*. This in turn may track caudad through the levators into the ischiorectal space. Crohn's

H. Abcarian, M.D., F.A.C.S (✉)
The University of Illinois at Chicago, Division of Colon and Rectal Surgery, John Stroger Hospital of Cook Country, IL 60612, USA
e-mail: abcarian@uic.edu

H. Abcarian (ed.), *Anal Fistula: Principles and Management*, DOI 10.1007/978-1-4614-9014-2_3,
© Springer Science+Business Media New York 2014

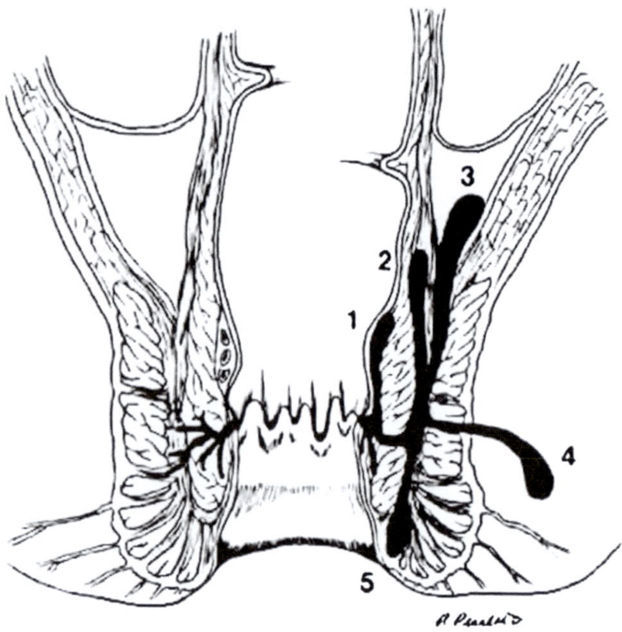

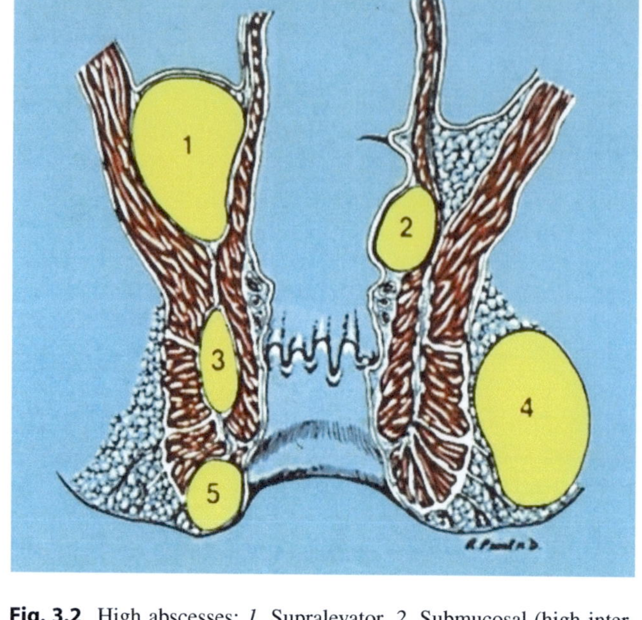

Fig. 3.1 (*Left*) Anal glands opening in the anal crypts and branching in intersphincteric space. (*Right*) Extension of abscess to adjacent spaces. *1*. Submucosal, *2*. High Intermuscular, *3*. Supralevator, *4*. Ischiorectal, *5*. Perianal. Provided courtesy of Russell K. Pearl, M.D., FACS, Department of Surgery, UIC

Fig. 3.2 High abscesses: *1*. Supralevator, *2*. Submucosal (high intermuscular). Low abscesses: *3*. Intersphincteric, *4*. Ischiorectal, *5*. Perianal. Provided courtesy of Russell K. Pearl, M.D., FACS, Department of Surgery, UIC

disease of mid and low rectum as well as the anorectum, by its transmural pathologic nature may extend to perirectal or perianal space as an abscess fistula. Similarly, ingested chicken and fish bones as well as swallowed toothpicks may puncture the wall of the rectum resulting in significant sepsis. External penetrating injuries (stab, gunshot, shot gun wounds) may result in an overt injury though at times more minor or subtle injuries gradually proceed to full-blown perirectal sepsis. Perforation of low rectal cancers may also present with large ischiorectal abscesses. It is important to biopsy the abscess well in order not to miss the underlying cancer. Specific infections such as tuberculosis have been covered in Chap. 19. Fungal infections, especially actinomycosis and oxyuris vermicularis infestation, have also been known to produce abscess fistulas in adults and children.

Clinical Manifestation

The clinical picture of anorectal abscess depends on the level (height) of the abscess. If an imaginary line is drawn across the anorectal ring, supralevator and high intermuscular abscess are located above this level. These will often manifest with systemic symptoms of fever, toxicity, etc., but are not always associated with pain and other local symptoms. Their diagnosis often relies on a thorough rectal examination which can be done under anesthesia in the operating room if needed. The intersphincteric, ischiorectal, and perianal abscesses are located caudad to the anorectal ring. They produce pain and swelling but are not associated with many systemic findings. These abscesses are easier to diagnosis and do not need any imaging modalities (Fig. 3.2).

Anorectal abscesses may drain spontaneously or may require surgical incision and drainage. Once the abscess is drained, there are three possible outcomes:

1. The abscess may completely heal without recurrence. This signifies possible lack of communication with the anal canal.
2. The abscess may heal and recur at the same site, weeks, months, or even years later. This signifies presence of communication to the dentate line, i.e., a fistula and
3. The abscess does not heal but continues to drain. Occasionally a thin film of epithelium may cover the external opening, causing collection of fluid, blood, or pus underneath it. This may give the patient a false sense of recovery until the area swells, causes pain or ruptures and the fistula reappears.

Anorectal fistulas are associated with preexisting abscesses in the majority of cases. In a study of 100 recurrent anorectal abscesses, an underlying fistula was demonstrated in the operating room in 68 % of the patients [12]. Conversely, fistulas may occur with less frequency from internal or external trauma, after anorectal surgery (hemorrhoidectomy, fissurectomy), infected episiotomies, repair of fourth-degree sphincter injury during delivery, infected anal fissure or Crohn's disease. These etiologies may cause a fistula, which

Table 3.1 Incidence of concomitant fistula in anorectal abscess

Type of abscess	No.	Fistula (%)
Intersphincteric	219	104 (47.4)
Supralevator	75	32 (42.6)
Perianal	437	151 (34.5)
Ischiorectal	233	59 (25.3)
High intermuscular	59	9 (15.2)
Total	1,023	335 (34.7)

does not necessarily originate from the anal glands at the anal crypt level but may seem to originate proximal or even distal to the dentate line.

In a study of a large cohort of patients ($n = 1,023$) Ramanujam et al. found 219 intersphincteric, 75 supralevator, 437 perianal, 233 ischiorectal, and 59 high intermuscular abscesses [1]. All patients underwent examination under anesthesia and an attempt was made to look for concomitant fistulas with gentle use of a fistula probe. The incidence of fistula in this subset classification of abscesses is depicted in Table 3.1.

It is interesting to note that the highest number of concomitant fistulas (47 %) was found in intersphincteric abscesses where the branches of anal glad terminate. With unroofing of abscess and primary fistulotomy when deemed appropriate and safe, the incidence of recurrent infection was only 3.7 % [1]. This is in stark contrast of the 68 % incidence of fistulas found in 100 patients with recurrent anorectal abscesses [12].

Conclusions

The association of abscess and fistulas is irrefutable. Aside from patients with small anorectal abscess treated with a minor incision and drainage in the outpatient setting, all others should be taken to the operating room for a formal examination under anesthesia. An experienced surgeon should be able to find communication with the anal canal with gentle probing using a blunt tipped fistula probe. If the fistula tract is easily identified, the surgeon may choose to perform a primary fistulotomy if the thickness of the overlying sphincter muscle is minimal. In all other cases with moderate to significant sphincter involvement, placement of a loose, draining Seton (braided suture or silastic vessel loop) will prevent future recurrent abscesses and allow for easy identification of internal and external openings of the fistula at the time of future definitive operative procedure.

References

1. Ramanujam PS, Prasad ML, Abcarian H, Tan AB. Perianal abscesses and fistulas: a study of 1023 patients. Dis Colon Rectum. 1984;27(9):593–7.
2. Scoma JA, Salvati EP, Rubin RJ. Incidence of fistulas subsequent to anal abscess. Dis Colon Rectum. 1974;17(3):357359.
3. Vassilevsky CA, Gordon PH. The incidence of recurrent abscess or fistula-in-ano following anorectal suppuration. Dis Colon Rectum. 1984;27(2):126–30.
4. Abcarian H. Anorectal fistulas: abscess-fistulas. Clin Colon Rectal Surg. 2011;24:14–21.
5. Hermann G, Desfosses L. Sur la muquese de la region cloacole de rectum. Compts Rend Acad Sci. 1880;90(III):1301–2.
6. Tucker CC, Hellwing CA. Histopathology of anal glands. Surg Gynecol Obstet. 1933;58:145–9.
7. Hill MR, Shryock EH, Rebell G. Role of anal gland in the pathogenesis of anorectal disease. JAMA. 1943;121(10):742–6.
8. Kratzer G. Anal ducts and their clinical significance. Am J Surg. 1950;79(1):32–9.
9. Eisenhammer S. The internal anal sphincter and the anorectal abscess. Surg Gynecol Obstet. 1956;103(4):501–6.
10. Parks AG. Pathogenesis and treatment of fistula in ano. Br Med J. 1961;1:463–6.
11. Goligher JC, Ellis M, Pissidis G. A critique of the anal glandular infection in the aetiology and treatment of idiopathic anorectal abscesses and fistulae. Br J Surg. 1967;54(12):977–83.
12. Charbot CM, Prasad LM, Abcarian H. Recurrent anorectal abscess. Dis Colon Rectum. 1983;26(2):105–8.

Adrian E. Ortega and Kyle G. Cologne

Introduction

Anorectal infections are classically categorized at specific versus nonspecific. Nonspecific infections are attributed to obstruction of a cryptoglandular structure with resultant propagation into the muscles and soft tissues surrounding the anorectum. Corman [1] credits the cryptoglandular "theory" to Herrmann and Desfosses [2] and Chiari [3] first elucidated in 1880s. Most of the literature credits Eisenhammer [4] and Parks [5]. While impossible to prove, the cryptoglandular theory as the origin of nonspecific anorectal infections is widely accepted by the world's surgeons. Specific causes are far less common and constitute a highly pleomorphic group. These involve an identifiable primary disease process (e.g., Crohn's disease) or other specific mechanism (e.g., previous surgery) and are not the main focus of this chapter.

The anal crypts reside at the base of the columns of Morgagni within the anal canal. These structures number between ten and 12 in individuals. Approximately half of all crypts will have an associated gland [6]. Collectively, they are considered cryptoglandular structures. The teleologic benefit of anal glands remains unknown. However, obstruction results in infection with propagation into and through the anal sphincters. Suppurative processes dissect through the tissues via three routes:

1. Superficially via a submucosal or subcutaneous pathway
2. Between the internal and external sphincters
3. Across the sphincters by either a transphincteric or extrasphincteric trajectory

As a result of these three basic routes of dissemination, five types of abscesses may be recognized according to the primary space occupied by the suppurative process. Spontaneous drainage may occur. Others resort to medical attention for evaluation and drainage. The literature is widely disparate with regard to the natural history of acute anorectal abscesses becoming chronic anal fistula. The incidence of abscesses forming anal fistula varies between 5 and 83 % according to one review [7].

In summary, five types of infections may result in essentially five types of anal fistula (Fig. 4.1). An understanding of the five types of abscesses and their potential to form five types of fistula is fundamental to the successful evaluation and treatment of nonspecific anorectal infections.

Clinical Evaluation

The routes of dissemination and primary space of occupation speak directly to the signs and symptoms presented by patients. Anatomy truly begets semiology—a patient's signs and symptoms. Perianal infections rarely pose a diagnostic problem. Patients present within a few days of onset of pain with obvious signs of an infection near the anal margin. Infections in this position are characterized by intense pain presumptively because these processes propagate from the sphincters through the micro-facial compartments formed by the corrugator cuti. A relatively small amount of suppuration can produce dramatic symptoms with obvious signs.

Abscesses in the ischioanal spaces behave quite differently. This compartment is comparatively large and comprised mostly by adipose tissue. Early abscesses may not demonstrate any overt physical signs. Many more days are generally required for detection by simple inspection. Before the evolution of obvious signs of rubor, dolor, calor, etc., ischioanal abscesses may be detected with a "bi-digital" rectal examination. With the examining index finger within the anorectum, the soft tissues are palpated by apposition of the thumb. Fullness of the ischioanal fossa is suggestive of an abscess in this position (Fig. 4.2).

Late presentation of ischioanal abscesses can be very dramatic especially in the setting of horseshoe abscesses, which occupy both fosse and one of the posterior spaces (Fig. 4.3).

A.E. Ortega, M.D. (✉) • K.G. Cologne, M.D.
Clinic Tower, 1200 N. State Street, A6231-A,
Los Angeles, CA 90033, USA
e-mail: ortega@med.usc.edu

H. Abcarian (ed.), *Anal Fistula: Principles and Management*, DOI 10.1007/978-1-4614-9014-2_4,
© Springer Science+Business Media New York 2014

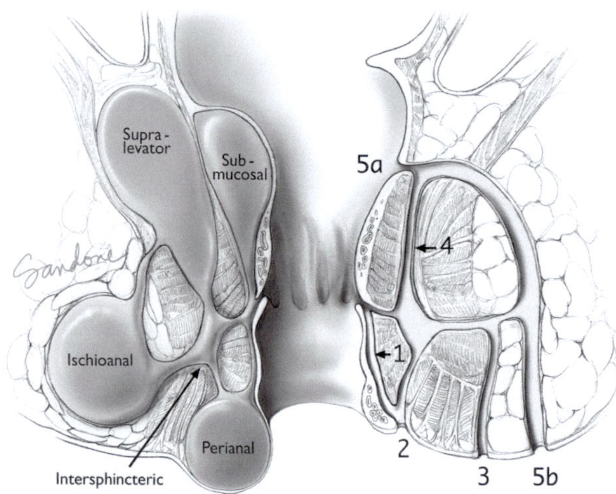

Fig. 4.1 Obstruction of anal gland at its crypt may result in infection disseminating via three pathways to form abscesses potentially in five anatomic locations (*left*). These abscesses may form fistulous trajectories, which mirror their initiating pathways and ending at their site of spontaneous versus surgical drainage (*right*)

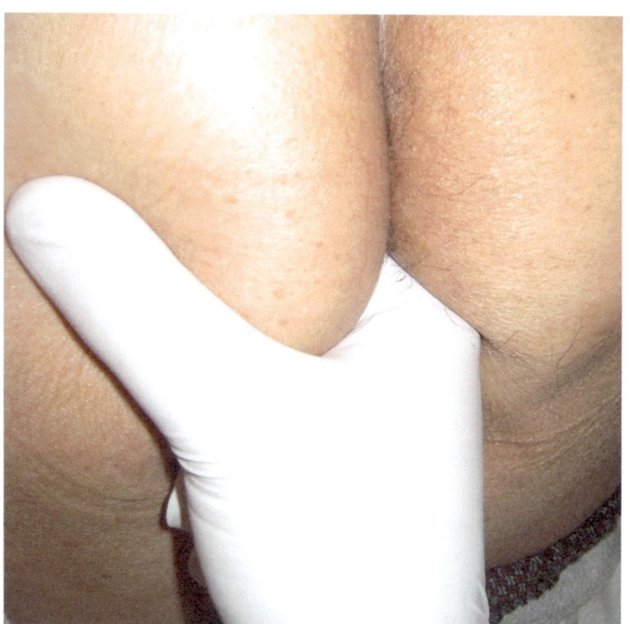

Fig. 4.2 Ischioanal space abscesses may be detected by palpation of the ischioanal fossa with the tissues palpated between the examiner's index finger and thumb ("bi-digital examination")

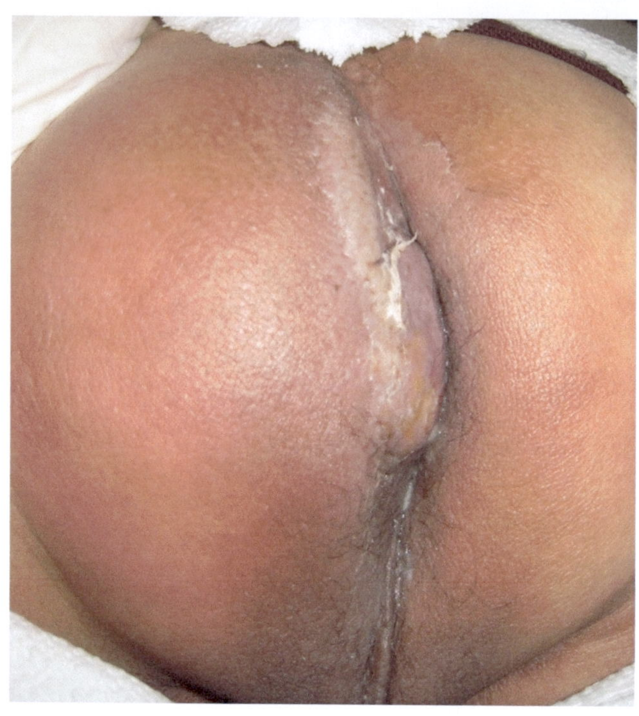

Fig. 4.3 A classic late presenting horseshoe abscess. Rubor and cellulitis are evident on both the left and right sides of the anal verge. The skin overlying the post-anal space is bulging with incipient epidermolysis

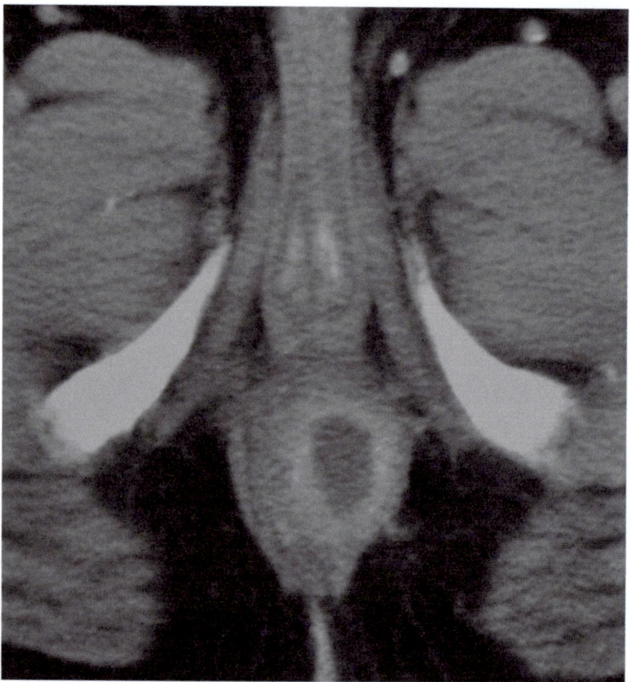

Fig. 4.4 A cystic fluid collection between the internal and external sphincter muscles of the mid-anal canal is evident on the CT scan. Note the incipient fat stranding in the bilateral ischioanal fossa. This is a classic appearance of a low-lying intersphincteric abscess

Intersphincteric abscesses may also pose a diagnostic challenge because of the relative paucity of physical signs. However, they represent a process, which is dissecting between the internal and external sphincters. Pain may in this scenario be amplified with bowel movements. Anorectal tenderness is the hallmark symptom. Many patients do not or will not tolerate an adequate examination. Imaging may be useful in this scenario (Fig. 4.4).

A patient's symptoms may provide other subtle clues regarding the anatomic configuration of an anorectal infection. Patients with abscesses above the sphincters may refer tenesmus, lower abdominal or pelvic pain. A primary abscess above the levators is confirmed by palpation of a boggy mass within the rectum on digital rectal examination. Palpation of rectal fullness in the setting of a patient with pain, possible fever and leukocytosis implies infection above the levator ani complex. There are three potential possible explanations:

1. A submucosal abscess
2. An intersphincteric supralevator abscess
3. An extrasphincteric supralevator abscess

Multiple space abscesses are not uncommon. The classic example is a horseshoe abscess arising from a posterior midline crypt. The propagation of infection arising from a posterior midline cryptoglandular complex may also propagate superficially, intersphincterically, or across the sphincters. Propagation of an infection across the sphincters into the ischioanal fossa is referred to as transphincteric. Those that cross the entire sphincter complex to reach the supralevator space are essentially extrasphincteric. Once an infection has reached one of these three posterior spaces, the process has a virtual free pathway to either or both ischioanal fossa—hence the pathogenesis of the horseshoe abscess. Suppurative processes originating in the abdomen or pelvis may dissect in the retro-rectal space. Once there, it has direct access to the ischioanal fossa via Alcock's canals bilaterally.

Effective evaluation of patients with anorectal infections requires an attentive history, which results in a directed physical examination. Inspection is the obvious first element, which may have in evidence obvious or visually imperceptible pathology. Bi-digital examination of the rectum confirms or excludes processes above the sphincters and/or the ischioanal fossa. An important component of the digital rectal examination includes palpation of the intersphincteric grove. This landmark physically is the step off palpable between the internal sphincter and the subcutaneous component of the external sphincter. It is a surrogate landmark for the dentate line within a 1–2 mm approximation. The originating crypt may be palpable on in this region. Pressure applied over the fluctuant process may decompress purulence into the offending crypt, which facilitates a definitive identification of the abscess and fistula. Examination of the rectum with either rigid or flexible sigmoidoscopy may be appropriate in selected cases where diagnostic uncertainty exists. All cases with perianal/perirectal necrosis should have an evaluation of the rectum as well as those demonstrating purulent drainage per rectum.

Imaging in Acute Anorectal Infection

Adjunctive imaging in the setting of cryptoglandular infections is rarely necessary with a careful clinical evaluation. However, it may be informative in the following settings:

- Suspicion of an intersphincteric abscess
- Patients with fluctuance or suppurative drainage within the rectum
- Evaluation of multiple space abscesses
- Consideration of an abdominopelvic etiology
- In cases of an inadequately drained or non-resolving infection

Figures 4.5 and 4.6 show clinical examples of selected imaging may be illustrative of the utility of imaging in acute anorectal infections.

Figure 4.7 shows the prevalence of the five types of infections based on pathway of dissemination and anatomic

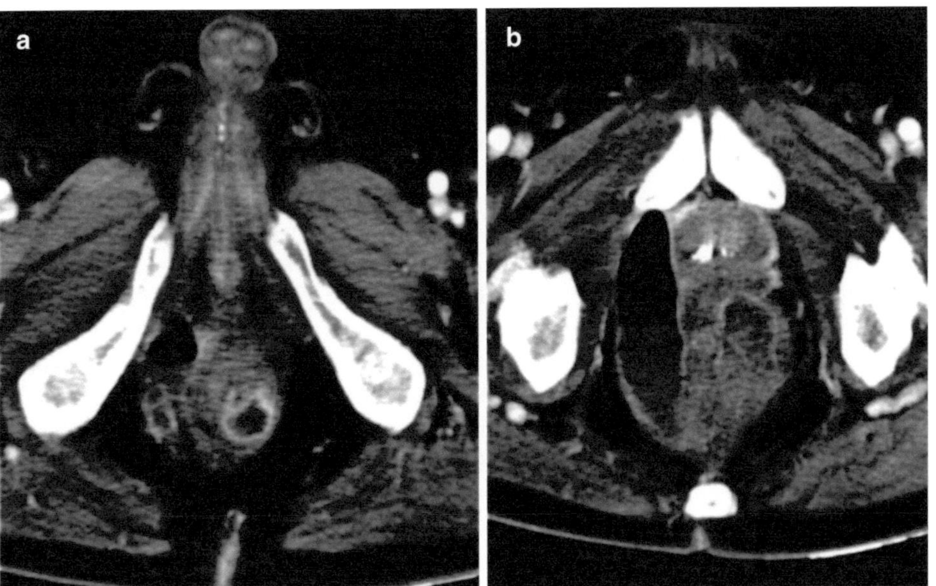

Fig. 4.5 (**a**) This CT scan image demonstrates fluid and gas within the sphincter complex at the level of the mid-anal canal. (**b**) A higher cut above the levator ani demonstrates an extensive fluid and gas collection. This scenario represents an intersphincteric supralevator abscess

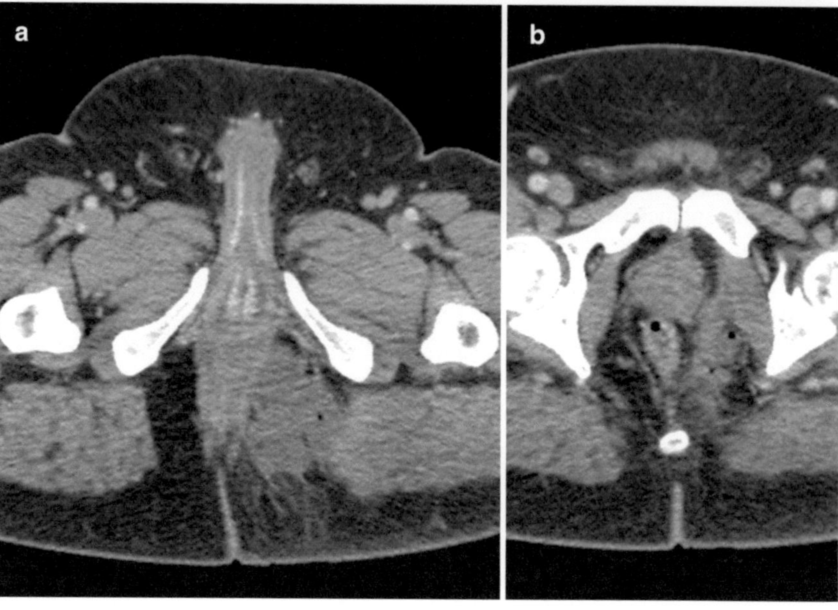

Fig. 4.6 (**a**) CT scan demonstrating a left-sided ischioanal abscess is in evidence. (**b**) A higher cut in the same case demonstrates an extrasphincteric extension of this abscess above the levators. Collectively, these two findings constitute an extrasphincteric supralevator abscess

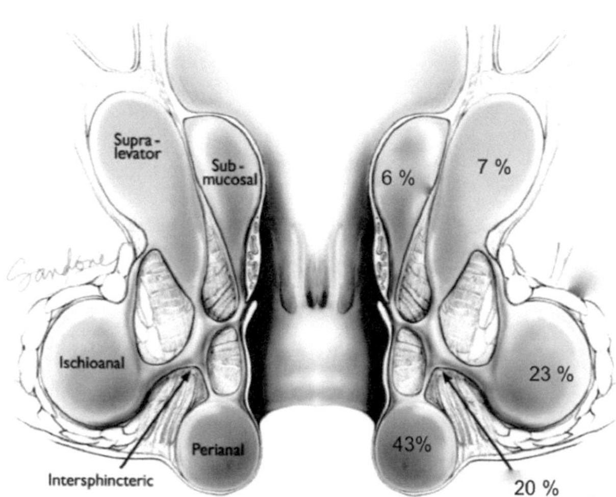

Fig. 4.7 Cryptoglandular anorectal infections occupy the perianal, ischioanal, intersphincteric, supralevator, and submucosal spaces in this order of frequency

location. It is readily apparent that majority of infections reside distally in the perianal, intersphincteric, or ischioanal spaces (86 %) [8].

Once supralevator infections are excluded by physical examination, it is generally acceptable to proceed with incision and drainage in the office or emergency department setting. The most important principle is to place a medial incision approximately 2.5 cm in length in a radial direction to the anal verge, which allows decompression of the suppurative process. The often-tempting impulse to place the incision over the greatest area of fluctuance may result in a very long resultant fistula. This tendency should be avoided at all cost. Instead, incision should be placed as medially as

possible while still over the abscess cavity. This approach minimizes the length of any subsequent fistula. Generally speaking, antibiotics are unnecessary except in immunocompromised patients and those with locally advanced and extensive soft-tissue infections. The authors prefer radial incisions over cruciate or circumanal because of their enhanced cosmetic result, i.e., radial incisions avoid a step off deformity once healing has occurred. Intersphincteric abscess confined to the distal anal canal can be simply managed with a stab-wound incision placed at the intersphincteric groove.

Infections above the levators and multiple space abscesses (horseshoes) are best managed in the operating room formally. Sedation and local anesthesia are generally sufficient in this setting, although general or regional anesthesia is also appropriate. Positioning is often the choice of the surgeon. However, the prone jackknife position is ideal in the teaching setting. Lithotomy and lateral decubitus positioning have their proponents. Once anesthetized, the surgeon is well advised to compress the area of fluctuance while simultaneously observing the crypts at the dentate line in order to identify the origin of the cryptoglandular infection. Compression of the abscess often results in purulent decompression of the abscess into the inciting crypt. Inflamed and infected crypts may also be palpable as a discreet divot or area of punctate induration at the base of the Morgagni columns. If the offending crypt is clearly identified, a probe may be passed very gently along the tract to identify the trajectory of the infection. Failure to identify the offending crypt and trajectory is a cause for pause. The surgeon is well advised to consider the type of fistula that may result from his or her intervention if the patient proceeds to the chronic phase (fistula formation). The ultimate goal is to provide satisfactory drainage and accept the potential formation of a fistula. A deliberate effort

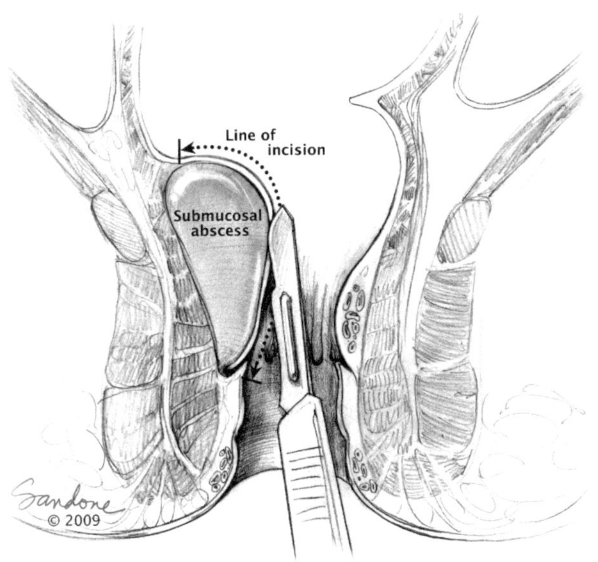

Fig. 4.8 Submucosal abscess drainage carries the incision from the dentate line to the apex of the collection within the anal canal and/or rectum

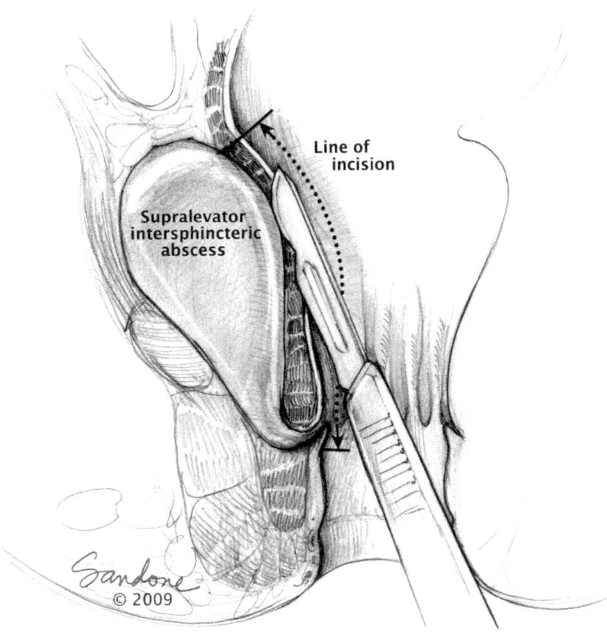

Fig. 4.9 A clearly demonstrated intersphincteric supralevator abscess is drained into the rectum in continuity with sectioning of the internal sphincter

is made to make the potentially resultant fistula as short and simple as possible. The debate over primary fistulotomy at the time of incision and drainage versus simple drainage remains operant but largely dependent on the surgeon's experience with this pathology.

The drainage of submucosal abscesses by extending an incision from the dentate line proximally through the anal canal and rectum is straightforward. An incision is made from the apex of the abscess within the rectum to the dentate line (Fig. 4.8). The abscess is drained into the rectum and anal canal in continuity. This procedure is facilitated greatly by performing it in a formal operating room.

Management of supralevator abscesses arising from an intersphincteric trajectory is slightly more complex. If the tract from the offending crypt to the abscess cavity is confidently identified, drainage is accomplished into the rectum and anal canal with a combined partial internal sphincterotomy (Fig. 4.9).

Extrasphincteric supralevator abscesses are by definition a multiple space infection, which traverse the sphincter process to ultimately dissect their way usually through the ischioanal fossa and into the supralevator spaces. These are categorically drained to perirectal skin just outside the anal margin with or without management of the primary cryptoglandular trajectory below. These are never drained into the rectum because of the complexity of the resultant fistula (Fig. 4.10).

The most commonly encountered multiple space abscess is the horseshoe comprising 15–20 % of all abscesses [9]. Its detection can be quite subtle or clinically quite dramatic. Inappropriate treatment may result from an overly cautious

intervention as well as from an overtly aggressive but imprecise surgical drainage (Figs. 4.4, 4.5, 4.6, 4.7, 4.8, 4.9, 4.10, and 4.11). An understanding of the underlying pathophysiology and anatomy is fundamental to the optimal management of horseshoe abscesses.

The underlying cause of the horseshoe abscess is the plugging of a posterior cryptoglandular structure. Like all others anal gland obstructions, the suppurative process dissects along the planes of the anorectum depending on the underlying relation of the anal gland to its surrounding musculocutaneous and tendinous structures. This propagation may proceed superficial to the sphincters, in-between the internal and external sphincters or across and potentially around and above the sphincters.

An obstructed posterior anal gland may propagate into theoretically one of four posterior spaces:
1. Superficial post-anal space
2. Deep post-anal space (of Courtney)
3. Supralevator space
4. Retro-rectal space

Direct spread to one or both ischioanal fossa may occur from any of these posterior spaces. The most common therapeutic mistake is the creation of bilateral counter incisions made over each ischioanal fossa and then connect these drainage sites with a penrose drain joining them passing through either the superficial or the deep post-anal spaces. This treatment usually results in a relatively challenging fistula (Fig. 4.12). Moreover, drainage may not be definitive.

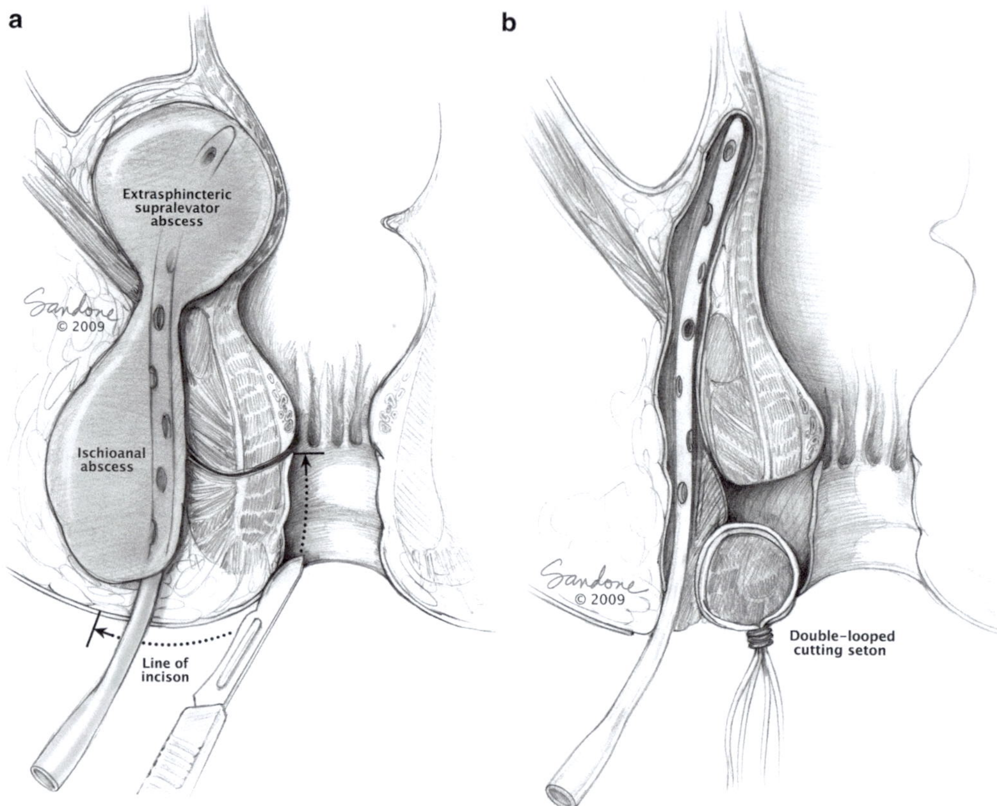

Fig. 4.10 (**a**) Incision and drainage of an extrasphincteric supralevator abscess requires drainage just outside the anal margin with a catheter. (**b**) Successful identification of the complicit cryptoglandular trajectory facilitates definitive treatment with a seton

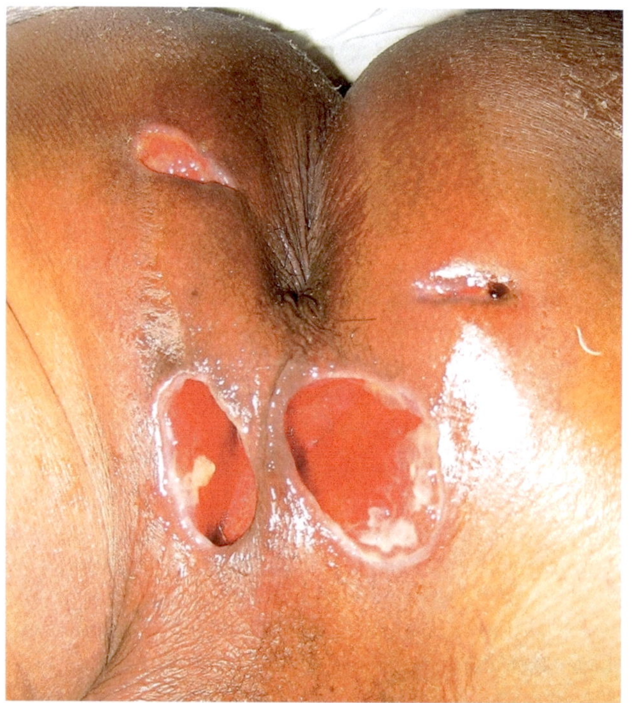

Fig. 4.11 Examination of a patient with a horseshoe abscess drained 1 week earlier with multiple incisions over the ischioanal fossa. The infection persists because of the absence of drainage of the post-anal space(s)

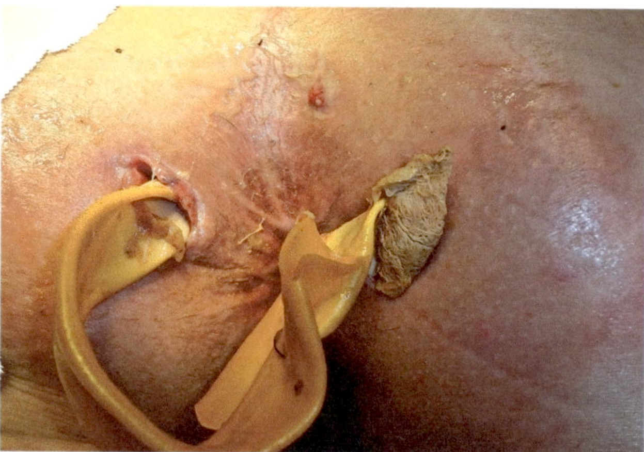

Fig. 4.12 A classic example of an inadequately treated horseshoe abscess is in evidence. A penrose drain was passed from one ischioanal fossa to the other via bilateral counter incisions days earlier. The surrounding cellulitis remains and an external opening is beginning to appear over the post-anal space in the posterior midline

The preferred approach in the management of the horseshoe abscess is exploration of the post-anal space. An incision is made from the posterior midline crypt to the tip of the coccyx. This maneuver exposes the superficial post-anal space. If the suppurative process is localized in this location, the bilateral ischioanal fossa should be explored digitally

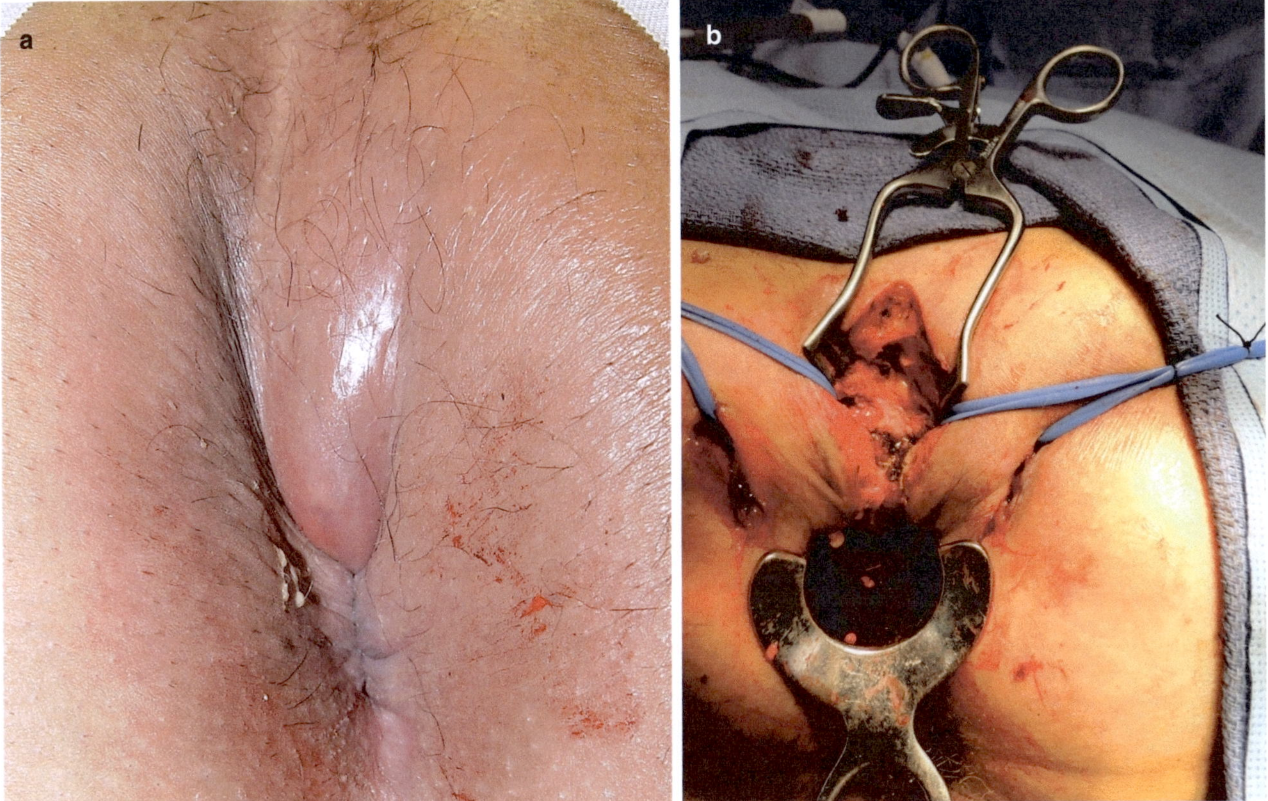

Fig. 4.13 Infection in the superficial post-anal space in continuity with both ischioanal fossa (**a**) is drained via a posterior midline incision and bilateral radial counter incisions with draining setons (**b**). The primary cryptoglandular trajectory appeared to be subcutaneous in this case

through this midline incision. If pus is encountered in either fossa, a radial counter incision is made either unilaterally or bilaterally (Fig. 4.13).

Once the superficial post-anal space is opened, it is often possible to delineate an intersphincteric trajectory of the cryptoglandular process. In this setting, some surgeons will elect to divide the internal sphincter unroofing the intersphincteric abscess into the superficial post-anal space. A reasonable alternative is the placement of a seton in this trajectory for management in a staged fashion (Fig. 4.14).

A normal exploration of the superficial post-anal spaced suggests a deeper infection in the deep post-anal space. There are three ways to gain surgical access into the deep post-anal space (Fig. 4.15):

1. Transanal division of the internal and the subcutaneous portion of the external sphincters.
2. Horizontal sectioning of the anococcygeal ligament disconnecting the sphincter from the coccyx;
3. Vertical sectioning of the anococcygeal ligament in its midline.

The first approach is that technique classically described by Hanley [10]. It is highly definitive in that it drains the primary abscess and the responsible cryptoglandular trajectory simultaneously. The disadvantage is that immediate

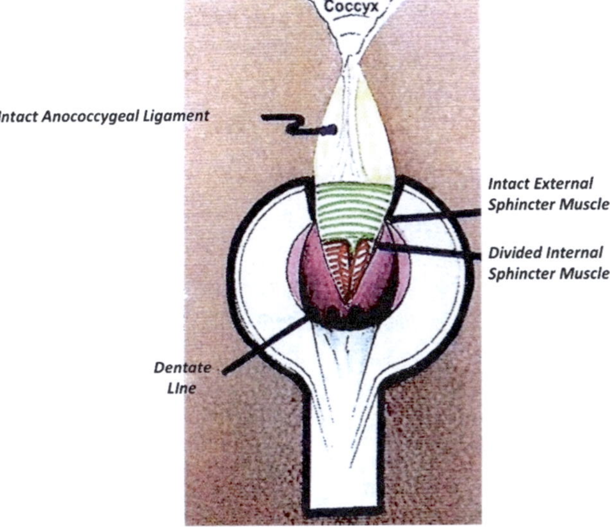

Fig. 4.14 Drainage of an intersphincteric superficial post-anal space abscess is accomplished with an incision from the midline posterior crypt to the tip of the coccyx in continuity with sectioning of the internal sphincter anterior to the culprit cryptoglandular trajectory

postoperative incontinence is the rule and not the exception. This complication appears to be relatively short-lived. However, it is particularly disturbing to the patient as well as

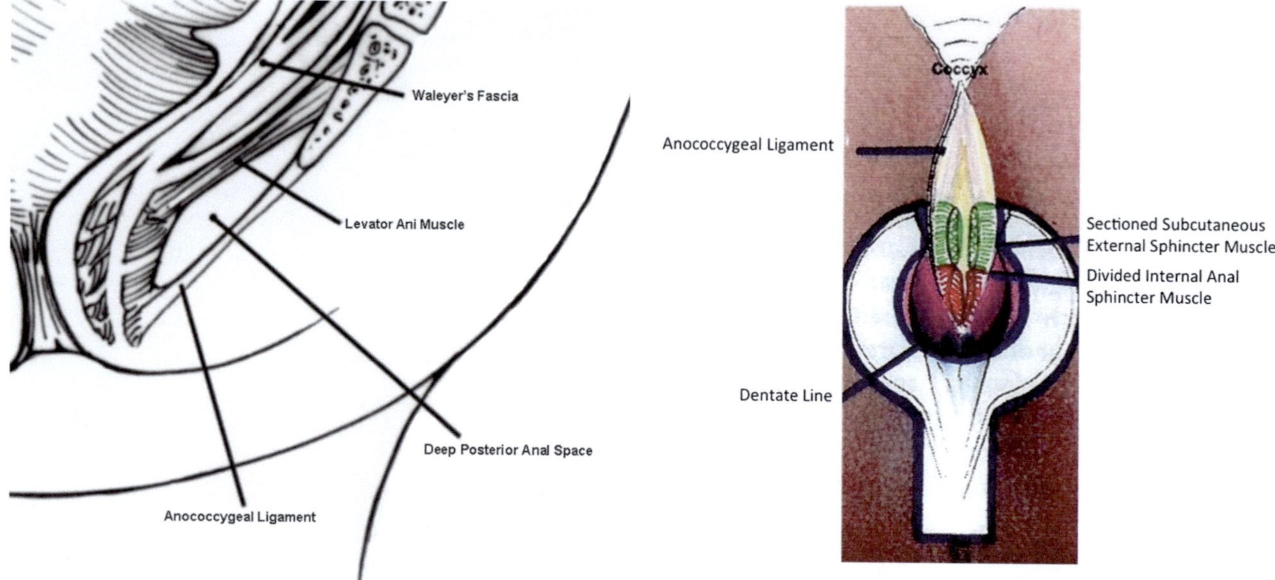

Fig. 4.15 Some form of sectioning of the anococcygeal ligament is required for access to the deep post-anal space. This approach also provides access to the supralevator space posteriorly as the pubococcygeus and ileococcygeus muscles insert onto to the sides of the tip of the coccyx. Adapted with permission from Kaiser and Ortega [6]

Fig. 4.16 The classic "Hanley" approach to the deep post-anal spaces divides the internal sphincter in continuity with the subcutaneous portion of the external sphincter. The anococcygeal ligament is functionally detached from the sphincter complex

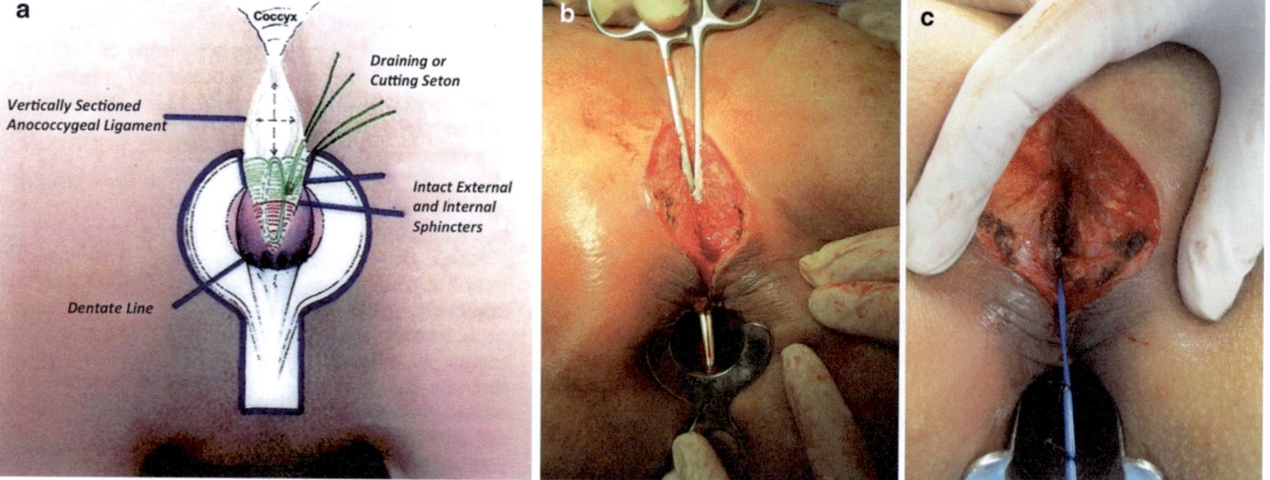

Fig. 4.17 (**a**) This technique exposes the post-anal space from posterior crypt to the tip of the coccyx. The anococcygeal ligament is incised vertically. (**b**) Once access to the deep post-anal space is established, the wound is explored gently to identify the responsible cryptoglandular trajectory. In essence, the primary infection has already accomplished this dissection. (**c**) A cutting or draining seton is left encircling the sphincters through the trajectory of the primary infected/obstructed cryptoglandular complex

the treating surgeon. This technique may also result in a long-term keyhole deformity (Fig. 4.16).

Transverse sectioning of the anococcygeal ligament also provides access to the deep post-anal space. In the short term, this maneuver is well tolerated. The long-term effect upon the sphincter is not precisely known.

The authors prefer entering the deep post-anal space by a vertical division of the anococcygeal ligament along its midline. This maneuver theoretically maintains the stability of the sphincter complex with respect to the coccyx. The primary cryptoglandular complex may be encircled with a seton for management in a staged fashion (Fig. 4.17).

It is important to note that horseshoe abscesses may not have overt skin changes early in their evolution. Moreover, the classic bilateral rubor over the ischioanal fossa may represent underlying frank suppuration *or* merely cellulitis emanating from the primary abscess. Therefore, counter incisions may be made on a more selective basis once a careful assessment is made from the posterior midline incision.

Postoperative management of cutting or draining setons affords a number of options. One option is to convert the draining seton encircling the sphincter mechanism into a cutting seton. However, a staged transphincteric fistulotomy in the posterior midline using a cutting seton may require 16–28 weeks [11]. Many surgeons prefer to await healing in the posterior midline wound. The shortened, well-defined fistula tract with an indwelling draining seton may then be managed at a later time generally with either a primary fistulotomy or an endorectal advancement flap.

References

1. Corman ML, editor. Colon and rectal surgery. 5th ed. Philadelphia: Lippincott, Williams & Wilkins; 2005. p. 279.
2. Herrmann G, Desfosses L. Sur la muqueuse la la region cloacale du rectum. CR Acad Sci. 1880;90:1301.
3. Chiari H. Ueber die analen Divertikel der Rectumsschleim-haut und ihre Beziehung zu den Analfisteln. Med Jahr. 1878;8:419.
4. Eisenhammer S. The internal anal sphincter and anorectal abscess. Surg Gynaecol Obstet. 1956;103:501–6.
5. Parks AG. The pathogenesis and treatment of fistula-in-ano. Br Med J. 1961;i:463–9.
6. Kaiser AM, Ortega AE. Anorectal anatomy. Surg Clin North Am. 2002;82:1125–38.
7. Rickard MJFX. Anal abscesses and fistulas. ANZ J Surg. 2005;75:64–72.
8. Ramanujam PS, Prasad ML, Abcarian H, Tan AB. Perianal abscesses and fistulas. A study of 1023 patients. Dis Colon Rectum. 1984;27:593–7.
9. Ustynoski K, Rosen L, Stasik J, Riether R, Sheets J, Khubchandani IT. Horseshoe abscess fistula. Dis Colon Rectum. 1990;33(7):602–5.
10. Hanley PH. Conservative surgical correction of horseshoe abscess and fistula. Dis Colon Rectum. 1965;8:364.
11. Gonzalez-Ruiiz C, Kaiser AM, Vukasin P, Beart RW, Ortega AE. Intraoperative diagnosis in the management of anal fistula. Am Surg. 2006;72(1):11–5.

Herand Abcarian

Introduction

A successful outcome from any type of fistula operation is dependent on accurate clinical assessment and classification. Generally, surgeons rely on a detailed history and careful physical examination.

The history of an anal fistula is often quite typical. The patient gives a history of a prior episode of perianal swelling and pain (low abscess) or deep rectal pain with fever and systemic symptoms (high abscess). The abscess either ruptures spontaneously and drainage of pus and blood is followed by resolution of acute pain or alternately the abscess may be drained by a surgeon to relieve the symptoms and prevent spreading sepsis. The spontaneously or surgically drained abscess will take one of three courses: (1) complete healing and no recurrence (less likely), (2) nonhealing and continuous drainage (more likely), or (3) healing and recurrence of the abscess (most likely).

The patient must be told that the infectious process begins in the anal canal and spreads outward and drainage of the abscess alone may not be adequate to eradicate the infection. Therefore, the patient should not blame the subsequent recurrent infections on the inadequacy of the original surgical drainage or the surgeon's skill.

This typical history can be found in the overwhelming majority of patients with fistula in ano. However, if the abscess is due to an ingested foreign body (e.g., fish bone, chicken bone, toothpick, needle, etc.), the sign and symptoms of anorectal abscess might be more muted and insidious until a full-blown abscess presents itself a few days later. On the other hand, the history of an infection caused by external penetrating injury is much clearer and the clinical course easier to follow. Abscesses due to inflammatory

bowel disease are often much less painful, contain very thin pus and the patient may present with some pain and drainage for weeks without a significant acute illness. Patients with hematologic disorders such as acute myelogenous leukemia (AML) often present with pain, erythema, fever, and tachycardia; but due to lack of leukocytosis (due to the original illness or as a result of chemotherapy) are unable to produce pus because of severe leukopenia. This is more likely to be seen in hematology–oncology units of major medical centers than in physician/surgeon's offices. When such patients are encountered, the surgeon must not rush into attempting to drain the abscess especially when in the majority of cases severe thrombocytopenia is part and parcel of pancytopenia. Aggressive board spectrum antibiotic therapy, patient isolation and supportive therapy including liberal use of granulocyte stimulating factor (GSF) should be instituted and the patient reexamined every few hours.

Recurrent fistulas appear at the exact same anatomic location after an abscess has apparently healed [1]. Intermittent swelling and pain followed by drainage and relief of pain are typical symptoms of anal fistulas. It should be noted that although horseshoe fistulas may drain on one side and later on the contralateral perianal space, their incidence are much less frequent than "regular" fistulas.

Assessment

The physical examination must be done with utmost gentleness and reassuring the patient that it should not cause any pain, especially if the acute abscess has already been dealt with. The patient may be examined on a tilt table in the knee chest position, but the same can be carried out in the Sims position if a prostoscopic table is not available. The first landmark is often readily visible to the secondary opening of the fistula, is often open and draining or has a telltale granulation tissue protruding from the opening. If a fistula opening is sealed, whether healed or temporarily closed with an epithelial layer, it is often seen as a small depression especially

H. Abcarian, M.D., F.A.C.S. (✉)
The University of Illinois at Chicago, Division of Colon and Rectal Surgery, John Stroger Hospital of Cook Country, IL 60612, USA
e-mail: abcarian@uic.edu

H. Abcarian (ed.), *Anal Fistula: Principles and Management*, DOI 10.1007/978-1-4614-9014-2_5,
© Springer Science+Business Media New York 2014

in chronic fistulas with fibrosis and retraction of the external opening.

The next step is to palpate the fistula tract. The Goodsall's rule illustrated in Chap. 2 often applies, especially if the fistula has not been operated on previously. Palpation of the soft tissue between the secondary opening and the anal canal often feels like a firm cord (much like the extensor tendons of the fingers) connecting the two. In deeper (higher) fistulas, this cord-like structure can be palpated only to the margin if the external sphincter as the tracts dips under the muscle to connect with the anal canal. The same finding can be elicited bilaterally in cases of horseshoe fistulas.

Rectal examination with bi-digital palpation may elicit induration in the perianal or ischiorectal fossa at the same side of the fistula. This signifies presence of an acute or chronic abscess cavity associated with the fistula. The primary opening may feel like small grain of rice or lentil. This is usually not painful unless there is active suppuration. In such cases, it is better to examine the patient under anesthesia and in the operating room. High fistula tracts will be felt as an indentation above the dentate line in the anorectal ring or lower rectal wall. Even then the primary opening is most often at the dentate line corresponding to Goodsall's rule, unless the patient has had previous surgery or the fistula is caused by perforation of the anorectal wall due to an ingested sharp foreign body as mentioned above.

Anoscopy, using an anoscope with side opening (e.g., Vernon-David or Ives) will allow visualization of the primary opening, which is often seen as a small dimple. Gentle pressure on the fistula track may result in discharge of pus from the primary opening, which confirms the diagnosis.

Examination under anesthesia (EUA) is undertaken with plans to address the fistula with curative intent. Due to the cost associated with EUA, this procedure should not be used routinely to clinically assess the fistula tract. The surgeon however may judiciously proceed to use a draining seton instead of definite surgical procedure if the fistula is considered to be too complex or undrained pus is encountered during EUA.

The best technique to delineate a fistula is gently advancing a blunt tipped probe (e.g., Pratt or S-shaped) from the secondary toward the primary opening while the latter is kept under vision with an operating anoscope or felt with the examining finger. If the fistula tract is torturous or curved, lateral traction using a Kocher clamp is often helpful to straighten the tract facilitating the passage of the fistula probe. If the fistula tract is very thin, lacrimal probes may be used instead of the regular fistula probes. If the fistula tract is very narrow, one may have difficulty delineating it even with lacrimal probes. In such cases slow injection of hydrogen peroxide alone or with the addition of 1–2 drops of methylene blue might result in bubbling of the injected material through the primary opening. A larger amount of methylene blue tends to stain the granulation tissue in dark blue color and obscure its ease of identification. This technique also is not fool proof and if a primary opening is not identified, it is best to terminate the procedure and try another EUA during a future symptomatic phase of fistula. It is not uncommon to be able to find the internal opening at a second or third try and the surgeon should avoid getting frustrated and persist to the point of causing a false passage. When the internal opening is found after some additional maneuvers, it is best to insert a loose marking seton to allow easy identification of the fistula tract during a subsequent definitive surgical procedure [2, 3]. Other helpful maneuvers in identification of the primary opening are covered in Chap. 9.

Ordinarily, a fistula being treated for the first time requires very little if any additional imaging. However with multiple operations resulting in scarring and distortion of the fistula tract, and in cases where there is more than one fistula encountered imaging might be helpful.

Imaging modalities are covered in Chap. 6, but essentially consist of the following:

1. Fistulography, which was popularized in the 1970s and 1980s but has fallen out of favor with advent of other imaging modalities. There were publications pro and con of fistulography but currently this procedure is rarely utilized [4].
2. Endoanal ultrasonography without or with injection of peroxide in the fistula tract. This modality is helpful not only in delineating the fistula tract and other potential associated tracts or abscess cavity but also as a road map for identification of fistula tracts during surgery.
3. Computerized tomography of pelvis and perineum with administration of contrast intravenously, intrarectally, orally, or injection through the fistula tract is helpful but more reserved for "high" fistulas originating in the pelvis or supralevator space.
4. Magnetic resonance imaging is quite helpful in diagnosing fistula and assessing the closure of the fistula after seemingly successful procedures, especially in Crohn's disease.

Much like preoperative staging of rectal cancer, interpretation of pelvic and perianal MRI requires expertise and is "operator dependent."

The purpose of the clinical assessment of fistula is twofold.

1. Identification of primary and secondary openings and the fistula tract itself which is described above.
2. Assessment of the complexity of fistula including clinical classification and the thickness of sphincter muscle involved. This is much harder than simple identification of the tract because it takes experience and judgment to decide which fistula is easily amenable to fistulotomy and which requires sphincter-sparing procedure. As Phillip suggests, it is more important to know how much sphincter will be left behind rather how much will be divided during fistulotomy (see Chap. 9). Reducing this to its simple form, it is

important for the surgeon to be sure whether the fistula is high or low and if the surgeon is inexperienced, unsure, or does not treat anal fistulas on regular basis, it is better to insert a loose marking seton (braided suture or vessel loop) in the tract and refer the patient to a specialist [3]. In other words, if in doubt, the surgeon must adhere to the policy of "primum non nocere."

Conclusion

Although fistula in ano is not a life-threatening disease, it is quite frustrating for the patient and the surgeon who goes through multiple procedures and get disappointed with the treatment failures and recurrences.

It is for this reason and medical/legal implications of treatment-related fecal incontinence that the involvement of a colon and rectal surgical specialist in the treatment of anal fistula is not only desirable, but most often mandatory.

References

1. Charbot C, Prasad ML, Abcarian H. Recurrent anorectal abscess. Dis Colon Rectum. 1983;26:105.
2. Ramanujam PS, Prasad ML, Abcarian H. Role of seton in fistulotomy of the anus. Surg Gynecol Obstet. 1983;419:157.
3. Pearl PK, Andrews JR, Orsay CP, et al. Role of seton in the management of anorectal fistulas. Dis Colon Rectum. 1993;36:573–9.
4. Kuipers HC, Shulpen TM. Fistulography for fistula-in-ano. Is it useful? Dis Colon Rectum. 1985;28(2):103–4.

Clinical Assessment and Imaging Modalities of Fistula in Ano

Kyle G. Cologne, Juan Antonio Villanueva-Herrero, Enrique Montaño-Torres, and Adrian E. Ortega

Introduction

Fistula disease is a frequent consequence of anorectal abscess. Up to 50 % of patients with an anorectal abscess progress to develop a chronic fistula. Cryptoglandular or idiopathic origin is the most frequent cause. Crohn's disease is the second most common [1].

The treatment of anal fistulas represents a significant problem in colorectal surgery. The first described treatment dates back to Hippocrates—the first to describe the use of a seton [2]. Hundreds of remedies have been proscribed to treat this disorder since. The difficulty in finding a universally successful treatment speaks to the pleomorphic nature of this disease entity. Clinical evaluation of fistulas becomes critical to determining the appropriate intervention. This chapter describes an approach to the assessment of fistulas and outlines the use of adjunctive imaging modalities.

Classification

Several classification schemes have been developed to better conceptualize fistulas. These are critical to understand. They portend implications important both in terms of defining anatomy and the likelihood of therapeutic success.

K.G. Cologne, M.D.
Keck School of Medicine at the University of Southern California, Los Angeles, CA, USA

J.A. Villanueva-Herrero, M.D.
Clinica Especializada en Colon, Recto y Ano (CECRA) and Hospital General de Mexico, Mexico DF, Mexico

E. Montaño-Torres, M.D.
Clinica Especializada en Colon, Recto y Ano (CECRA) and Hospital General Regional de Iztapalapa, Mexico DF, Mexico

A.E. Ortega, M.D. (✉)
Keck School of Medicine at the University of Southern California, Los Angeles, CA, USA

LAC+USC Medical Center, Los Angeles, CA, USA
e-mail: ortega@med.usc.edu

David Henry Goodsall is credited with the first "topographical" description of anal fistula. He divided the perianal region into posterior and anterior hemispheres. Goodsall's rule states that fistula having an external orifices situated behind (posterior) to a transverse line drawn through the center of the anus usually have their internal orifice in the posterior midline. It further states that fistula with an external opening in front (anterior) of this line generally have an internal opening directly in line with this, forming a straight, radial fistulous trajectory (Fig. 6.1) [3]. In a series examining the accuracy of this dictum in 216 patients with fistulas, it appears to be more accurate for posterior fistulas. Anterior fistulas less often follow this straight course described, with an average of 49 % following the proposed path [4]. Therefore, Goodsall's rule serves as an imperfect guide to identify the course of fistula tracts.

Park's classification of fistulas represents the de facto description of fistulas today [5]. His initial classification scheme was slightly more elaborate, but included the following four basic fistula types (with percentages based on his preliminary series of 400 patients): intersphincteric (45 %), transphincteric (29 %), suprasphincteric (20 %) and extrasphincteric (5 %). Today, these percentages have changed slightly based on larger series to represent the scope of clinical disease as follows: intersphincteric (70 %), transphincteric (20–25 %), suprasphincteric (1–3 %), and extrasphincteric (1–2 %) (Fig. 6.2) [6].

Intersphincteric fistulas are the most common. They traverse a minimal distance and extend from an internal opening near the intersphincteric groove to an external location typically located outside the anal margin. The intersphincteric groove represents the palpable step off between the internal sphincter and the subcutaneous portion of the external sphincter. Within a few millimeters, it represents a surrogate landmark for the dentate line where the anal crypts reside. Intersphincteric fistula is a result of a drained perianal abscess originating from a gland that did not extend beyond the external sphincter. The fact that this is the most common type of fistula is consistent with the anatomic description that 80 % of glands are submucosal, 8 % extend to the internal

H. Abcarian (ed.), *Anal Fistula: Principles and Management*, DOI 10.1007/978-1-4614-9014-2_6,
© Springer Science+Business Media New York 2014

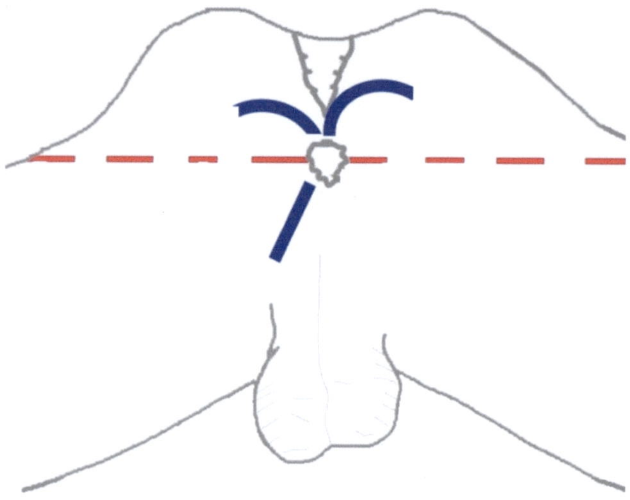

Fig. 6.1 Goodsall's rule states that anal fistula with anterior secondary openings tend to follow a straight radial trajectory to a primary opening in the anal canal at the level of the dentate line. Posterior secondaries follow a curvilinear trajectory into a posterior midline primary. Anterior secondary openings found greater than 3 cm from the anus also tend to follow a curvilinear path into the posterior midline crypt

sphincter, 8 % course to the longitudinal external muscle, and only 3 % penetrate the internal sphincter extending beyond the intersphincteric space [7].

Transphincteric fistulas are the next commonest. These involve both the internal and external sphincters and pass into the ischioanal fossa. These typically result from a peri-rectal abscess. The length of the fistula is determined by the location of the previous incision and drainage or site of spontaneous decompression.

Suprasphincteric fistulas are relatively rare. These curvilinear fistula tracts originate at the level of the dentate line but traverse cephalad above the puborectalis before turning downward through the ischioanal fossa to reach the perianal skin.

Extrasphincteric fistulas are usually caused by overzealous probing and creation of false fistula tracts. These result in an internal opening above the sphincter complex that passes through the levators rendering them amongst the most difficult types to treat.

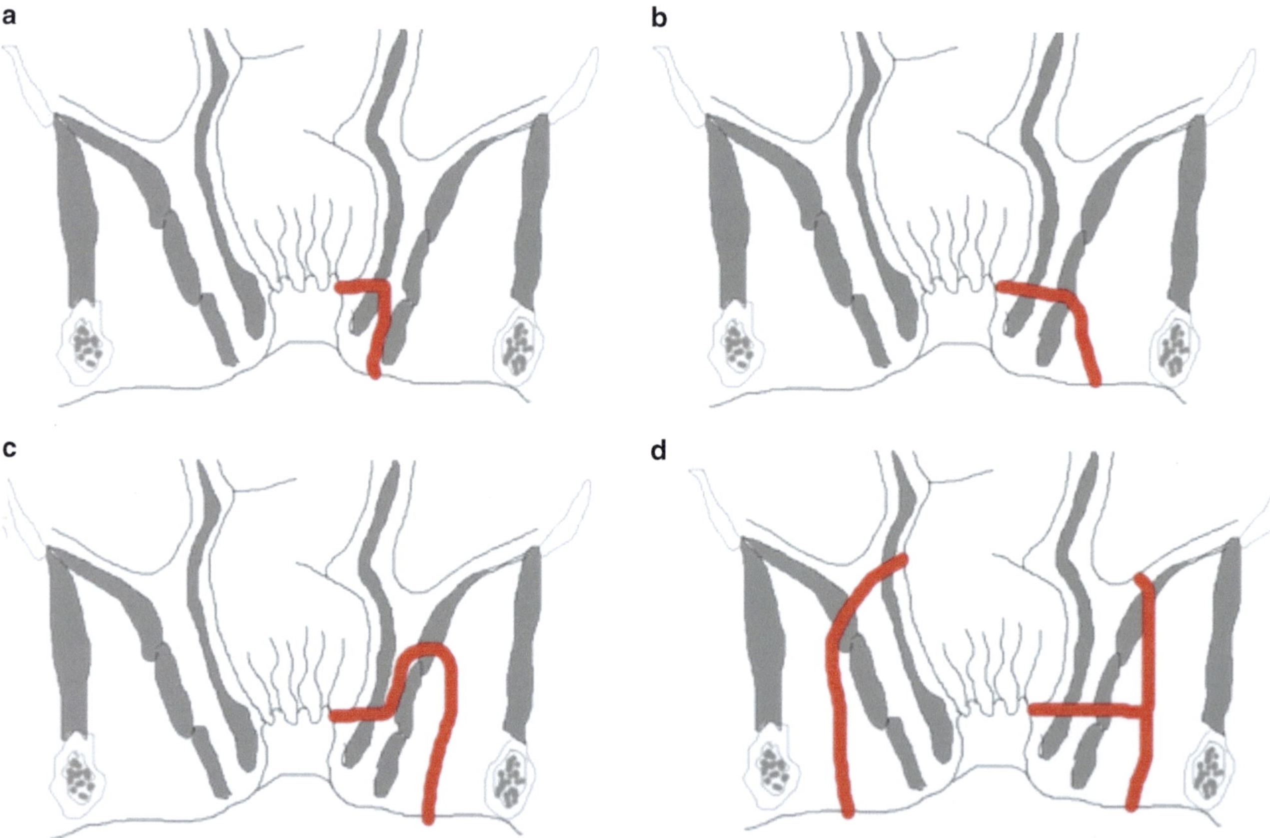

Fig. 6.2 Park's classification of anal fistulas: (**a**) low intersphincteric; (**b**) low transphincteric; (**c**) supralevator; (**d**) two variations of extrasphincteric fistula. On the left is a variant seen in iatrogenic recurrent fistulas or associated with Crohn's disease. On the right is an uncommon variant of cryptglandular origin

The concept "complex fistula" is a common term in the surgical vernacular, albeit not a part of Park's classification. A useful definition of "complex fistula" is any fistula other than a simple intersphincteric or low transphincteric configuration. The term further may be used to describe those that include multiple tracks, anterior location in females, recurrent fistulas, those with preexisting incontinence, previous radiation, or in the setting of another disease process (such as Crohn's disease) [8]. It is termed complex because the treatment requires a more complicated approach and cannot be treated by simple fistulotomy. The "complex fistula" has been a catalyst of much innovation, although no single approach has proven superior at adequately eradicating this disease process. Infections tracking above the levator muscles may ultimately form suprasphincteric or extrasphincteric fistula. The former course between the sphincter muscles; the latter course lateral to the external sphincter muscle. Abdominal pelvic infections may disseminate into the retrorectal and supralevator spaces as well as the ischioanal fossae via Alcock's canals acutely. Drainage lateral to sphincter complex is recommended but may result in an extrasphincteric fistula.

One additional type of fistula includes the horseshoe fistula. These originate most commonly from either bilateral intersphincteric or transphincteric fistula tracts arising from a single posterior midline crypt. They are important to recognize, because they are often mismanaged due to a failure to identify the underlying source—infection in one of the postanal or posterior space(s): superficial, deep, supralevator, and rarely retrorectal.

Clinical Evaluation

Anal fistula arising in the setting of specific diseases should be investigated according to the clinical context in which they present. The classic example is chronic inflammatory bowel disease—particularly Crohn's. Evaluation includes the documentation of the state of the rectal mucosa assessed by endoscopic examination prior to any attempt at fistulotomy. Satisfactory results are much lower with the success rates of definitive surgery often below 50 % when active proctitis is present [9]. Moreover, sphincter function should be assessed and clearly documented. If appropriate, an incontinence score should be assigned to these patients. All procedures for the surgical correction of anal fistula have the potential of altering fecal continence. However, preexisting alterations in continence are important to document preoperatively. Finally, investigation into any imunocompromised state, such as HIV, should be a part of the history. There is conflicting evidence whether low CD4+ counts affect wound healing. Patients on Highly Active Antiviral Therapy (HAART) with normal CD4+ counts should be treated no differently than non-immunosuppressed patients [10–12].

In the absence of any complicating factors, most colorectal surgeons will proceed with an exam under anesthesia (EUA) and definitive surgical eradication of the fistula by a variety of surgical techniques currently available. The role of preoperative imaging has been debated. It remains unclear that this adds any additional information to the skilled practitioner. Arguments for the preoperative use include that it aids in operative planning and counseling the patient as well as allowing the practitioner to proceed with an appropriate definitive procedure at the first operation [13, 14]. Opponents argue that even with complex fistula tracts, definitive management at the first procedure is not always possible. The primary goal should be control of anorectal sepsis, with definitive procedure reserved for a time when there is decreased infection and inflammation of surrounding tissues [15]. Although imaging can serve to correctly identify the course of the fistula tract in the majority of patients, it remains unclear whether the time and expense to perform these studies is justified, especially since most patients will have low-lying, simple fistulas. The true advantages of these imaging techniques come in delineating high, multiple, or recurrent tracts. It is the authors' preference to always perform EUA and definitive fistula management at the time of the first surgery if possible. Adjunctive imaging techniques are reserved for those whose anatomy is unclear at the time of surgery. A review of 101 patients showed that primary crypt identification was possible 93 % of the time with surgery alone. Hydrogen peroxide was seen to drain through the internal opening of 83 % of those who underwent injection through the external opening of the fistula [16].

There are other useful techniques during EUA for anal fistula. Palpation of the intersphincteric groove with an index finger often reveals palpable induration or a divot in the area of the originating crypt. Superficial fistula tracts can also be palpable from their external opening into the anal canal. Some authors employ a crochet-type hooked probe to identify the internal opening. Others apply a clamp lateral to the external opening in order "to straighten" the tract. The safety and efficacy of these last two maneuvers is unknown.

The authors' practice is ritualistic and regimented in the following fashion during the course of EUA for anal fistula:

1. Topographical inspection of the perianal region
2. Palpation of the intersphincteric groove and the tissues surrounding the external opening(s)
3. Examination of the anal canal with a Parks retractor
4. Injection of the external opening(s) with hydrogen peroxide ± dilute methylene blue; multiple external openings are injected from furthest away to those most medial to the anal verge
5. Passage of a silver probe gently from the external opening to the internal opening.

Of note, multiple external openings are common. However, more than one internal opening is also known to

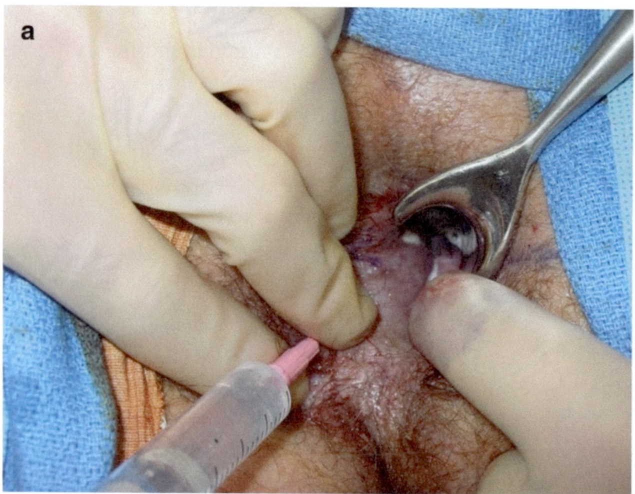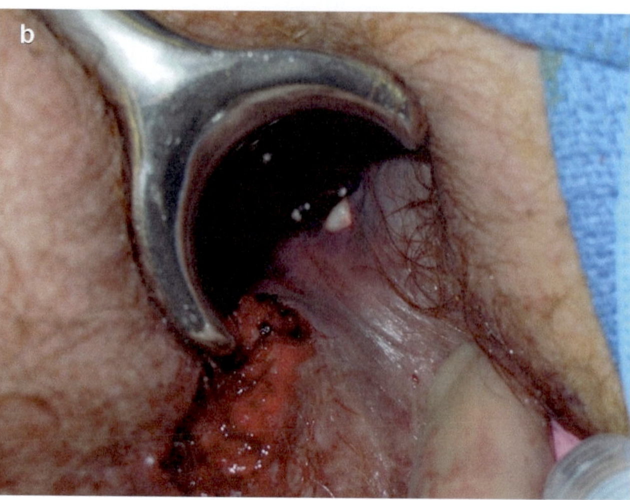

Fig. 6.3 (**a**) Injection of a left anterolateral external opening. Hydrogen peroxide emanates from two adjacent cypts via radial trajectories. (**b**) Injection of a right second anterolateral external opening a third independent radial tract in this same patient. This case underscores the importance of a stepwise, regimented approach for the evaluation of anal fistula at the timer of EUA

occur. Therefore, passage of the probe as an initial maneuver may be misleading as well as potentially iatrogenic if a false opening is created. A case in point is evident in Fig. 6.3.

Failure to identify a primary internal opening is not uncommon. The most traditional approach in this setting is to sequentially follow the tract from the external opening hopefully to its origin at the internal opening. This approach has inherent risks especially when following a deep fistulous trajectory. It is eminently reasonable to back out and obtain either an ultrasound or MRI. Another potential promising alternative in this setting is the video-assisted anal fistula treatment (VAAFT) technology platform. Further experience is necessary.

Radiologic Evaluation

In cases of complex fistulas or recurrent anal fistulas, the use of imaging techniques should be strongly considered. It should be noted that the most common reason for extrasphincteric fistula tract development is iatrogenic probing and creation of false fistula tracts. Therefore, if it is not possible to delineate or control the entire fistula tract at the time of the index operation, it is advisable to control what can be identified and investigate the anatomy further with advanced imaging. There exist numerous options for imaging of fistulas. These include CT, MRI, ultrasound, and fistulography.

Fistulography using fluoroscopy and computed tomography (CT) are regarded as obsolete because of the radiation burden, and suboptimal visualization of fistulas using contrast media [17]. An exception may be in the acute setting with suspected abscess. CT scanning is useful acutely to define the location of an infection where there is a paucity of clinical findings. This allows the practitioner to define any deeper areas of infection and suggest an origin (such as a supralevator, pure intersphincteric, extrasphincteric, or horseshoe abscesses). This additional information is useful to know before proceeding to the operating room to deal with an abscess with appropriate aggressiveness. CT imaging plays little or no role in the evaluation of chronic fistula tracts.

Endorectal ultrasound (US) provides excellent definition of the fistula tract anatomy, especially with fistula tract enhancement using hydrogen peroxide. Correlation with intraoperative examination is better than 90–94 %. [13, 18–20]. Although endorectal ultrasound provides excellent definition of anatomy, it does depend to a large degree on the examiner's experience. 3D imaging has enhanced further the accuracy of ultrasound examination, and has been used since the late 1990s [21]. The ultrasound probe may be used with two frequency settings: 7 or 10 MHz. Higher frequency (e.g., 10 MHz) does not penetrate as deeply, but gives higher resolution images close to the probe. For this reason, it is ideally suited for ultrasound within the anal canal, but may not be as well suited for deeper fistula tracks passing at some distance from the rectum [22]. The authors consider that single image, 2D ultrasonography is difficult to interpret. Moreover, situations in which the interpreter may not have been present at the time of the examination implies an additional and significant handicap. Fistula tracts are 3D structures and their course is difficult to convey on a single images. As a result, 3D ultrasound allows a more thorough evaluation of the fistula anatomy outside of the time of examination. This feature is extremely useful for the practitioner who does not do his/her own ultrasonography (Fig. 6.4).

There are several "tricks" to properly performing injection of hydrogen peroxide at the time of EUS. Gas bubbles can create artifact and obscure anatomy. Therefore, a minimum amount of hydrogen peroxide should be used during the

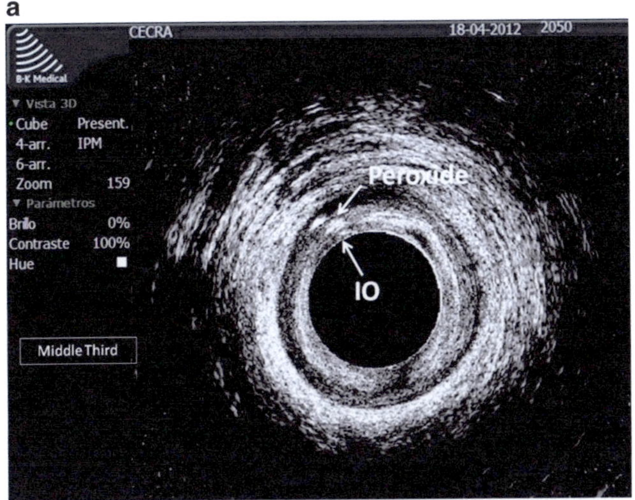

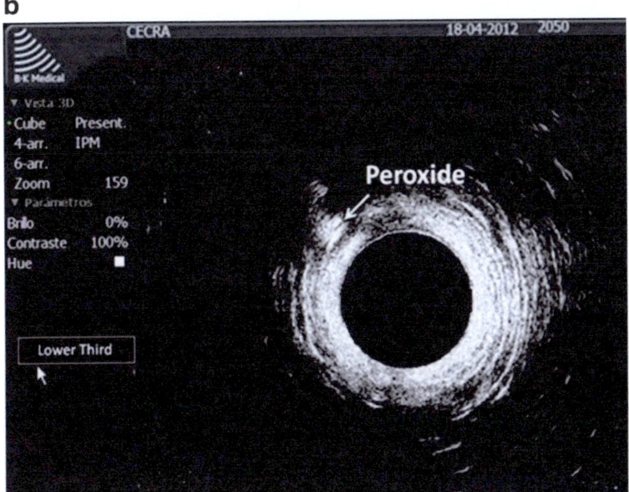

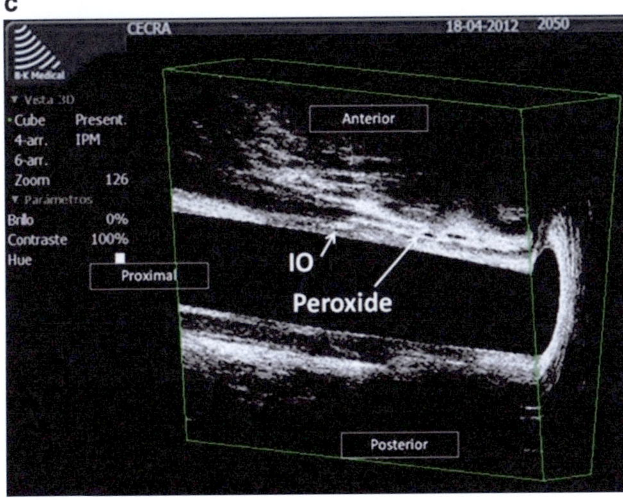

Fig. 6.4 2D Ultrasonography (**a, b**). (**a**) The internal opening (IO) of an intersphincteric fistula at the level of the middle third of the anal canal. (**b**) The same trajectory at the border of the external sphincter in the lower thrid of the anal canal. (**c**) 3D reconstruction of the same study evidences the length of the intersphincteric fistula ending at the internal opening in the middle third of the anal canal

examination. The authors prefer to use 12 mL of 1.5 % hydrogen peroxide injected after first clearing the fistula tract of any debris by flushing with saline. Pressure must be applied to the external opening at the time of injection to prevent retrograde extravasation and increased bubbling. This maneuver may require help by an assistant. The fistula probe is then passed into and out of the fistulous trajectory following the tract. If 3D ultrasound is used, it may be cycled at this point. The internal opening of a fistula tract is defined by the presence of a hyperechoic breach at the level of the internal sphincter. 3D US may fail to detect the primary orifice when there is more than one internal opening (IO) [23]. Suprasphincteric fistulas are more difficult to identify than other types. Table 6.1 describes the sensitivity and specificity of various studies evaluating the use of ultrasound to define fistula anatomy. It varies by fistula type, and is most accurate for intersphincteric and transphincteric trajectories. More complex fistulas are more difficult to interpret, and require greater skill on the part of the endosonographer. A distinct advantage of ultrasosund is its portability. Intraoperative ultrasound is commonly utilized in specialized centers.

Magnetic resonance imaging (MRI) is another valuable tool for the elucidation of fistula anatomy. It has the advantage of not being user-dependent for interpretation, as well as the ability to evaluate fistula tracts that course distant from the anus. It may be performed with or without contrast medium, and/or using an endorectal coil. One problem with the endorectal coil is that it requires transanal insertion. Some patients cannot tolerate the coil. Moreover, the field of view is limited compared to surface-phased array coils [24]. In general, MRI has the disadvantages of being relatively expensive, not always available, and its diagnostic value depends on technical conditions. In complex cases, MRI can correctly identify the fistula tract in up to 90 % of patients. This observation is especially valid in recurrent fistulas, where MRI can have an impact on therapeutic decision making in up to 75 % of cases [25–27].

There are a number of technical aspects of MRI that are worth mentioning. In order to best visualize any fistula tract, the field should be tilted forward and centered along the anal canal. The axial and coronal images obtained should be relative to this axis [28]. Specific characteristics that may be seen were outlined by Buchanan et al. who showed that acute angulation from the internal opening tended to be found in high transphincteric tracts, whereas those exhibiting obtuse angulation tended to be lower fistulas [29]. In addition, different weighted images on MRI give varying information. Selective, fat-saturated (T2WI) images provide excellent special resolution and increase the hyperintense nature of fistulous tracks and fluid collections. Alternatively, single tau inversion recovery (STIR) sequence images may be used in patients with significant artifact from hip replacement or postsurgical suture. Finally, contrast-enhanced (gadolinium)

Table 6.1 Accuracy of ultrasound to detect fistula act (by fistula classification)

Authors	Patients	Intersphincteric	Transsphincteric	Suprasphincteric	Extrasphincteric
Pomerri et al. [30]	99	100	80	NR	84.2
Ortiz et al. [31]	128	80	93	50	NR

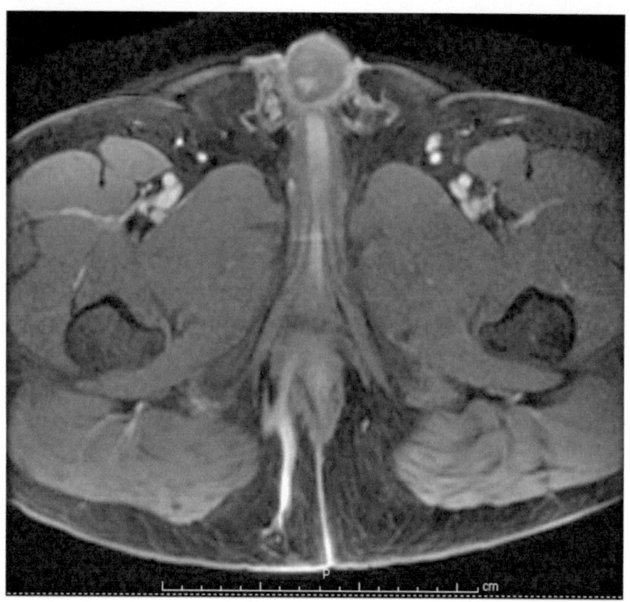

Fig. 6.5 MRI in a patient who underwent an unsuccesful EUA. This axial view shows a long fistula tract ending a considerable distance from the anal verge and originating on the right anterolateral aspect within the anal canal

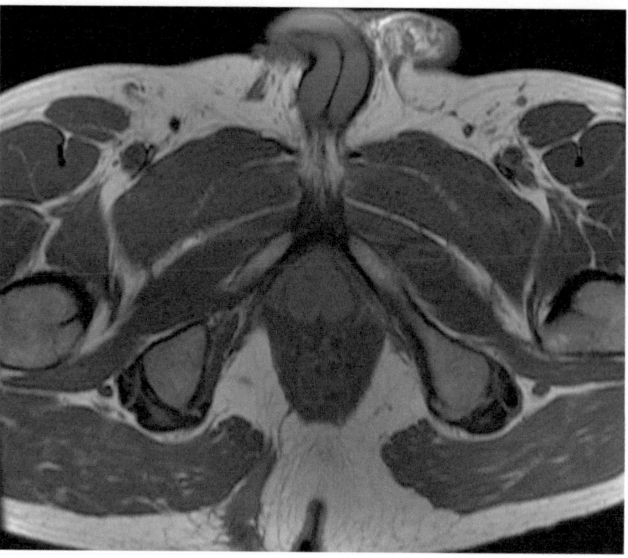

Fig. 6.6 Axial MRI view of a patient with a recurrent fistula ending at a secondary opening in the gluteal tissues with its primary opening at the level of the puborectalis muscle—probably the consequence of an iatrogenic primary exploration

T1WI helps differentiate scarring and granulation tissue or inflammation in patients with equivocal fat saturation. This modality also may show seton positioning better [28]. MRI may be more difficult to fully assess fistulous tracts in the setting of an acute abscess secondary to the high signal intensity on T2-weighted images of pus, which may obscure the true nature of any underlying fistula tracks. Figures 6.5 and 6.6 are excellent examples of MRI delineation of problematic fistula in ano.

Summary and Treatment Strategies

The most important factor in evaluating a fistula in ano is an EUA by an experienced clinician. EUA for anal fistula is a subtle art form that serves to establish a correct diagnosis, and leads to the successful resolution in a majority of cases. In the event the fistula tract cannot be identified, or safely connected to an identified internal opening, an appropriate drainage procedure should be done and advanced imaging pursued. MRI, 2D, and 3D ultrasound allow the practitioner to gain an understanding of a 3D structure that may be difficult to gain in the operating room in these circumstances. This information is difficult to convey with 2D images, and the surgeon is well advised to review the images at the time of the examination with ultrasound, or review the whole series of MRI images in conjunction with a radiologist to gain a full understanding of the anatomy. This information may serve to better guide further therapy.

Summary

- Physical diagnosis of anal fistula requires a systematic approach.
- Failure to elucidate fistula anatomy is an important indication for adjunctive imaging.
- Both ultrasound and MRI have individual advantages in the evaluation of anal fistula.

References

1. Davies M, Harris D, Lohana P, et al. The surgical management of fistula-in-ano in a specialist colorectal unit. Int J Colorectal Dis. 2008;23(9):833–8.
2. Adams F. On fistulae. In: The genuine works of Hippocrates translated from the Greek with a preliminary discourse and annotation. New York: William Wood; 1849.
3. Goodsall DH, Miles WE. Ano-rectal fistula. In: Miles WE, Goodsall DH, editors. Diseases of the anus and rectum. London: Longmans, Green & Company; 1900. p. 92–137.

4. Cirocco WC, Reilly JC. Challenging the predictive accuracy of Goodsall's rule for anal fistulas. Dis Colon Rectum. 1992;35(6): 537–42.

5. Parks AG, Gordon PH, Hardcastle JD. A classification of fistula-in-ano. Br J Surg. 1976;63:1–12.

6. Vasilevsky CA, Gordon PH. Benign anorectal: abscess and fistula. In: Wolff BG et al., editors. The ASCRS textbook of colon and rectal surgery. New York: Springer; 2007.

7. Seow-Choen F, Ho JMS. Histoanatomy of anal glands. Dis Colon Rectum. 1994;37:1215–8.

8. Whiteford MH, Kilkenny III J, Hyman N, et al. Practice parameters for the treatment of perianal abscess and fistula-in-ano (revised). Dis Colon Rectum. 2005;48:1337–42.

9. Marchesa P, Hull TL, Fazio VW. Advancement sleeve flaps for treatment of severe perianal Crohn's disease. Br J Surg. 1998;85: 1695.

10. Consten CJ, Siors FJM, Noten HJ, et al. Anorectal surgery in human immunodeficiency virus-infected patients. Dis Colon Rectum. 1995;38:1169–75.

11. Savafi A, Gottesman L, Dailey TH. Anorectal surgery in the HIV+ patient: update. Dis Colon Rectum. 1991;34:299–304.

12. Aleali M, Gottesman L. Anorectal disease in HIV-positive patients. Clin Colon Rectal Surg. 2001;14:265–73.

13. Ratto C, Grillo E, Parello A, et al. Endoanal ultrasound-guided surgery for anal fistula. Endoscopy. 2005;37(8):722–8.

14. Poen AC, Felt-Bersma RJ, Eijsbouts QA, et al. Hydrogen-peroxide enhanced transanal ultrasound in the assessment of fistula-in-ano. Dis Colon Rectum. 1998;41(9):1147–52.

15. Sileri P, Cadeddu F, D'Ugo S, et al. Surgery for fistula-in-ano in a specialist colorectal unit: a critical appraisal. BMC Gastroenterol. 2011;11:120.

16. Gonzalez-Ruiz C, Kaiser AM, Vukasin P, et al. Intraoperative physical diagnosis in the management of anal fistula. Am Surg. 2006;72(1):11–5.

17. Sahni VA, Ahmad R, Burling D. Which method is best for imaging of perianal fistula? Abdom Imaging. 2008;33:26–30.

18. Malik AI, Nelson RL. Surgical management of anal fistulae: a systematic review. Colorectal Dis. 2008;10:420–30.

19. Soltani A, Kaiser AM. Endorectal advancement flap for cryptoglandular or Crohn's fistula-in-ano. Dis Colon Rectum. 2010;53:486–95.

20. Rizzo JA, Naig AL, Johnson EK. Anorectal abscess and fistula-in-ano: evidence-based management. Surg Clin North Am. 2010;90:45–68.

21. Gold DM, Bartram CI, Halligan S, et al. Three-dimensional endoanal sonography in assessing anal canal injury. Br J Surg. 1999; 86(3):365–70.

22. Saclarides TJ. Anorectal ultrasound. In: Machi J, Staren ED, editors. Ultrasound for surgeons. 2nd ed. Philadelphia: Lippincott Williams & Wilkins; 2005.

23. Buchanan GN, Bartram CI, Williams AB, et al. Value of hydrogen peroxide enhancement of three-dimensional endoanal ultrasound in fistula-in-ano. Dis Colon Rectum. 2005;48(1):141–7.

24. de Souza NM, Gilderdale DJ, Coutts GA, et al. MRI of fistula-in-ano: a comparison of endoanal coil with external phased array coil techniques. J Comput Asst Tomogr. 1998;22(3):357–63.

25. Buchanan GN, Halligan S, Bartram CI, et al. Clinical examination, endosonography, and MR imaging in preoperative assessment of fistula in ano: comparison with outcome-based reference standard. Radiology. 2004;233(3):674–81.

26. Buchanan G, Halligan S, Williams A, et al. Effect of MRI on clinical outcome of recurrent fistula-in-ano. Lancet. 2002; 360(9346):1661–2.

27. Buchanan GN, Halligan S, Williams AB, et al. Magnetic resonance imaging for primary fistula in ano. Br J Surg. 2003;90(7):877–81.

28. Gage KL, Deshmukh S, Macura KJ, et al. MRI of perianal fistulas: bridging the radiological-surgical divide. Abdom Imag. 2012;38(5):1033–42.

29. Buchanan GN, Williams AM, Bartram CI, et al. Potential clinical implications of directions of a trans-sphincteric anal fistula track. Br J Surg. 2003;90(10):1250–5.

30. Pomerri F, Dodi G, Pintacuda G, Amadio L, Muzzio PC. Anal endosonography and fistulography for fistula-in-ano. Radiol Med. 2010;115(5):771–83.

31. Ortiz H, Marzo J, Jiménez G, DeMiguel M. Accuracy of hydrogen peroxide-enhanced ultrasound in the identification of internal openings of anal fistulas. Colorectal Dis. 2002;4(4):280–3.

Herand Abcarian

Introduction

Frederic Salmon in 1847 founded a specialty unit for proctology, i.e., the St. Mark's Hospital for Fistulae, etc. in City Road, London. Many surgeons studied and worked at St. Marks and the specialty spread through Europe and across the Atlantic. Joseph P. Matthews studied under Allingham in the UK prior to establishing the first proctology section and unit at the University of Kentucky in Louisville. The specialty gained recognition in the US leading to the incorporation of the American Proctologic Society in Columbus Ohio in 1899 with Dr. Matthews as its first President. Surgical texts were published on the sole subject of proctology and preceptorships led to propagation the specialty in the US. Over the ensuing decades St. Marks' remained a Mecca for education of surgeons in proctology and despite many successes in treatment of many proctologic condition, cure of fistulas remained much more elusive than any other condition.

Classification of Anal Fistula

From the beginning, it was obvious that all fistulas were not the same. Therefore to be able to discuss treatment strategies, operations (to be done and to avoid), a systematic classification utilized across all borders was needed. Each major institution in the UK and the US embarked on its own classification. Even though this was helpful in reporting the results of therapy, it was difficult if not impossible to compare results of surgical therapy amongst various institutions due to lack of a standard classification and common nomenclature.

H. Abcarian, M.D., F.A.C.S. (✉)
The University of Illinois at Chicago, Division of Colon and Rectal Surgery, John Stroger Hospital of Cook Country, IL 60612, USA
e-mail: abcarian@uic.edu

Goligher's classification and incidence of various fistulas is shown in Table 7.1. He classified 10–15 % of fistulas as subcutaneous, 60–70 % as low, and 15 % as high anal, 5 % as anorectal and the submuscular or high intermuscular variety was noted to be very rare [1]. Since 1976, when Parks et al. published their comprehensive classification of anal fistulas, this has become the most utilized classification [2] (Fig. 7.1). A modification of the original classification is depicted in Fig. 7.1. The advantage of this classification is threefold: (1) It accurately places the fistula in the known and accepted anorectal anatomy; (2) it assists the surgeon in assessing the simplicity or complexity of the fistula and the choice of the surgical approach; and (3) it allows the surgeon to discuss with the patient success or failure rate of the operation, the extent of the procedure, the postoperative sick days and disability, and the potential incidence of postsurgical anal incontinence. This information is critical in the process of informed consent.

The four main classes of fistulas are:

1. *Intersphincteric*: The fistula originates at the dentate line and tracks caudad between the internal and external sphincter opening in the perianal region close to the anal verge. This fistula is seen following a perianal abscess and is typical of the ones seen in fistulizing midline anal fissures.

2. *Transsphincteric*: The fistula originates at the dentate line and traverses the internal and external sphincter opening in the ischiorectal fossa. Depending on the height of the fistula varying degrees of sphincter involvement may be encountered. Treatment of high transsphincteric fistulas is more challenging due to increased risk of incontinence.

3. *Suprasphincteric*: Originates at the dentate line and tracks cephalad to the external sphincter mechanism before opening into the skin at the ischiorectal fossa. These fistulas are not amenable to simple fistulotomy due to high risk of total incontinence

4. *Extrasphincter*: Traverses the entire sphincter mechanism including puborectalis, opening proximally either at the dentate line (secondary to supralevator abscess) or in the lower rectal wall (secondary to internal or external

H. Abcarian (ed.), *Anal Fistula: Principles and Management*, DOI 10.1007/978-1-4614-9014-2_7,
© Springer Science+Business Media New York 2014

Table 7.1 Classification and incidence of fistulas [1]

Type	Percent
Subcutaneous	10–15
Low anal	60–70
High anal	15
Anorectal ischiorectal pelvic rectal	5
Submucosa, high intermuscular	Very rare

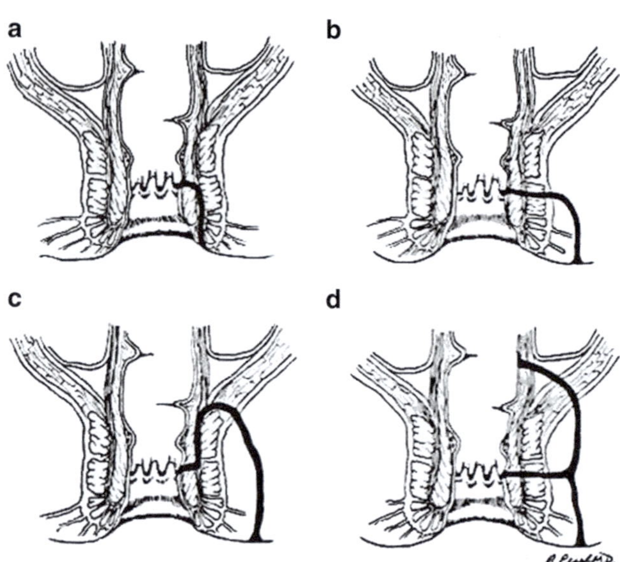

Fig. 7.1 The classification of anal fistulas. (**a**) Intersphincteric. (**b**) Transsphincteric. (**c**) Suprasphincteric. (**d**) Extrasphincteric (With permission Parks et al. [2])

penetrating trauma) and distally in the ischiorectal fossa or in the buttocks. This type of fistula is often secondary to trauma or Crohn's disease.

Management Strategies in Fistula-in-Ano

The aim of surgery for anal fistula is to cure the patient with minimal or no sequela. If the surgeon is too conservative, the fistula may persist or recur after a short period of "healing" but the patient's continence is preserved. On the other hand, if the surgeon is too aggressive, a false passage may be created, or the fistula may heal with varying degrees of disturbance of continence (Fig. 7.2). So to follow the dictum of "primum non nocere," it takes an accurate assessment of the fistula and an experienced surgeon who deals with fistulas on a daily basis to perform the appropriate operation and prevent postsurgical incontinence (Fig. 7.3).

Fistulotomy or Fistulectomy

There has been and continues to be a basic controversy whether fistulotomy or fistulectomy should be performed for anal fistulas. There has been only one randomized trial com-

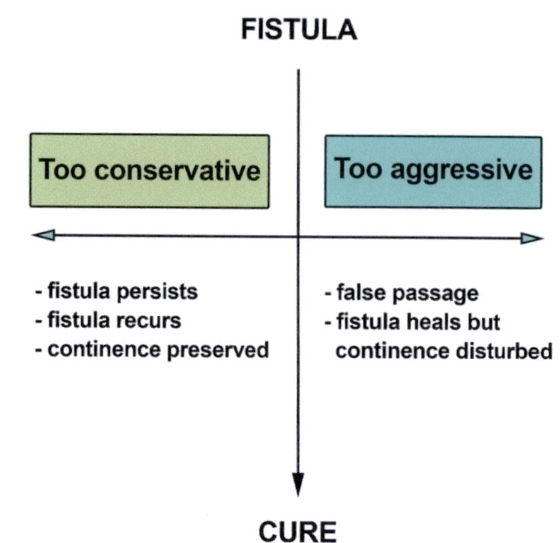

Fig. 7.2 Management goal in fistula surgery

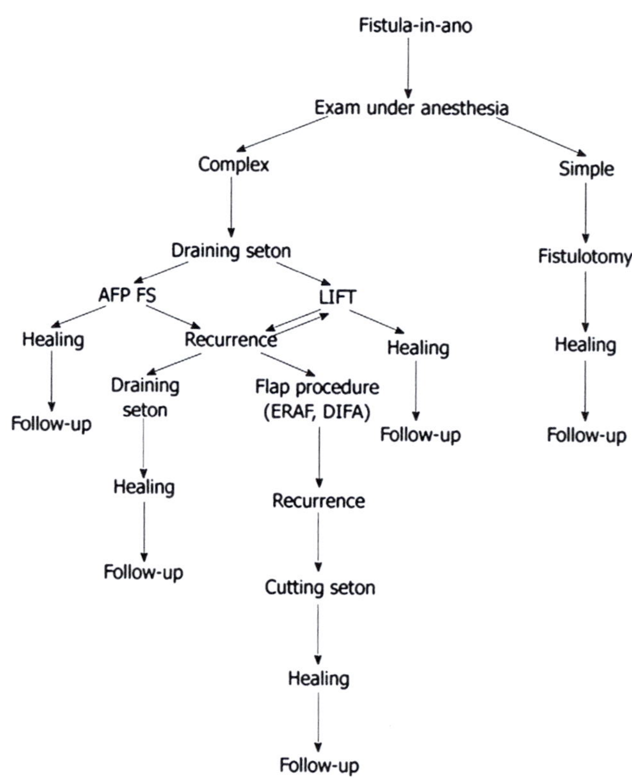

Fig. 7.3 Treatment algorithm for simple and complex fistula-in-ano

paring the two techniques by Kronborg [3] who alternately assigned patients to one or the other procedure. Fistulotomy fared better due to prolonged healing time associated with fistulectomy. A small section of the tract can be excised (biopsied) if there is concern for Crohn's disease or malignancy, in cases of long-standing fistulas. Nelson and colleagues stressed the need for taking a biopsy from recurrent abscess wall or fistula tract to exclude malignancy. Low rectal or anal cancer (adenocarcinoma) may penetrate tissue and manifest as a recurrent abscess fistula. On the other hand, a very long-standing fistula in ano may develop into a squamous cell cancer [4]. The presence of mucus in fistulous abscess should raise the index of suspicion of malignancy [5].

Primary Fistulotomy

At the time of drainage of an abscess, the surgeon may find a fistula right away or after gentle probing with a blunt tipped probe. Primary fistulotomy was reported to be safe and with no adverse consequences in 1,000 consecutive cases [6]. Ramanujam et al. reported on 1,023 anorectal abscesses. Where the fistula was identified at the time of the incision and drainage and the experienced surgeon felt comfortable with primary fistulotomy, the results of primary fistulotomy were excellent and the recurrence rate was 3.4 % (Table 7.2) [7]. However, Vasilevsky and Gordon found fistulas in only a third of drained abscesses and argued against primary fistulotomy [8]. In any case primary fistulotomy requires an experienced surgeon exercising good judgment and extreme care in order

to avoid postsurgical fecal incontinence and worse yet, recurrence due to creation of an inadvertent false passage.

Staged Fistulotomy implies that a high or complex fistula is treated in stages. At the first operation a portion of the sphincter mechanism is incised and a loose (marking) seton is placed around the remaining (undivided) external sphincter. After a period of 6–8 weeks the patient is reexamined under anesthesia and if the first stage sphincterotomy is healed by fibrosis, the remainder of sphincter is divided and the setons removed. In a study of 480 fistulotomies, Ramanujam and colleagues reported excellent healing with minimal (2 %) impairment of continence [9]. However; this report preceded the development of anorectal physiologic studies. In a larger study of staged fistulotomy using seton from the same institution Pearl and colleagues reported recurrence rate of 3 % and major incontinence, defined as the need to wear a pad, in 5 % of 110 patients treated in this fashion (Fig. 7.4) [10]. This is in contradistinction of the incidence of incontinence in cutting setons, which is reported to be as high as 12 % in a meta-analysis [11].

Inpatient or Outpatient Fistulotomy

Outpatient fistulotomy is the standard of care for majority of fistulas. A straight local anesthesia, local anesthesia with conscious sedation or local anesthesia with monitored anesthesia care may be utilized depending on patient's emotional state and tolerance of pain. Spinal and general anesthesia can be utilized for more complex cases needing longer operative times. Ambulatory surgery was also recommended by the

Table 7.2 Incidence of fistulas in 1,023 abscesses [7]

Type of abscess	Number of abscesses	% of Fistulas
Intersphincteric	219	47.4
Suprasphincteric	75	42.6
Intersphincteric	437	24.5
Ischiorectal	233	25.3
High Intermuscular	59	15.2

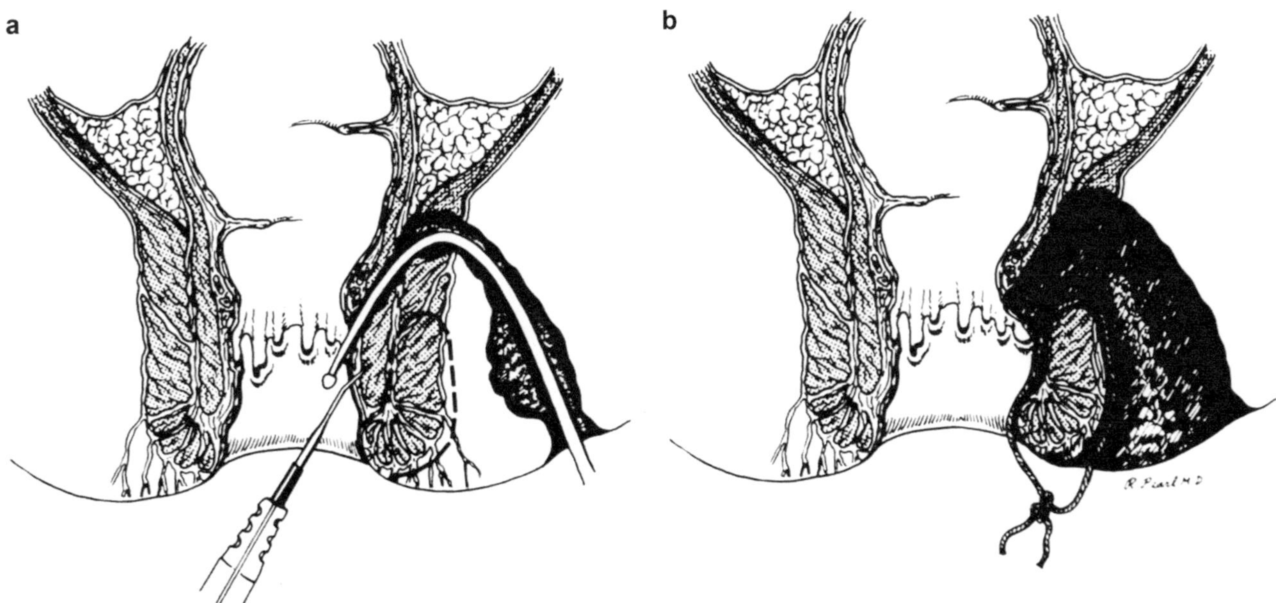

Fig. 7.4 Staged fistulotomy for transsphincteric fistulas. (**a**) Primary fistulotomy with seton (Courtesy of Dr. Russell Pearl). (**b**) Second fistulotomy (Courtesy of Dr. Russell Pearl)

Standard Task Force of the American Society of Colon and Rectal Surgeons [12].

A more recent American Society of Colon and Rectal Surgeons Practice Parameters for fistula surgery recommends:

- Outpatient surgery if the fistula, fistulous abscess, or limited anorectal pathology warrants ambulatory care.
- Inpatient care when fistulas involve adjacent organs (rectovaginal, rectourethral, horseshoe) often needing extensive surgery.
- Inpatient surgery when extensive cellulitis or an associated abscess necessitates intravenous antibiotic therapy [13].

Surgical Alternatives in Fistula-in-Ano

Intersphincteric Fistulas

Fistulas can be laid open with minimal internal sphincterotomy. The extent of this operation is no different than that of lateral internal sphincterotomy, i.e., division of the internal sphincter distal to the dentate line. This procedure is equally indicated in midline fissures which have fistulized and is the procedure of choice rather than lateral internal sphincterotomy.

Transsphincteric Fistulas

These involve varying degrees of external sphincter involvement. Therefore a fistulotomy requiring division of the external sphincter, as of necessity, will result in some disturbance of continence estimated in one study to be in the range of 17–33 % [14]. The lay-open technique including transsphincteric fistulas (low and high) is covered in a separate chapter. All nonsphincerotomy or sphincter-sparing techniques including seton, fibrin sealant, endorectal advancement flaps, dermal advancement flap, biologic and synthetic plugs and ligation of intersphincteric fistula tracts have been developed to avoid sphincterotomy and prevent fecal incontinence. These techniques are discussed in separate chapters.

Suprasphincteric Fistulas

The same principals in selection of treatment alternatives used in transsphincteric fistulas are also applicable (with more significant importance) in suprasphincteric fistulas. It is critical to employ sphincter-sparing operations to prevent postsurgical incontinence. Alternative techniques are addressed in other chapters.

Extrasphincteric Fistulas

With the internal opening cephalad to the levators, extrasphincteric fistulas are not amenable to the usual fistula operations. If the internal opening is low enough to allow an endorectal advancement flap, this technique may be employed. Otherwise or in case the flap advancement fails, transsphincteric (Mason) approach may be employed with or without a covering colostomy. This technique was advocated by Mason and Kilpatrick for the treatment of rectourethral fistulas [15]. The advantage of this approach for extrasphincteric fistulas is that it affords the surgeon an excellent exposure in a virgin field [16]. With the patient in the jackknife position an incision is made beginning at the posterior anal verge and carried for 10–12 cm just off midline, 1 cm away from the coccygeal border. Skin, subcutaneous tissue, and the fascia and distal 5 cm of gluteus maximus fibers are divided to reach the pelvic floor. The levator plate, puborectalis, external and internal sphincters are sharply divided and marked with paired colored sutures for ease of identification during closure. The posterior rectal wall lies at the depth of the wound and the primary opening of the fistula can be approached directly. This is excised and closed with a vest over pants rectal advancement flap. The rectal wall is closed and the muscular layers are approximated individually (with the aid of colored suture) using absorbable sutures. The gluteus fascia, subcutaneous tissues and skin are then closed. A suction drain may be placed in deeper to the gluteus if necessary (Fig. 7.5). The external tract of the fistula is curetted and kept open for two weeks using a mushroom or Malecot or catheter. This technique is used only rarely, therefore the success rate of the operation is not well documented [17]. In my personal series of nine patients, eight healed and one recurred secondary to breakdown of the internal opening repair. This patient was treated with a draining Seton for 3 months and the fistula was closed subsequently with fibrin sealant. His diverting stoma was then reversed 3 months later (Abcarian H, unpublished data). Transsphincteric approach is ideal for access to the mid-rectum for fistulas and also for excision of retrorectal crysts [18].

Horseshoe Fistula

This type of fistula is often an extension of a midline transsphincteric fistula to one or both ischiorectal fossae through the deep postanal space. The classic treatment of primary posterior fistulotomy and the lay open of both arms of the horseshoe results in a large open wound with delayed healing and prolonged disability. In 1965 Hanley described a more conservative technique which included unroofing of deep postanal space, widening of the secondary openings and curettage of the intervening subcutaneous horseshoe tracts without laying them open [19]. Hanley and colleagues reported the long-term results of 41 horseshoe fistulas treated in this manner with no recurrence or incontinence [20]. Hamilton reported 4 recurrences in 57 patients [21]. Pezim stressed the importance of drainage (deroofing) of deep postanal space and reported 92 % healing rate in 24 patients [22].

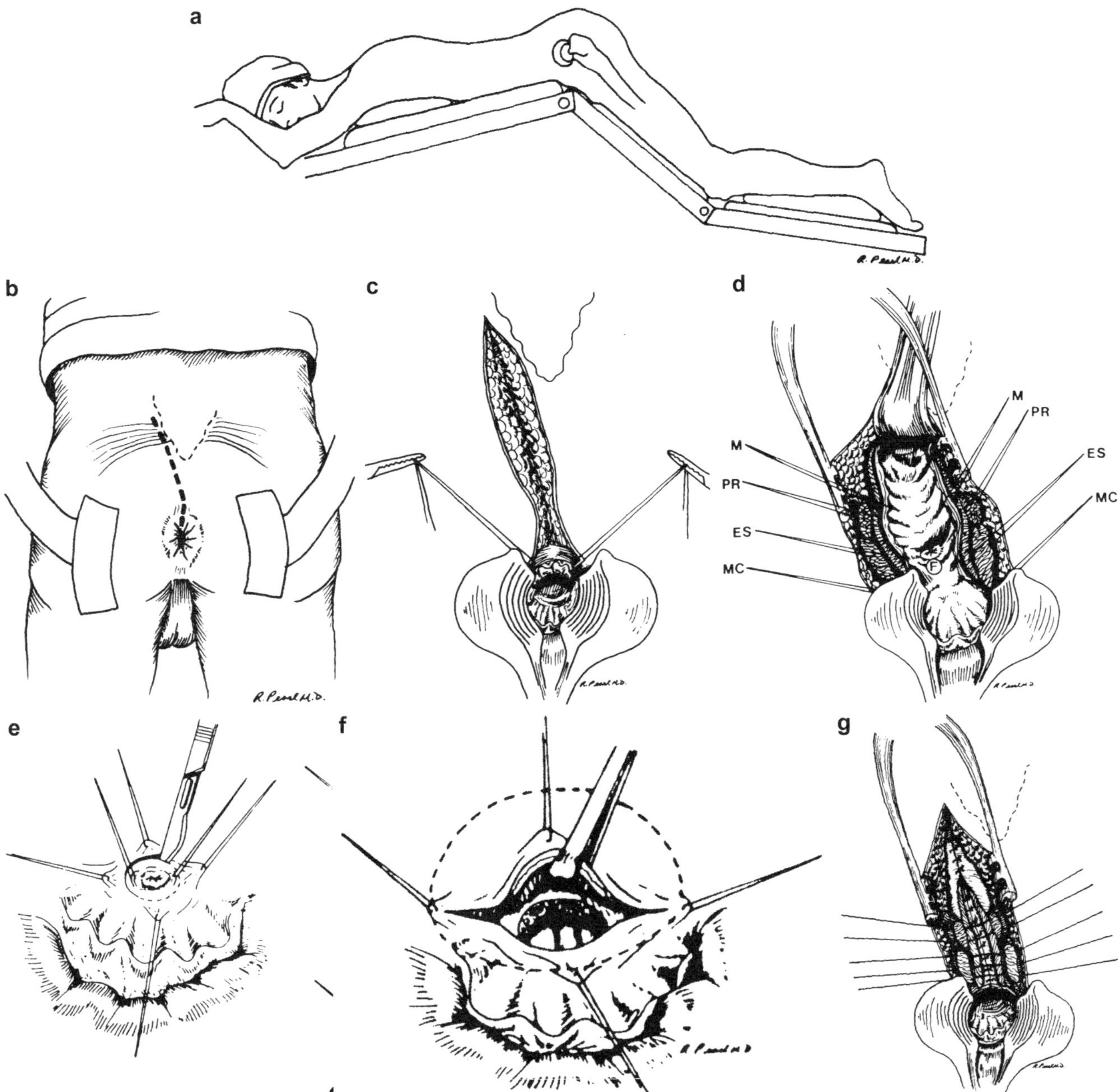

Fig. 7.5 Mason procedure for exposure of mid-rectum. (**a**) Patient placed in prone jackknife position (Courtesy of Dr. Russell Pearl). (**b**) Incision beginning at midline posterior of anus and extending 10–12 cm cephalad adjacent to coccyx (Courtesy of Dr. Russell Pearl). (**c**) Skin and subcutaneous layers are opened. All muscles are divided between paired colored sutures (Courtesy of Dr. Russell Pearl). (**d**) Depiction of complete posterior exposure to fistula (Courtesy of Dr. Russell Pearl). *M* mucosa, *PR* puborectalis, *ES* external sphincter, *IS* internal sphincter, *MC* mucocutaneous junction, *F* fistula. (**e**) excision of fistula (full thickness) (Courtesy of Dr. Russell Pearl). (**f**) Vest over pants closure of rectal wall (Courtesy of Dr. Russell Pearl). (**g**) Layered closure of rectal wall and sphincter muscles (Courtesy of Dr. Russell Pearl)

Summary

Safe and effective treatment of anal fistulas depends on:

1. Accurate classification of the fistulas, i.e., understanding the exact anatomy.
2. Good judgment regarding choice of seton vs. fistulotomy.
3. When appropriate or in doubt, choosing conservative over aggressive approach.
4. Familiarity with multiple alternatives to fistulotomy.
5. Tailoring the operations to the patient rather than the reverse.
6. Always adhering to the old adage, "First do no harm." One of John Alexander Williams' famous quotes was:

"More sphincters are injured by aggressive surgeons rather than by aggressive disease."

7. Any finally, never hesitate to refer the patient to a more experienced specialist.

References

1. Goligher JC. Surgery of the anus, rectal and colon. 2nd ed. New York: McMillan; 1961.
2. Parks AG, Gordon PH, Hardcastle JD. A classification of fistula-in-ano. Br J Surg. 1976;63(1):1–12.
3. Kronborg D. To lay open or excise fistula-in-ano: a randomized trial. Br J Surg. 1985;72(12):970–2.
4. Nelson RL, Prasad ML, Abcarian H. Anal carcinoma presenting as a perirectal abscess or fistula. Arch Surg. 1985;120:632–5.
5. Kulaylat MN, Doerr RJ, Karamanoukian H, Barrios G. Basal cell carcinoma arising in a fistula-in-ano. Arch Surg. 1996;62(2):1000–2.
6. McElwain JR, McLean MD, Alexander RM, et al. Anorectal problems: experience with primary fistulectomy for anorectal abscess, a report of 1000 cases. Dis Colon Rectum. 1975;18(8):646–9.
7. Ramanujam PS, Prasad ML, Abcarian H, Tan AB. Perianal abscesses and fistulas: a study of 1023 patients. Dis Colon Rectum. 1984;27:593–7.
8. Vasilevsky CA, Gordon PH. The incidence of recurrent abscesses or fistula-in-ano following anorectal suppuration. Dis Colon Rectum. 1984;27(2):126–30.
9. Ramanujam PS, Prasad ML, Abcarian H. Role of seton in fistulotomy of the anus. Surg Gynecol Obstet. 1983;157:419–22.
10. Pearl RK, Andrews JR, Orsay CP, Weismann RI, Prasad ML, Nelson RL, Cintron JR, Abcarian H. Role of the seton in the management of anorectal fistulas. Dis Colon Rectum. 1993;36:573–9.
11. Ritchie RD, Sackier JM, Hodde JP. Incontinence rates after cutting seton treatment for anal fistula. Colorectal Dis. 2009;11(6):564–71.
12. Standards Task Force, American Society of Colon and Rectal Surgeons. Practice parameters for ambulatory anorectal surgery. Dis Colon Rectum. 1991;34(3):285–6.
13. Stelle SR, Kumar R, Feingold DL, et al. Practice parameters for the management of perianal abscess and fistula-in-ano. Dis Colon Rectum. 2001;54(12):1465–74.
14. Parks AG, Stitz RW. The treatment of high fistula-in-ano. Dis Colon Rectum. 1976;19(6):487–99.
15. Kilpatrick FR, Mason AY. Post-operative recto-prostatic fistula. Br J Urol. 1969;41:649–54.
16. Mason AY. Surgical access to rectum – a transsphincteric exposure. Proc R Soc Med. 1970;63 Suppl 1:91–4.
17. Prasad ML, Nelson R, Hambrick E, Abcarian H. York mason procedure for repair of postoperative rectoprostatic urethral fistula. Dis Colon Rectum. 1983;26:716–20.
18. Abel ME, Nelson RL, Prasad ML, Pearl RK, Orsay CP, Abcarian H. Parasacrococcygeal approach for the resection of retrorectal developmental cysts. Dis Colon Rectum. 1985;28:855–8.
19. Hanley PH. Conservative surgical correction of horseshoe abscess and fistula. Dis Colon Rectum. 1965;8(5):364–8.
20. Hanley PH, Ray JE, Pennington EE, et al. Fistula-in-ano: a ten-year follow-up study of horseshoe-abscess fistula – in-ano. Dis Colon Rectum. 1976;19(6):505–15.
21. Hamilton CH. Anorectal problems: the deep postanal space—surgical significance in horseshoe fistula abscess. Dis Colon Rectum. 1975;18(8):642–5.
22. Pezim ME. Successful treatment of horseshoe fistula requires deroofing of the deep postanal space. Am J Surg. 1994;167(4):513–5.

Seton (Loose, Cutting, Chemical)

8

Vamsi R. Velchuru

Introduction

Fistula-in-ano is a common surgical condition with a high incidence and a prevalence of 1.2 to 2.8/10,000 in the western world [1]. Management depends on the etiology, such as cryptoglandular pathology (commonest), Crohn's disease, HIV, malignancy, tuberculosis, and ileo-anal pouch anastomosis. Patients present as an emergency with anorectal abscesses needing surgical drainage. Twenty-six to thirty-seven percent develop a fistula at follow-up after anorectal abscess drainage [2]. Management of fistula-in-ano has changed over millennia, with seton placement to sphincter-cutting techniques to recent muscle saving procedures. Management of anal fistulae is complex and few patients can have recalcitrant fistulae leading to perennial quandary.

Ayurvedic-medicated setons have been described for anal fistula in Sushruta Samhita [3], a compilation of surgical procedures by a Sushruta an Indian Surgeon as early as sixth century BC. Hippocrates in fourth century BC has described the use of horsehair and lint to cut the muscle to achieve cure for anal fistulas. In the last few decades, sphincter-saving procedures have been increasingly used for this complicated disease. However, initial drainage of sepsis and seton placement as a temporary or a permanent remedy still has a role.

High trans-sphincteric fistula remains a challenge even in the twenty-first century, as curative treatment involves muscle cutting leading to potential incontinence. Interestingly in a 25-year single-institutional review of 2,267 fistula operations, the incidence of sphincter-cutting procedures such as fistulotomy decreased from 98.7 % in 1975 to 50.4 % in 2009; during the same period non-cutting procedures increased from 1.3 to 49.6 %, a substantial increase. This might well be due to tangible evidence of incontinence following sphincter-sacrificing procedures with anorectal physiology testing and anal ultrasonography. This conservative approach might be the factor for the increase in more than one procedure in patients from 1.3 % during 1975–1979 to 32.9 % three decades later during 2005–2009 [4].

The aim of fistula management is to drain the sepsis, define the anatomy (EUA and imaging), rule out associated conditions (Crohn's, tuberculosis), obliteration of fistulous track with preservation of continence. Setons can be employed as cutting and a non-cutting seton, i.e., divider or a marker [5]. The Ayurvedic seton is a medicated cutting seton [6]. In this chapter we discuss, a cutting seton, non-cutting seton (or a loose seton) and a chemical seton. Setons are usually inserted following drainage of abscess, to relieve residual sepsis and prevent collections and encourage fibrosis, this in turn creates a fibrosed track for a definite procedure on a later date. In the case of the cutting seton and the ksharasutra, the aim is to facilitate controlled transection of the sphincter muscle to heal the fistula.

Seton Material

The type of seton used is usually typical to the individual surgeon. Seton means "thick, stiff hair" in Latin in the Webster's dictionary. A few of the type of setons used are the Ayurvedic-medicated thread [6], braided sutures [7], thread, rubber band [8], penrose drains [9], cable tie seton [10], etc. Seton material should be non-absorbable, non-slippage material, comfortable and less irritant to the patient and equally effective in causing focal reaction of the track leading to fibrosis.

V.R. Velchuru, M.B.B.S, F.R.C.S. (Edin.), F.R.C.S. (Gen. Surg.) (⊠)
James Paget University Hospitals Foundation Trust, Lowestoft Road, Gorleston, Great Yarmouth, Norfolk, UK NR31 6LA
e-mail: velchuru@hotmail.com

H. Abcarian (ed.), *Anal Fistula: Principles and Management*, DOI 10.1007/978-1-4614-9014-2_8,
© Springer Science+Business Media New York 2014

Technique of Seton Insertion

Patient can be prone (North America) or lithotomy (United Kingdom) depending on the surgeon's preference. Evaluating the exact anatomy preoperatively with MRI or Endoanal Ultrasonography helps identify the level of fistula, deep-seated collections, and identify the fistulous tracts particularly in complex and redo fistulas [11–16]. Hydrogen peroxide injection into the external opening can help to identify the track during Examination under Anesthesia [17]. In the same study, hydrogen peroxide-enhanced ultrasound increased the accuracy from 62 to 95 % compared to a standard conventional ultrasound. Grooved Lockhart–Mummery or malleable lacrimal probes have been used to negotiate and identify the track. Sepsis is drained, track is curetted, secondary tracks are identified and again curetted. Railroad technique has been employed both to insert the seton [18] or changing the medicated seton weekly [19] and for regularly tightening the cutting seton.

It is vital to document a detailed and exact anatomy in the pictorial form in the operative note for future reference. Sitz baths are advised in the immediate postoperative period to keep the area clean.

Loose Seton

The purpose of a loose seton is not to damage or cut the sphincter and as the name implies it is placed in the tract and tied loosely. Its benefits range from primary treatment in simple abscess and fistulae to final recourse in complex intractable fistulas. Loose setons can be used:

1. At the time of initial drainage of abscess. It acts as a drainage and prevents further recurrence of sepsis. This can act as a marker for surgery in the future [20].
2. For definitive treatment of trans-sphincteric fistula without transecting either sphincters.
3. In complex fistulas, to promote healing of secondary tracks and to help mature the primary track before definitive surgery such as LIFT.
4. Two staged fistulotomy. The sphincter is divided in two stages, and the seton is used to allow the healing of the divided sphincter segment before further division [5].
5. Long-term drainage for complex cases such as Crohn's perineum.

At the initial presentation of perianal abscess, an experienced colorectal surgeon can identify the track and consider primary treatment of the fistula. Primary fistulotomy can be undertaken with good success rates if the fistula is superficial [21]. If it is a high fistula, or the sphincter muscle thickness unclear, which is often the case due to acute suppuration a seton should tied loosely for drainage and as a marker for definitive surgery in the future [20].

Loose Seton and Staged Fistulotomy

A staged fistulotomy is carried out in high trans-sphincteric or supra-sphincteric fistulas, when single stage fistulotomy is thought to carry high risk of incontinence [22, 23]. The principles are drainage of sepsis and deep sphincter division or internal sphincterotomy was initially undertaken, this was followed by division of distal sphincter. Loose seton was left in situ for the remaining track to prevent it from closing and forming a source of sepsis. Ramanujam et al. presented their results for 45 patients with supra-sphincteric tracks. Initially, the deep sphincter complex was divided and a loose seton placed at the remainder distal sphincter. When the wound healed forming a track around the seton, laying open of the track was undertaken with fair results. One had a recurrence and only one patient had mild incontinence [20].

Another large series ($n=89$) with the same technique in patients with complex fistula and anterior fistula in women concluded that staging fistulotomy was preferable to cutting seton method for complex fistulas [5]. In another series ($n=34$) of patients with trans-sphincteric and extra-sphincteric fistulas, recurrence was seen in 6 %, however nearly 60 % had abnormal incontinence [24]. A study of ten patients with extra-sphincteric fistula, there was no recurrences with the technique, mild incontinence was noted in six patients and one patient had major incontinence [23]. Similar technique was employed in 47 patients, the recurrence rates was 9 %, with an overall incontinence of 66 %, with 25 % having major incontinence [25]. The healing rates of staged fistulotomy are acceptable, however the incontinence rates are high.

Loose Seton Alone

Seton placement alone with no transection of either sphincter has also been reported. In a small series of 12 patients, 25 % had recurrence and 8 % had mild incontinence [26]. Similarly, in a study with patients ($n=79$) having low trans-sphincteric and inter-sphincteric fistula long-term setons were placed. Average treatment duration was 54.8 weeks, and the seton was left to migrate out spontaneously, or if the track was superficial a fistulotomy was performed. Recurrence was 3.7 %, with a low incontinence of 0.9 % [27]. This technique preferably works with inter-sphincteric and low trans-sphincteric fistulas.

Seton and High Fistulas

Few studies have shown that high trans-sphincteric fistulas can be treated with drainage of inter-sphincteric space, internal sphincterotomy, complete preservation of external sphincter with loose seton placement [22, 28–30]. Recurrence rates ranged from 15 to 56 % in these studies. In Thomson's study [29], recurrence (56 %) was treated with laying open of fistulas leading to significant major incontinence (47 %). Incontinence when external sphincter is completely preserved is usually mild (36–62 %) [28, 30].

Seton and Sphincter-Saving Procedures

Setons have been used preceding definite surgery such as LIFT or Advancement flap [31–33]. Seton helps both in draining sepsis and maturing the track due to fibrosis. There were no increased recurrence rates because of seton [32]. It was thought that low recurrence rates following LIFT and advancement flap in an RCT was probably due to prior seton placement, leading to drainage of sepsis [31]. Further large-scale studies are needed to evaluate this advantage.

Seton in Crohn's

Crohn's anal fistulae can be onerous to manage. A third of Crohn's patients present with fistulas [34]. Anterior fistulas are more frequent with Crohn's disease [35]. Acute suppurative abscess should be treated with incision and drainage. Seton placement is done to identify the track, drain sepsis, and most importantly stabilize the disease [5, 28, 36–38]. Medical therapy should only be instigated when there is minimal residual sepsis. In severe refractory disease, defunctioning the bowel might be necessary. Crohn's proctitis is a contraindication for any local procedures such as rectal advancement flaps and LIFT. Fistulotomy [39], flap procedures [40], and fistula plug [41] have been tried with varied success. Two-thirds of Crohn's fistula healed with a combined approach with seton insertion following drainage of sepsis, infliximab, and maintenance with azathioprine [42]. Another study in the UK evaluated the role of drainage of sepsis, loose seton placement, fistulotomy, flap procedures followed by infliximab therapy. Setons were removed following second dose of therapy. Complete response was seen in 29 % of patients and 42 % had partial response [43]. In complex cases particularly in Crohn's perineum, long-term seton treatment preserves sphincter function and manages sepsis [44]. It is to be noted that complex Crohn's fistulae can be difficult to treat and a long-standing loose setons aid in drainage of deep pelvic collections and prevents new ones to form. Final option would be a proctectomy for recalcitrant Crohn's fistulas.

Evidence and Recommendation

Evidence for the efficacy of loose setons for fistulae are in the form of case series. Over the years, a loose seton has become an important tool in the surgeon's armamentarium from the initial management of fistula-in-ano to complex cases where other modalities have been unsuccessful. As discussed it can be used at the time of initial drainage of abscess to prevent recurrence of sepsis, help in maturing the track, complex high anal fistula fistulas, moreover in Crohn's disease where all treatments have failed. Loose setons as a staged fistulotomy have good healing rates, however the incontinence rates can be high. Most of the studies are case series and hence level of evidence and recommendation would be Level 2C. Only a few case studies have used loose setons without transection of muscle, with good healing rates and less incontinence. This technique is useful in patients with low trans-sphincteric and inter-sphincteric fistula. Again the level of evidence and recommendation is Level 2C.

Cutting Seton

The main objective of fistula-in-ano treatment is to get rid of fistulous tract with a good functional outcome. This depends on the etiology, extent of muscle involvement, and proportionate sphincter division. Cutting seton as the name implies is used for a controlled division of the sphincter to aid in healing of the fistula. Inflammatory reaction and fibrosis of the transection site prevents retraction of the sphincter continuity during the cutting process [45] which probably help in reducing incontinence.

Appropriate patient selection and identifying the type of fistula is important [46], as a fistulotomy will help heal the fistula, nevertheless this will lead to incontinence. Typically low trans-sphincteric fistulas involving the distal third to one-half of external sphincter are ideal for a sphincterotomy [7]. A balance should be maintained between healing of the fistula and the level of incontinence accepted by the patient. This can be only achieved by understanding the patients' expectations and having a forthright dialogue. Hence, fistula management should always be tailored to individual patients.

Sphincterotomy can be undertaken by a staged fistulotomy [20], partial external sphincterotomy [7], and a cutting seton. A cutting seton gradually cuts through the enclosed muscle, with aim to cure the fistula with good functional outcome. Different types of setons have been used to achieve this effect. Silastic [47], braided silk [48], nylon [49], rubber band [8, 25, 50], cable tie [10], and penrose drain [9] are among a few used by the surgeons as a cutting seton.

Seton tightening was again undertaken depending upon the materials used and the surgeon's preference. Setons were changed weekly [51] and tightened depending on the material and surgeon's preference. Seton tightening ranged from 2 to 30 days [48, 52, 53]. In a few patients the seton was not tightened after initial placement [54], particularly elastic [55] setons. Numerous other techniques [56] have been described, such as leg strap and tourniquet [57], hangman's tie [58], cable tie [10], tight ligature knots, split-shot sinker [59], rubber band seton with progressive ligatures between previous knot and the muscle [8] and silk [60].

Complex fistulae are investigated with MRI to delineate the track. Under anesthesia, the fistulous track is identified with hydrogen peroxide, with or without endoanal ultrasound, any deep abscess drained, track probed and internal opening identified, side tracks are curetted, the skin overlying the fistula along with the fibrosis excised [7], and the seton is inserted. Initially, a loose seton might be considered to drain sepsis before changing to a tight seton later.

Randomized Controlled Trials

Most studies involving cutting seton are of Level 2B. Only four randomized controlled trials have been described. Two large studies, where the chemical cutting setons were used, are discussed in the next section [6, 19]. A randomized trial compared a modified cutting seton (internal anal sphincter preserving seton) insertion to conventional cutting seton in high trans-sphincteric fistulas. The modified cutting seton procedure entailed closure of the internal opening of the fistula by a small mucosal flap, repair of the IAS muscle and rerouting the seton through the inter-sphincteric space, to encourage external anal sphincter cutting. A total of 34 patients were randomized. Prospective continence score measurements and anorectal manometry were undertaken. Incontinence was seen in two patients in the cutting seton group compared to one in the IAS preserving group. There was no difference in incontinence scores, recurrence rates, or healing time among both the groups, at a mean follow-up of 12 months [49]. In a Cochrane review, the technique of IAS-preserving seton was thought to be cumbersome with no benefit [61].

A randomized prospective crossover trial of fibrin glue and cutting seton for trans-sphincteric fistula showed significant healing rates in the seton group compared to the fibrin glue group ($p=0.0007$). The 60 % failures in the glue group were again randomized to have a second glue injection or a seton treatment. In spite of the better healing rates with seton insertion, there was higher fecal incontinence and significantly worsening of anal manometry in these patients [62].

Cutting Seton and Incontinence

Incontinence rates with cutting setons can vary from 0 to 67 % [25, 45, 63]. This depends on the level and type (simple or complex) of the fistula and the extent of sphincter cutting. The slow division of the sphincter muscle is expected to cause less damage and preserve sphincter function. In a review [45] the average incontinence rate was 12 %; however

it was observed that there was no standardization of incontinence among studies. Incontinence rates in both high and low trans-sphincteric fistulas was 31–53 % with an average of 20.5 %. Rates with supra-sphincteric and extra-sphincteric fistulas were significantly higher with 67 % and 37 % respectively. When studies with poor data concerning type of incontinence were excluded, the incontinence rate was 32 %. Nearly 6 % were incontinent to solid stool. When etiology was considered, the median incontinence rate with cryptoglandular fistula was 20 %. This review included the chemical seton studies (46 %) in the analysis.

Another systematic review evaluated the recurrence and incontinence rates after seton treatment with or without internal anal sphincter division. Only six articles out of 18 studies analyzed incontinence scores. The median overall postoperative FI was 5.6 % (range; 0–52.4) in the preserved internal anal sphincter group compared to 25.2 % (range: 0–75). In spite of the heterogeneity in reporting and end-points, the review revealed importance of preservation of the IAS during seton placement. The recurrence rates were not significantly different in both groups [60].

Cutting Seton and High Complex Fistulas

The role of cutting seton for high and complex (extra-sphincteric and supra-sphincteric) fistulae has been evaluated with varied results. Recurrence rates ranges from 0 to 29 % [28, 49, 50, 53, 55, 64–67]. Huge discrepancy exists with incontinence rates as there has been no standardization in assessment. Incontinence rates from mild soiling to significant symptoms range from 0 to 64 % [66, 68]; however most are minor symptoms. In a review, median rate of incontinence to flatus was 9.75 % and to liquid stool was 18 % and solid stool was 5 % [45]. Ten percent of patients can develop major incontinence [63]. Significant incontinence has been reported in women and a cutting seton for anterior fistulas should be avoided in patients with previous vaginal delivery [67]. This might well be due to the short sphincter in women which has been damaged during normal labor.

Cutting Seton in Horseshoe Fistulas

Management of complex horseshoe fistulae can be challenging. In a retrospective review, 23 patients with posterior horseshoe fistula were treated with modified Hanley procedure with drainage of post anal space and a cutting seton. Most patients male. Cutting setons were tightened monthly. Complete healing was seen in 91.3 %, at follow-up (6–25 months). None had incontinence [69]. Use of a hybrid seton (elastic surgical glove with less tension) on 21 cases for this complex condition showed healing rates of 95 %, with no significant change in incontinence score postoperatively [70]. Success rates with cutting seton for complex high and horseshoe fistulas have recurrence rates of 0–21 % [28, 71].

Evidence and Recommendations

Small randomized controlled trials have been conducted. Incontinence rates with cutting seton are high, this rises further when the level of internal opening is farther away. Major incontinence can occur in nearly 10 % of patients. Healing rates are acceptable. A cutting seton can be used in trans-sphincteric fistula management (Level of Evidence and recommendation: 2B) and in selected extra-sphincteric fistula on a clear understanding that there is high risk of incontinence. In a Cochrane review, the technique of IAS preserving seton for fistula was thought to be of no benefit.

Chemical Seton

Ksharasutra or chemical seton for fistula-in-ano (Bhagandara) is a cutting seton which has been used since many centuries in the Indian subcontinent for both low and high fistula-in-ano [3]. The Ayurvedic seton is a linen thread embedded with various Ayurvedic and plant extracts to give better outcomes. The aim is to cause sustained chemical reaction, removing debris, and promote growth of healthy granulation tissue to aid healing. The medicinal extracts can stimulate lymphocyte growth [72] and demonstrates antiseptic and antihistaminic properties [73].

The technique of insertion is akin to a regular seton with few modifications by individual surgeons. Examination under anesthesia [74] is undertaken, track is identified, probed and curetted, abscess drained, and the ksharasutra placed. As in all cases of fistula-in-ano, the exact anatomical location of the fistula is documented and the type of fistula is identified. The length of the fistula and the thread is documented. It is tied snugly or tight and the principle is similar to a cutting seton. The patient is reviewed regularly in the outpatient department preferably weekly [6, 19] and the seton changed through a railroad technique [75] and tightened. Incontinence rates, recurrence and burning in [6] the postoperative period have been analyzed along with unit cutting time (UCT). UCT is the average time (in days) to cut and heal 1 cm of the fistula. This predicts the average time for treatment [76], however the exact clinical relevance is unknown apart from a guide to length of treatment. Few authors have analyzed for speed of effect of particular medicated thread [77].

Numerous medicinal extracts have been used to cure fistula-in-ano with varied results [75, 77, 78]. Ksharasutra preparation can be laborious with numerous coatings of Ayurvedic abstracts [75, 77], to achieve a particular pH. As in the case of Srivastava et al., the linen thread is coated 11 times with the latex of *Commiphera mukul*, seven coatings of alkaline *Achyranthes aspera* and finally three coatings of *C. longa* to achieve an alkaline pH of 9.75 [75]. A non-randomized clinical trial comparing medicated seton to a thread showed a quicker healing rate with the chemical seton (7 weeks vs. 11 weeks). Recurrence rates over 4 years follow-up were 3.33 % in the chemical seton group compared to 13.33 % in the thread group [75].

Randomized Controlled Trials

Interestingly, large randomized controlled trials have included chemical setons. In an RCT ($n = 100$) [6], Ayurvedic seton was compared to conventional fistulotomy, no recurrences were seen in the Ayurvedic seton group at 2 months follow-up. Patients were evaluated with pre and post-procedure manometry and endoanal ultrasonography. Three of the 46 patients in the chemical seton group had incontinence episodes however none had solid stool incontinence. The limitation of this study was the short 68 days follow-up.

A large multicentric RCT randomized patients into conventional surgery ($n = 237$) and chemical seton ($n = 265$). Complete wound healing was seen in all patients; however this was significantly longer in the ksharasutra group (8 vs. 4 weeks). In spite of the higher drop out rates (40 %) at 1 year follow-up across both groups, the recurrence rates were significantly lower with the chemical seton group (4 % vs. 11 %, $p = 0.03$). At 1 year FU, mild anal incontinence was observed in eight patients in the chemical seton group compared to 13 patients treated with surgery. The authors conclude that the chemical seton is a safe and effective alternative treatment to conventional surgery [19].

In other large study of 114 patients, none had recurrence and incontinence at over a median follow-up at 9 months. In this series, a loose seton was applied initially before changing to the ksharasutra. Interestingly, in cases where the internal opening was not identified, the external wound was packed with ksharasutra and the authors claim that the internal opening was visualized in 3–4 days [73].

Outcomes

The healing time with medicated seton ranged from 8 to 16 weeks [19, 73, 79] compared to conventional surgery (4 weeks). No recurrences were noted in high anal fistulae patients treated with chemical seton [19, 75, 76, 80]. Overall average recurrence was 0–5.88% (Table 8.1). None had major incontinence. Minor incontinence ranged from 0 to 14 %.

Table 8.1 Outcomes following chemical seton treatment for anal fistula

Authors	Type of study	Chemical seton (n)	Follow-up months	Minor incontinence (n/%)	Recurrence %
Ho et al. [6]	RCT	46	2	3/6.5	0
Shukla et al. [19]	RCT	155	12	8/5.1	4
Mohite et al. [73]	Prospective	114	6–30	0	0
Srivastava et al. [75]	Clinical trial	30	24	2/6.6	3.33
Panigrahi et al. [76]	Prospective	50	9–12	7/14	5.88

Most of the incontinence was transient [75]. The cure rates are between 94 and 100 % (Table 8.1) [74, 80]. However, most studies report fistula heterogeneity.

Complications

Complications following ksharasutra usually are severe burning pain, redness and induration, abscess [73], and slippage of thread. Transient burning pain is the commonest complication and is seen in most patients [19] following ksharasutra probably due to alkaline extracts in the thread. Severe burning pain was seen in over 30 % of patients [73]. Post-procedure abscesses needing drainage have been described [73, 75] needing drainage.

Evidence and Recommendations

Ksharasutra is a safe and effective method to treat fistula-in-ano of cryptoglandular origin. It can be carried out in the outpatient setting and patients can be ambulatory soon. Recurrence rates and incontinence rates are low, with complications such as abscess and burning pain after the procedure. The mode of action is by drainage of pus, slow and constant cutting through of the fistulous tract and the sphincter, and most importantly chemical action on the unhealthy tissue and antiseptic effect of the medicinal extracts. Analysis of a single RCT in a Cochrane review did not reveal any benefit compared to a fistulotomy (Evidence: 2A). It is extensively used in the Indian Subcontinent however not in the Western world.

References

1. Zanotti C, Martinez-Puente C, Pascual I, et al. An assessment of the incidence of fistula in ano in four countries of the European Union. Int J Colorectal Dis. 2007;22(12):1459–62.
2. Nelson R. Anorectal abscess fistula: what do we know? Surg Clin N Am. 2002;82:1139–51.
3. Sushruta Samhita: Chikitsasthanam. Chapter 17, Shlokas 29-33;5th Ed.(Motilal Banarasi Das, Varanasi, India), 1975; p456.
4. Blumetti J, Abcarian A, Quinteros F, et al. Evolution of treatment of fistula in ano. World J Surg. 2012;36(5):1162–7.
5. Pearl RK, Andrews JR, Orsay CP, et al. Role of seton in the management of anorectal fistulas. Dis Colon Rectum. 1993;36(6):573–9.
6. Ho KS, Tsang C, Seow-Choen F, et al. Prospective randomised trial comparing Ayurvedic cutting seton and fistulotomy for low fistula-in-ano. Tech Coloproctol. 2001;5:137–41.
7. Abcarian H. Anorectal infection: abscess-fistula. Clin Colon Rectal Surg. 2011;24(1):14–21.
8. Hanley PH. Rubber band seton in the management of abscess anal fistula. Ann Surg. 1978;187(4):435–7.
9. Culp CE. Use of Penrose drains to treat certain anal fistulas: a primary operative seton. Mayo Clin Proc. 1984;59:613–7.
10. Memon AA, Murtaza G, Azami R, et al. Treatment of complex fistula in ano with cable tie seton: a prospective case series. ISRN Surg. 2011; Article ID 636952
11. Buchanan GN, Halligan S, Bartram CI, et al. Clinical examination, endosonography, and MR imaging in preoperative assessment of fistula in ano: comparison with outcome-based reference standard. Radiology. 2004;233:674–81.
12. Beets-Tan RG, Beets GL, van der Hoop AG, et al. Preoperative MR imaging of anal fistulas: does it really help the surgeon? Radiology. 2001;218:75–84.
13. Lindsey I, Humphreys MM, George BD, et al. The role of anal ultrasound in the management of anal fistulas. Colorectal Dis. 2002;4:118–22.
14. Lunniss PJ, Barker PG, Sultan AH, et al. Magnetic resonance imaging of fistula-in-ano. Dis Colon Rectum. 1994;37:708–18.
15. Siddiqui MR, Ashrafian H, Tozer P, et al. A diagnostic accuracy meta-analysis of endoanal ultrasound and MRI for perianal fistula assessment. Dis Colon Rectum. 2012;55(5):576–85.
16. Deen KI, Williams JG, Hutchinson R, et al. Fistulas in ano: endoanal ultrasonographic assessment assists decision making for surgery. Gut. 1994;35:391–4.
17. Poen AC, Felt-Bersma RJF, Eijsbouts QAJ, et al. Hydrogen peroxide-enhanced transanal ultrasound in the assessment of fistula-in-ano. Dis Colon Rectum. 1998;41:1147–52.
18. Seow-Choen F, Nicholls RJ. Anal fistula. Br J Surg. 1992;79(3):197–205.
19. Shukla NK, Narang R, Nair NGK, et al. Multicentric randomized controlled clinical trial of Ksharassotra in the management of fistula-in-ano. Indian J Med Res. 1991;94:177–85.
20. Ramanujam PS, Prasad ML, Abcarian H. The role of seton in fistulotomy of the anus. Surg Gynecol Obstet. 1983;157(5):419–22.
21. Ramanujam PS, Prasad ML, Abcarian H, et al. Perianal abscesses and fistulas. A study of 1023 patients. Colon Rectum. 1984;27(9):593–7.
22. Parks AG, Stitz RW. The treatment of high fistula-in-ano. Dis Colon Rectum. 1976;19(6):487–99.
23. Kuypers HC. Use of the seton in the treatment of extrasphincteric anal fistula. Dis Colon Rectum. 1984;27:109–10.
24. Van Tets WF, Kuijpers JH. Seton treatment of perianal fistula with high anal or rectal opening. Br J Surg. 1995;82:895–7.
25. Garcia-Aguilar J, Belmonte C, Wong DW, et al. Cutting seton versus two stage seton fistulotomy in the surgical management of high anal fistula. Br J Sociol. 1998;85:243–5.
26. Joy HA, Williams JG. The outcome of surgery for complex anal fistulas. Colorectal Dis. 2002;4:254–61.

27. Lentner A, Wienert V. Long-term, indwelling setons for low trans-sphincteric and inter sphincteric anal fistulas. Experience with 108 cases. Dis Colon Rectum. 1996;39(10):1097–101.
28. Williams JG, MacLeod CA, Rothenberger DA, et al. Seton treatment of high anal fistulae. Br J Surg. 1991;78(10):1159–61.
29. Thomson JP, Ross AH. Can the external anal sphincter be preserved in the treatment of trans-sphincteric fistula-in-ano? Int J Colorectal Dis. 1989;4(4):247–50.
30. Kennedy HL, Zegarra JP. Fistulotomy without external sphincter division for high anal fistulae. Br J Surg. 1990;77:898–901.
31. Mushaya C, Bartlett L, Schulze B, et al. Ligation of intersphincteric fistula tract compared with advancement flap for complex anorectal fistulas requiring initial seton drainage. Am J Surg. 2012;204(3):283–9.
32. Aboulian A, Kaji AH, Kumar RR. Early results of ligation of the inter-sphincteric fistula tract for fistula-in-ano. Dis Colon Rectum. 2011;54(3):289–92.
33. Yassin NA, Hammond TM, Lunniss PJ, Phillips RK. Ligation of the intersphincteric fistula tract in the management of anal fistula. A systematic review. Colorectal Dis. 2013;15(5):527–35.
34. Singh B, Mortensen NJ, Jewell DP, et al. Perianal Crohn's disease. Br J Surg. 2004;91:801–14.
35. Coremans G, Dockx S, Wyndaele J, et al. Do anal fistulas in Crohn's disease behave differently and defy Goodsall's rule more frequently than fistulas that are cryptoglandular in origin? Am J Gastroenterol. 2003;98(12):2732–5.
36. White RA, Eisenstat TE, Rubin RJ, et al. Seton management of complex anorectal fistulas in patients with Crohn's disease. Dis Colon Rectum. 1990;33:587–9.
37. Makowiec F, Jehle EC, Becker HD, et al. Perianal abscess in Crohn's disease. Dis Colon Rectum. 1997;40:443–50.
38. Faucheron JL, Saint-Marc O, Guibert L, et al. Long-term seton drainage for high anal fistulas in Crohn's disease – a sphincter-saving operation? Dis Colon Rectum. 1996;39:208–11.
39. Morrison JG, Gathright JB, Ray JE, et al. Surgical management of anorectal fistuals in Crohn's disease. Dis Colon Rectum. 1989;32:492–6.
40. Ozuner G, Hull TL, Cartmill J, et al. Long-term analysis of the use of transanal rectal advancement flaps for complicated anorectal/vaginal fistulas. Dis Colon Rectum. 1996;39(1):10–4.
41. O'Connor L, Champagne BJ, Ferguson MA, et al. Efficacy of anal fistula plug in closure of Crohn's anorectal fistulas. Dis Colon Rectum. 2006;49:1569–73.
42. Topstad DR, Panaccione R, Heine JA, et al. Combined seton placement, infliximab infusion, and maintenance immunosuppressives improve healing rate in fistulizing anorectal Crohn's disease: a single center experience. Dis Colon Rectum. 2003;46:577–83.
43. Antakia R, Shorthouse AJ, Robinson K, et al. Combined modality treatment for complex fistulating perianal Crohn's disease. Colorectal Dis. 2013;15(2):210–6.
44. Takesue Y, Ohge H, Yokoyama T, Murakami Y, Imamura Y, Sueda T. Long-term results of seton drainage on complex anal fistulae in patients with Crohn's disease. J Gastroenterol. 2002;37(11):912–5.
45. Ritchie RD, Sackier JM, Hodde JP. Incontinence rates after cutting seton treatment for anal fistula. Colorectal Dis. 2008;11:564–71.
46. Parks AG, Gordon PH, Hardcastle JD. A classification of fistula in ano. Br J Sociol. 1976;63(1):1–12.
47. Charua-Guindic L, Mendez Moran MA, Avendano Espinosa O, et al. Seton de corte en el tratamiento de la fistula anal compleja. Cir Cir. 2007;75:351–6.
48. Durgun V, Perek A, Kapan M, et al. Partial fistulotomy and modified cutting seton procedure in the treatment of high extrasphincteic peri-anal fistulae. Dig Surg. 2002;19:56–8.
49. Zbar AP, Ramesh J, Beer-Gabel M, et al. Conventional cutting vs internal anal sphincter preserving seton for high transsphincteric fistula: a prospective randomized manometric and clinical trial. Tech Coloproctol. 2003;7:89–94.
50. Dziki A, Bartos M. Seton treatment of anal fistula: experience with a new modification. Eur J Surg. 1998;164:543–8.
51. Deshpande PJ, Sharma KR, Sharma SK, et al. Ambulatory treatment of fistula-in-ano—results in 400 cases. Indian J Surg. 1975;37:85–9.
52. Christensen A, Nilas L, Christiansen J, et al. Treatment of trans-sphincteric anal fistulas by the seton technique. Dis Colon Rectum. 1986;29:454–5.
53. McCourtney JS, Finlay JG. Cutting seton without preliminary internal sphincterotomy in management of complex high fistula in ano. Dis Colon Rectum. 1996;39:55–8.
54. Flich Carbonell J, Diaz Fons F, Bolufer Cano JM, et al. Fistula peri-anal. Seccion de esfinteres con seton. Rev Esp Enferm Apar Dig. 1987;72:339–42.
55. Mentes BB, Oktemer S, Tezcaner T, et al. Elastic one stage cutting seton for the treatment of high anal fistulas: preliminary results. Tech Coloproctol. 2004;8:159–62.
56. Subhas G, Bhullar JS, Al-Omari A, et al. Setons in the treatment of anal fistula: review of variations in material and techniques. Dig Surg. 2012;29:292–300.
57. Thompson Jr JE, Bennion RS, Hilliard G. Adjustable seton in the management of complex anal fistula. Surg Gynecol Obstet. 1989;169:551–2.
58. Loberman Z, Har-Shai Y, Schein M, et al. Hangman's tie simplifies seton management of anal fistula. Surg Gynecol Obstet. 1993;177:413–4.
59. Awad ML, Sell HW, Stahfield KR, et al. Split-shot sinker facilitates seton treatment of anal fistulae. Colorectal Dis. 2009;11:524–6.
60. Vial M, Pares D, Pera M, et al. Faecal incontinence after seton treatment for anal fistulae with and without surgical division of internal anal sphincter: a systematic review. Colorectal Dis. 2010;12:172–8.
61. Jacob TJ, Perakath B, Keighley MR. Surgical intervention for anorectal fistula. Cochrane Database Syst Rev. 2010;5:CD006319.
62. Altomare DF, Greco VJ, Tricomi N, et al. Seton or Glue for trans-sphincteric anal fistulae: a prospective randomized crossover clinical trial. Colorectal Dis. 2010;13:82–6.
63. Williams JG, Farrands PA, Williams AB, et al. The treatment of anal fistula: ACPGBI position statement. Colorectal Dis. 2007;9 Suppl 4:18–50.
64. Ege B, Leventoglu S, Mentes BB, et al. Hybrid seton for the treatment of high anal fistulas: results of 128 consecutive patients. Techniques in Coloproctology. 2013. DOI - 10.1007/s10151-013-1021-z.
65. Isbister WH, Al Sanea N. The cutting seton: an experience at King Faisal Specialist Hospital. Dis Colon Rectum. 2001;44(5):722–7.
66. Hämäläinen KP, Sainio AP. Cutting seton for anal fistulas: high risk of minor control defects. Dis Colon Rectum. 1997;40(12):1443–6.
67. Hasegawa H, Radley S, Keighley MR. Long-term results of cutting seton fistulotomy. Acta Chir Iugosl. 2000;47(4 Suppl 1):19–21.
68. Gurer A, Ozlem N, Gokakin AK, et al. A novel material in seton treatment of fistula in ano. Am J Surg. 2007;193:794–6.
69. Browder LK, Sweet S, Kaiser AM. Modified Hanley procedure for management of complex horseshoe fistulae. Tech Coloproctol. 2009;13(4):301–6.
70. Leventoğlu S, Ege B, Menteş BB, et al. Treatment for horseshoe fistula with the modified Hanley procedure using a hybrid seton: results of 21 cases. Tech Coloproctol. 2013;17(4):411–417.
71. Pezim ME. Successful treatment of horseshoe fistula requires deroofing of deep postanal space. Am J Surg. 1994;167(5):513–5.
72. Gewali MB, Philapitiya U, Hattori M, et al. Analysis of a thread used in the ksharasootra treatment in Ayurvedic medicinal system. J Ethnopharmacol. 1990;29:199–206.

73. Mohite JD, Gawia RS, Rohondia O, et al. Ksharasootra treatment for fistula-in-ano. Indian J Gastroenterol. 1997;16(3):96–7.

74. Faujdar HS, Mehta GG, Agarwal RK, et al. Management of fistula in ano. J Postgrad Med. 1981;27:172–7.

75. Srivastava P and Sahu M. Efficacy of Ksharasutra therapy in the management of fistula-in-ano. World J Colorectal Surg. 2010; 2(1):Article 6.

76. Panigrahi HK, Rani R, Padhi MM, et al. Clinical evaluation of Kshara Sutra therapy in the management of fistula-in-ano – a prospective study. Ancient Sci Life. 2009;28(3):29–35.

77. Rao SD. Efficacy of kshara sutra made from papaya and snuhi latex in the treatment of fistula-in-ano. Ancient Sci Life. 1998;18(2):145–51.

78. Lobo SJ, Bhuyan C, Gupta SK, et al. A comparative clinical study of Snuhi Ksheera Sutra, Tilanala Kshara Sutra and Apamarga Kshara Sutra in Bhagandara (Fistula in Ano). Ayu. 2012;33(1):85–91.

79. Deshpande PJ, Sharma KR. Treatment of fistula-in-ano by a new technique, review and follow up of 200 cases. Am J Proctol. 1973;24:49–60.

80. Deshpande PJ, Sharma KR. Successful nonoperative treatment of high rectal fistula. Am J Proctol. 1976;24:39–47.

Philip Tozer and Robin K.S. Phillips

Introduction

Fistulotomy involves laying open a fistula tract and allowing the resultant wound to heal by secondary intention. A fistula fully laid open is very unlikely to recur, but in cases of higher tracts where a significant proportion of the external sphincter would be divided, and therefore (and more importantly) little functioning sphincter would be left intact, there is a risk of lack of bowel control. Patient selection, counselling and consent are key.

Few worry about fistulotomy for low anal fistulas (submucosal, intersphincteric and low transsphincteric); most decry the technique in higher fistulas and reach for sphincter preserving albeit much less successful methods. Yet published series of carefully selected higher fistulas treated by fistulotomy reveal considerable success with good patient satisfaction and surprisingly little disturbance in bowel control.

High quality evidence is lacking across the board in anal fistula management. A Cochrane review of anal fistula surgery identified few studies comparing methods of fistula surgery and fewer still high quality randomised controlled trials ($n = 10$), suggesting that there remains significant scope for further research in this area [1]. Studies represent a mixed bag of all sorts of fistulas, not standardised for aetiology, the presence of horseshoeing or secondary extensions and with varied ascertainment of healing and follow-up. Ortiz et al. [1] argue 1 year follow-up is enough. They found that all 18 recurrences following fistulotomy or advancement flap repair ($n = 115$ and 91, respectively) arose within 1 year. No additional recurrences arose during the remaining median 42 months follow-up. Yet there clearly are cases

who re-present much later [22]—but how rare are they? Is 1 year follow-up without MRI validation of the endpoint really sufficient?

Addressing the Compromise

Patients with anal fistulas are faced with a dilemma: any procedure they choose will have either a higher failure rate or a higher risk of functional impairment. Sphincter preserving techniques offer a lower risk of functional impairment but the risk of recurrence is higher than for laying open.

The degree of impairment depends on a number of factors, only one of which is the amount of good quality contracting external sphincter left intact following fistulotomy. Determining what matters most to the patient depends on how the question is posed. The fistula already renders the patient technically 'incontinent', with inadvertent leakage of pus, added to which are smell, pain and concern lest the fistula strike again at some inconvenient time in the future (when on holiday, travelling and so on). Ellis [2] has asked patients the question one way and unsurprisingly has arrived at an answer preferring recurrence over minor functional disturbance. Like with a referendum, choice of wording is crucial; slightly altered wording can result in opposite answers.

What Is Incontinence?

The term 'incontinence' is a very bad and misleading term, covering as it does every eventuality from a minor stain in the underwear through inadvertent breaking of wind to stool running down the legs in public. On hearing the word, patients worry about the latter, when in fact the former is more likely. It is true that even minor flatus incontinence or mucus leakage may be abhorrent to some patients for personal, social or cultural reasons, but it is equally true that the word can be used in a bully's sense; to browbeat, unfairly win an argument or frighten into acquiescence.

P. Tozer, M.B.B.S., M.D. (Res.), M.R.C.S., M.C.E.M.
R.K.S. Phillips, M.B.B.S., M.S., F.R.C.S. (✉)
St. Mark's Fistula Research Unit, St. Mark's Hospital, Watford Road, Harrow, London, UK HA1 3UJ
e-mail: robin.phillips@nhs.net

H. Abcarian (ed.), *Anal Fistula: Principles and Management*, DOI 10.1007/978-1-4614-9014-2_9,
© Springer Science+Business Media New York 2014

The word 'incontinence' is probably best not used when talking with patients, having as it does images of horses and colostomy bags. But discussing potential inadvertent escape of wind or the odd 'skid mark' in the underwear is very important so that the patient can make a fair and informed choice. To do this, the surgeon must estimate the risk and extent of any impairment of continence which may occur based on the anatomy of the fistula tract to be laid open and on pre-existing bowel function and the presence or absence of irritable bowel syndrome (IBS).

Incontinence Scoring

Several scoring systems for assessing continence exist and can be used to assess and describe the degree of impairment of continence a patient experiences. The Wexner [3] and Vaizey [4] (Table 9.1) incontinence grading systems, which latter was based on the former and included three modifications, attempt to objectify patient experience of continence impairment. But the utility of such scores not only in counselling patients but also in reporting outcomes may be limited. For example, daily incontinence to flatus and daily incontinence to solid stool are valued with an equal weight. Inadvertently breaking wind and seeing the odd daily 'skid mark' in the underwear if coupled with wearing a protective lining would score 12/20 on the Wexner score, which according to the description might be accepted to be minor functional disturbance yet through looking at the number appears pretty significant. Even so, these incontinence scores are widely used in publications, reviewers demanding them. Misleading clinically as they may be, the scoring systems do permit statistical analysis of changes in incontinence score pre- and post-surgery, for example. But when talking to patients and even when publishing results, more descriptive language adds clarity.

The Anatomy of Incontinence

Historically, Milligan and Morgan suggested the anorectal ring was key to continence following fistulotomy, indicating as long as a complete ring of muscle is left intact 'all the anal sphincter muscles below this ring may be divided [...] without

harmful loss of control' [5]; but social niceties were likely different in those days. Impairment of continence following fistulotomy is well recognised and factors affecting this impairment are increasingly understood.

Whereas the external sphincter was once considered the more important in maintaining continence, we have argued recently that internal sphincter division, seen when even low fistulas are laid open, determines most functional disturbance after either high or low fistulotomy—except where Milligan and Morgan's anorectal ring is cut, when frank and devastating incontinence will result. Others dispute this [6, 7].

Our two studies examined incontinence following fistulotomy in patients who underwent either internal sphincterotomy for intersphincteric tracts or internal and external sphincterotomy for transsphincteric tracts and demonstrated a similar level of minor continence disturbance [8, 9]. In addition, anal manometry following sphincterotomy was performed in the Lunniss et al. study which found that while all patients undergoing fistulotomy had a reduced maximum resting anal tone, there was no difference in this reduction after division of both sphincters when compared with IAS division alone [9]. Division of the EAS did lower squeeze pressures in the lower canal whereas IAS division alone did not, but without functional consequence. Combining the manometric and clinical data suggests that IAS division, which reduced maximum resting anal tone, was associated with a minor impairment of continence, whereas additional division of the EAS reduced the voluntary squeeze pressure but did not influence functional outcome. Complete division of the EAS was not performed in any patients. Higher thresholds of anal electrosensitivity in the area of the divided anoderm were also noted.

Similar findings in 148 patients who underwent fistulotomy for intersphincteric fistulas (and therefore IAS division alone) were published by Toyanaga et al. in 2007. They found that resting tone and length of the high pressure zone were reduced following fistulotomy but voluntary contraction was not affected and of the 30 patients (21 %) who suffered impairment of continence, only four suffered a higher degree than flatus incontinence [10]. Likewise Chang et al. found similar manometric results in a study of 45 patients who underwent fistulotomy for intersphincteric tracts in whom resting pressures were reduced but voluntary squeeze was unaffected [11].

Table 9.1 Vaizey incontinence score [4]

	Never	Rarely	Sometimes	Weekly	Daily
Incontinence for solid stool	0	1	2	3	4
Incontinence for liquid stool	0	1	2	3	4
Incontinence for gas	0	1	2	3	4
Alteration in lifestyle	0	1	2	3	4
				No	Yes
Need to wear a pad or plug				0	2
Taking constipating medicines				0	2
Lack of ability to defer defecation for 15 min				0	4

Further support for the idea that IAS division is the main factor leading to minor disturbance in bowel control after fistulotomy comes from Kennedy et al. who described a technique to preserve the EAS by encircling it with a seton after laying open the fistula through the IAS [12]. Despite a completely preserved EAS, at least a third of patients developed minor incontinence.

Internal sphincterotomy for other conditions, such as fissure, also disturbs continence. Bennett and Goligher in 1962 found that 34 % of 127 patients undergoing internal sphincterotomy for fissure suffered flatus incontinence, although this rate diminished with longer follow-up [13]. In another study published in 1989, Khubchandani et al. found impairment of continence in as many as 35 % of patients who had undergone sphincterotomy for fissure [14]. Refinements to the technique, including the position and length of the sphincterotomy as well as more careful selection (given effective medical alternatives), have seen incontinence rates falling in recent reports, but the association between IAS injury and minor incontinence remains clear.

In a study of patterns of incontinence after anal surgery (including sphincterotomy, fistulotomy and others), Lindsey et al. examined 93 patients with incontinence and considered the nature of their sphincteric injuries [15]. Ninety-eight percent of the patients had an IAS injury on endoanal ultrasound, whereas only a third had an EAS injury. Most patients had defects in the high pressure zone of the anal canal which led to a reverse of the normal resting pressure gradient.

In addition to the quantity of muscle divided, Zbar has argued that specific factors, such as the rectoanal inhibitory reflex or a recognisable distal sphincter deficiency noted in some patients before surgery, as well as other measurable parameters from anal manometry or MR imaging, may all contribute to incontinence after surgery and that assessment of these factors may reduce predictable post-operative functional impairment summarised in [16], adding that preservation of the IAS is vital for pristine continence. However, without an evidence-based systematic approach to preoperative anal sphincter assessment, perhaps using manometry and imaging (but see below), and without an understanding of the influence of such an approach on the outcomes of surgery, the place of these techniques in preoperative decision making is unclear. What is more, for all its apparent objectivity anorectal physiology testing is not that objective: the same test repeated by the same operator on different occasions gives different results; the same test by different operators on the same occasion gives different results.

Assessment Before Fistulotomy

In the office/outpatient setting assessment of pre-existing bowel function and continence is important, along with a history of previous sphincter surgery or potential injury (e.g. complicated vaginal delivery). IBS is a relative contra-indication to lay open.

The key is the ability to feel the internal opening in a conscious patient and to estimate the likely chance and degree of disturbance were that fistula to be laid open. This should then be put to the patient who can make an informed choice.

The internal opening feels like a small grain of sand or piece of rice and is slightly tender when pushed. As in all bodily systems, there is considerable redundancy: normal renal function with half of one kidney, the ability to resect more than half the liver or remove a lung; likewise with the anal sphincter quite a lot can be cut with little consequence. As a ball park figure, a consenting patient with normal bowel habit and without IBS could have 2 cm of cephalad anal sphincter left behind: two thirds would not notice continence disturbance, and one third would experience only inadvertent loss of flatus and occasional 'skid marks' on the underwear [8, 17]. In referral centres and with much experience of assessment that distance can be reduced to 1 cm and with some patients with a weekly bowel habit to 0.5 cm.

Any continence deficit noted at presentation is clearly also crucial. In a study of 84 patients, 50 of whom underwent fistulotomy and the rest permanent loose seton insertion, continence at referral was the only factor which predicted continence at discharge; 84 % of those continent at referral maintained full continence at discharge compared with 27 % of those with a continence impairment at referral ($P < 0.001$) [17]. There may also be a defect in the EAS distal to the internal opening from previous fistulotomy, leading to a 'step-down' or 'keyhole' deformity, which enables further fistulotomy to this level with impunity.

Understanding the Potential Anatomy

The key anatomical features proposed by Goodsall and Miles include location of the internal and external openings, the course of the primary tract and the presence of secondary extensions. Difficult cases include those with high tracts, secondary extensions and anterior fistulas in women, as well as those with inflammatory bowel disease.

There is no accepted definition of what constitutes a high fistula. In practice the key determination is not how much sphincter will be cut, but how much contracting sphincter will be left behind (just as in liver surgery, it is not how much liver is removed, but how much is left behind). Perhaps the word 'complex' is better than 'high', as it takes into account secondary extensions and the presence of inflammatory bowel disease or previous failed surgery.

We have previously defined a low fistula as one with a primary tract which is subcutaneous, intersphincteric or low transsphincteric (involving no more than the most distal 1 cm of external anal sphincter), and high fistulas as those with higher transsphincteric, suprasphincteric or extrasphincteric primary tracts [8]. By this definition, we would lay open many high fistulas as well as almost all low ones.

We would be cautious about anterior fistulas in women as the anterior sphincter can be very short.

Fistulotomy Technique

The surgeon needs a clear idea of bowel function and the patient's consent before starting. Where there is doubt about fistula anatomy, MRI scanning using well-described techniques will help plan the approach and give a strong indication as to the likely site of the internal opening and of the presence of any secondary extensions. Mechanical bowel preparation and antibiotic prophylaxis are not normally employed. Some surgeons prefer an enema shortly before surgery.

Light general anaesthesia is preferred. Local anaesthesia, spinal/epidural anaesthesia and deep general anaesthesia with endotracheal intubation all end up with a paralysed external anal sphincter muscle which can make intra-operative judgment difficult. Under light general anaesthesia the anaesthesia can be lightened further leading to minor struggling or coughing, all of which contract the external anal sphincter and permit easy intra-operative identification of what length of external anal sphincter would be left behind were the fistula to be laid open.

Patient positioning is up to an individual surgeon's preference. The authors prefer the lithotomy position with the ischial tuberosities on the end of the operating table and 120° of flexion at the hip (where possible). Illustrations used have adopted that orientation.

First, the area between the anus and the external opening is firmly palpated with a lubricated finger (Fig. 9.1). A superficial tract is easily felt, giving a clue as to where in the anus to find the internal opening. With a deep tract, nothing will be felt.

The internal opening will usually be found at the dentate line and Goodsall's rule usually applies. Injection of hydrogen peroxide (or a variety of other agents) may facilitate its identification, but is not fool proof, failing to demonstrate the internal opening when there is an epithelialised internal opening.

Supralevator induration takes experience to identify. The levator muscle should feel soft, like a fillet steak, but when there is sepsis in the vicinity it feels hard, like bone. The problem is that bone is expected when performing rectal examination—the sacrum, ischial tuberosities, coccyx and so on, so induration may be overlooked. It helps to compare the 'softness/boniness' of mirror images on the clock face of the anus (Fig. 9.2). Thus 4 o'clock with 8 o'clock, 1 o'clock with 11 o'clock. Prior MRI in such cases is extremely useful.

If supralevator induration is found having already palpated a more superficial tract, this heralds a secondary extension. On the other hand, having failed to palpate a superficial tract (Fig. 9.1), induration at the anorectal junction would be expected, denoting a high tract in the roof of the ischioanal fossa, as seen in most horseshoe fistulas.

The set of instruments needed are shown in the figure (Fig. 9.3). The partially curved Lockhart–Mummery fistula probe is perhaps the most useful. All probes must be handled gently, guided by knowledge already gained as to the site of the internal opening and a finger in the anus at that point. As with negotiating a bend at colonoscopy, slight pull-back while negotiating a bend prevents the tip impacting in the fistula wall and creating a false passage.

Some fistula tracts are very narrow or tend towards an hourglass shape, such that the portion passing through the sphincter complex is not sufficiently wide to accept the probe (Fig. 9.4). In these cases hydrogen peroxide injected from the external opening may not exit the internal opening. A lacrimal probe will often negotiate such a tract. Once the probe has been passed through the tract and has entered the anal canal a further assessment can be made of the level

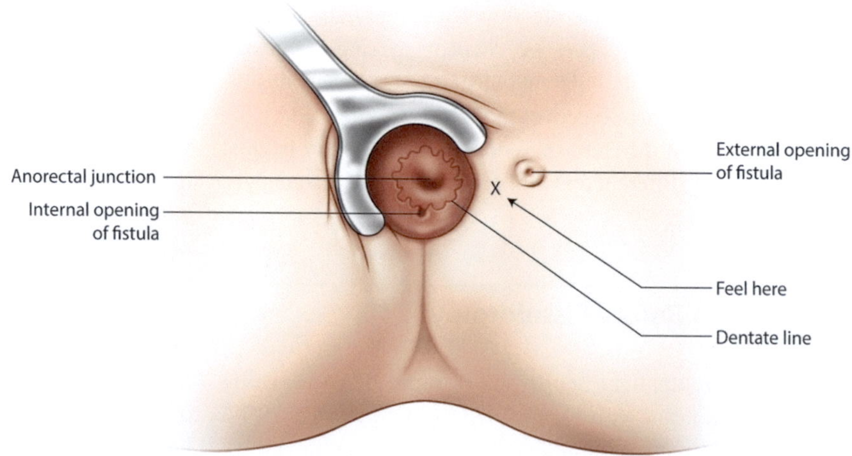

Fig. 9.1 Superficial palpation to detect the depth and direction of the fistula tract

Fig. 9.2 Palpation of the supralevator area to detect induration indicative of a high primary tract or secondary extension

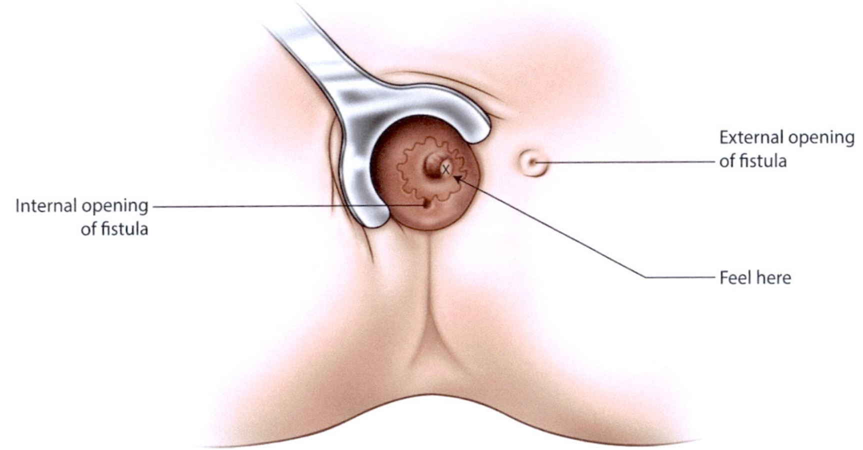

Fig. 9.3 Lacrimal probes (*left*), the Eisenhammer retractor and Lockhart–Mummery probes

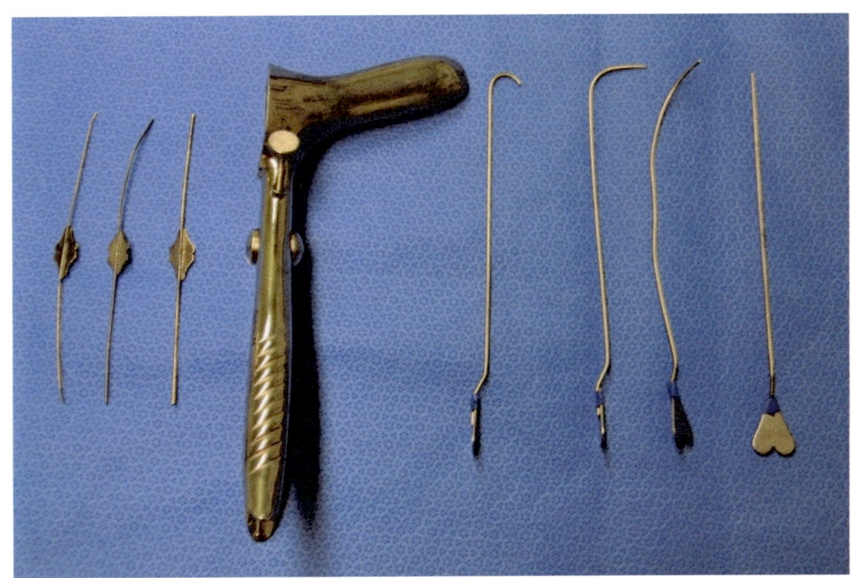

Fig. 9.4 Narrowing of the fistula tract with an hourglass deformity. A lachrymal probe may pass through if the Lockhart–Mummery probes do not

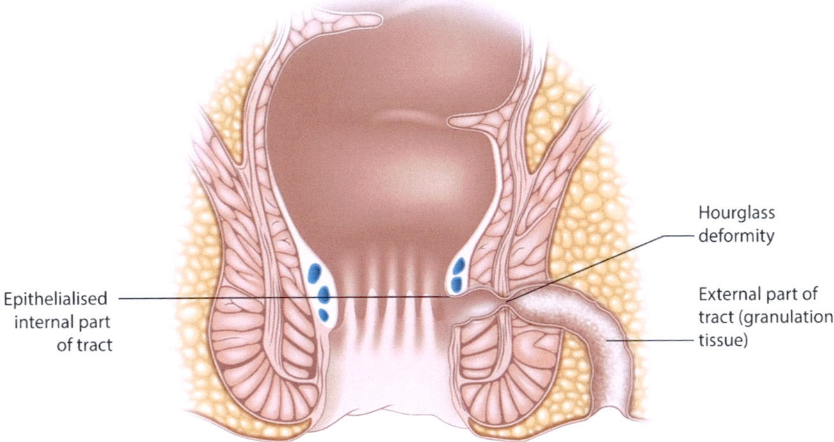

Fig. 9.5 Horseshoe fistulas may travel to the roof of the ischioanal fossa before running posteriorly towards the midline and then turning caudad before entering the anal canal

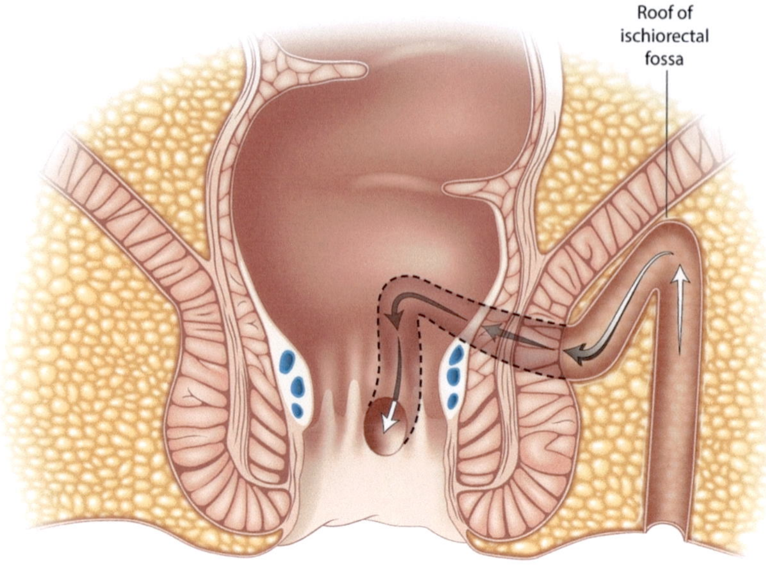

Fig. 9.6 A curved incision is made tracking the edge of the darkened anal pigment (which marks the outer boundary of the EAS) and this incision is deepened into fat. The tract is then laid open into this wound, avoiding damage to the EAS. Granulation tissue is curetted

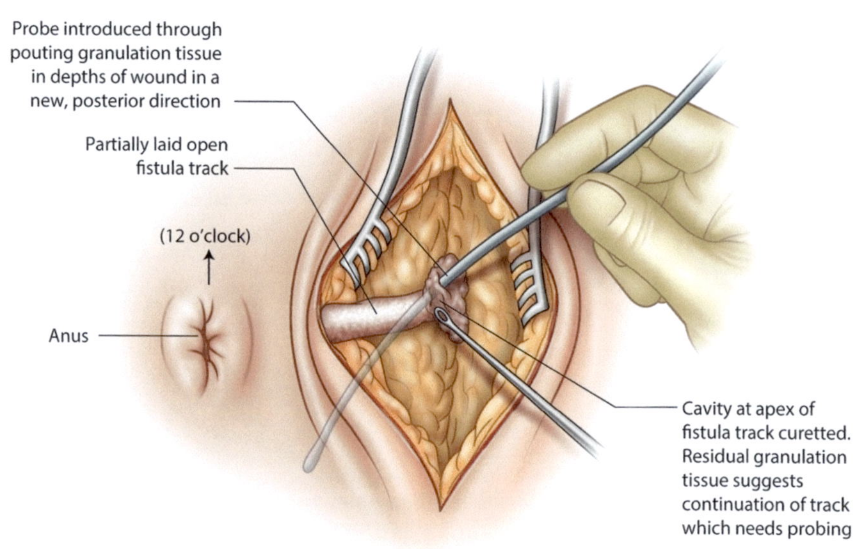

of the fistula and the risk to function encountered if fistulotomy is performed. (Mostly, this judgment has already been made from the outpatient/office assessment. But to be able to make such a judgment in that setting requires a learnt ability to feel the internal opening in the conscious patient already described above. If not sure at this stage as to how much sphincter would be left behind were the fistula to be laid open, then the anaesthetist can be asked to lighten the anaesthesia, resulting in the anal sphincter contracting as outlined earlier. Alternatively, a loose seton may be placed and the patient re-examined when awake to determine the same.)

Some tracts cannot be negotiated with a fistula probe. The classic case is with a horseshoe fistula (Fig. 9.5). The strategy in these circumstances is depicted in Fig. 9.6.

Once the fistula has been negotiated a decision is taken whether or not to lay it open, mark it with a seton or adopt one of the other techniques covered in this book. The decision has already often been taken in the office/outpatient setting as described earlier, influenced by bowel habit, lack of IBS, patient's wishes and so on. Suffice it to say that the important consideration is how much sphincter to leave behind, not how much to cut. To repeat: as a ball park figure, a consenting patient with normal bowel habit and without IBS could have 2 cm of cephalad anal sphincter left behind: two thirds would not notice continence disturbance, and one third would experience only inadvertent loss of flatus and occasional 'skid marks' on the underwear [8, 17]. In referral centres and with much experience of assessment that distance can be reduced to 1 cm and with some patients with a weekly bowel habit to 0.5 cm.

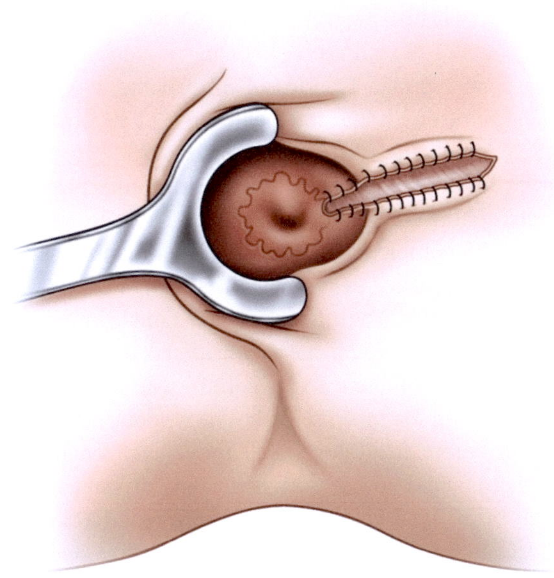

Fig. 9.7 Marsupialisation involves suturing the skin to the edge of the fistula tract with absorbable sutures to reduce wound size

Once the fistula has been laid open, granulation tissue is curetted away meticulously. Any point where it is difficult to curette away granulation tissue heralds the possibility of a secondary extension and needs careful probing.

Where possible, the wound can be marsupialised (Fig. 9.7).

Post-operative Care

The first 2 weeks with a large wound can be uncomfortable, but once lined with granulation tissue pain eases. There will be discharge and pus and blood and the patient will worry about infection, particularly when stools pass through the wound. Infection is actually rare. The wound can take 8 weeks or longer fully to heal, depending on its size and depth. Premature wound closure can lead to recurrence and can be prevented by regular wound digitation (which the patient or partner can be taught to do themselves once the wound is comfortable after the first fortnight). Sitz baths and various dressings are frequently used, but there is little evidence as to their efficacy.

Outcomes of Fistulotomy

The principle late complications are recurrence and impairment of continence, the latter not necessarily equating with dissatisfaction [6]. For example, Garcia-Aguilar reported in 2000 more dissatisfaction in patients suffering recurrence (61 %) than impairment of continence (24 %) [18].

Early complications relate to wound healing and discomfort. A randomised controlled trial of fistulotomy with and without marsupialisation from Thailand published in 2011 demonstrated reduced pethidine use in the marsupialised group but not improved healing [19]. Pescatori et al. showed the obvious, that marsupialised wounds were significantly smaller afterwards, and stayed smaller for 4 weeks [20]. They also found that bleeding was less but there was no difference in pain or septic complications. Ho et al. also found faster healing with marsupialisation (at a mean of 6 weeks compared to 10 weeks without) [21]. In a Cochrane review, the Ho and Pescatori studies were combined showing a small benefit in terms of recurrence and also, perhaps surprisingly, that incontinence was lower in the marsupialised group [1]. The review did not consider pain or wound healing.

Recurrence and Incontinence Rates After Fistulotomy

Several studies have examined fistulotomy in the context of case series and some as trials comparing fistulotomy with other techniques. Lindsey et al. published a trial in 2002 which included seven patients with low fistulas treated by fistulotomy, none of whom experienced recurrence or impairment of continence [22]. There was also no recurrence found in 54 patients with low fistulas laid open in a study comparing this with an Ayurvedic chemical seton [23]. Three patients experienced (mostly minor) deterioration in their continence. Van der Hagen et al. published results of fistulotomy in 62 patients with low tracts (although 15 % had Crohn's disease and 30% were recurrent fistulas and so might be considered 'complex') [24]. They found the longer the follow-up the higher the recurrence: 7 % at 1 year rising to 39 % at 3 years (although it might be argued that some in Crohn's disease might have been new rather than recurrent fistulas). Five percent developed minor staining after surgery.

In a very large series, Rosa et al. undertook fistulotomy in 70 % of 844 cases of anal fistula, the remainder treated by fistulectomy alone or a combination of both techniques [25]. Overall recurrence and incontinence rates were similar; 5 % and 7 % (mostly flatus/staining), respectively. A prospective multicentre study was published by Hyman in 2009 [26]. There were 13 hospitals and 245 patients, Crohn's disease in 10 %, recurrent tracts in almost a third, multiple tracts in a fifth and smoking in a quarter. In 120 patients the fistula was laid open and 87 % healed at 3 months. Both women and those who had already experienced recurrence were more likely to develop recurrence, and there was a tendency for a higher risk in smokers. In 2008 van Koperen et al. reported 109 patients undergoing fistulotomy for low fistulas with 7 % recurrence but minor staining in 41 % [27]. No factors significantly associated with recurrence were found.

It would seem that in most studies, the majority of which examined low fistulas but some also considering higher tracts, fistulotomy produced a recurrence rate of around 5 %.

Fistulotomy in Complex, Recurrent or High Fistulas

Fistulotomy in high fistulas should be undertaken with more caution, but with careful patient selection, some surgeons, often with tertiary referral practices and acknowledged expertise in fistula management, have demonstrated good results in this setting.

We have recently published two small series of fistulotomy including high, complex and recurrent tracts. In 2011 we reported a mixed series of mostly complex, recurrent and/or high anal fistulas treated surgically of which 48 were high fistulas treated by fistulotomy [8]. The recurrence rate was 4 % and the operation-induced continence disturbance was 36 %, the majority to flatus or with minor staining. This rate was similar to the low fistulas laid open in the same series. In 2012 we reported a separate, mixed series of 50 patients with mostly high, complex and/or recurrent fistulas who underwent fistulotomy [17]. The overall recurrence rate was 7 % including 9 % of those patients referred by another colorectal surgeon. We found that the presence of secondary extensions identified at fistulotomy was significantly associated with the risk of recurrence. Mostly minor deterioration in control was experienced by 40 %.

As with low, simple fistulas, fistulotomy remains the most effective way of healing high or recurrent fistulas; the risk of (albeit mostly minor) incontinence is probably around one in four to one in three patients and similar to that seen with low fistulas similarly laid open. This group of patients often have a chronicity and severity of symptoms as well as experience of failure which means they may be even more willing to tolerate flatus incontinence or minor staining for the chance of a cure.

Fistulotomy with Immediate Sphincter Reconstruction

In order to obtain the high cure rate of fistulotomy but obviate the risk of continence impairment associated with sphincter division, some surgeons have advocated immediate sphincter repair at the time of fistulotomy or fistulectomy. An early series of 120 almost exclusively low fistulas reported rapid wound closure following fistulotomy and immediate reconstruction with three patients (4 %) suffering recurrence and all patients satisfied with their functional outcome [28]. Higher and recurrent fistulas have also been examined. In 1995

Christiansen et al. reported a series of 14 patients with recurrent high anal fistulas treated with fistulectomy and immediate reconstruction [29]. Two (14 %) recurred and three patients (21 %) suffered minor incontinence. In 2009 Jivapaisarpong reported a series of 33 patients, 94 % with high transsphincteric tracts, and achieved a 12 % recurrence rate with no continence disturbance reported [30]. In a study comparing endoanal advancement flap with fistulectomy and immediate sphincter repair published in 2010, Roig et al. reported on 75 complex anal fistulas with a recurrence rate of 11 % and continence disturbance in 21 % [31].

Two recent series from the same unit (and with slightly overlapping study periods) have considered the impact of this technique on continence very carefully. In 2012 Arroyo et al. reported on 70 patients with and without continence impairment before fistulotomy and immediate repair [32]. Fistulas were medium/high transsphincteric or suprasphincteric in all cases. More than 40 % were recurrent. Recurrence occurred in 9 % of patients and the overall post-operative incontinence rate was 21 %. Of the 48 patients fully continent before the study procedure, eight (17 %) developed minor incontinence. Of the 22 who presented to the study with impairment of continence, 15 (70 %) gained significantly improved continence, although no corresponding improvement in anal manometry was seen.

Earlier, Perez et al. reported a very similar set of results in a series of 35 mostly high transsphincteric fistulas, 16 of them recurrent, with a recurrence rate of 6 % [33]. Of the 24 patients fully continent on entering the study, 3 (13 %) developed minor incontinence. Of the 11 with impairment of continence before the study procedure, function improved in 9 (70 %) and remained static in the other two. In these studies patients were given IV antibiotics for 3 days after surgery, allowed oral intake on the second post-operative day and were discharged on day 4 with instructions to return to normal diet on day 6.

We balance acknowledgment of these results with a degree of scepticism. Experience of secondary anal sphincter repair after obstetric injury showed many wound failures and deteriorating results over time [34].

Fistulotomy vs. Fistulectomy

Some surgeons advocate fistulectomy as an alternative to fistulotomy. In 1985 Kronborg compared the two techniques in a randomised controlled trial and found that while complications and recurrence were similar, the fistulectomy patients took around a week longer to heal [35]. Lewis favoured core out fistulectomy and stated with some truth that since the tract is followed under direct vision and without probing, false passages are not created, secondary tracts are transected and more easily seen and the exact relation of the tract to the sphincter can be identified before division [36].

Toyonaga and colleagues undertook a prospective but not randomised observational study comparing fistulotomy with core out fistulectomy in high transsphincteric fistulas in 2007 [37]. Of the 70 patients recruited, three suffered recurrence with no difference seen between the two groups (1 of 35 fistulotomy, 2 of 35 fistulectomy, ns) but continence impairment was more common in the fistulotomy group. The impairment was mostly to flatus or staining of undergarments in both groups and occurred in 43 % after fistulotomy compared to 17 % after fistulectomy. All patients were satisfied by their outcome.

A randomised trial of 40 patients with low, simple fistulas reported by Jain et al. in 2012, compared core out fistulectomy with fistulotomy and marsupialisation [38]. All but two fistulas were very low, being subcutaneous or intersphincteric. Follow-up was only 12 weeks during which time there were no recurrences and no impairment of continence. The fistulectomy wounds took 2 weeks longer to heal but there was no difference in post-operative pain or return to social or sexual activity.

No clear advantage of fistulectomy over fistulotomy has been demonstrated. Although the Toyonaga study suggested a better functional outcome, the non-randomised nature of the study limits its impact.

Incontinence After Surgery

As discussed above, the degree of continence impairment seen after fistulotomy depends on a combination of factors including the amount of contracting muscle (IAS and EAS) left after division, anorectal and perineal sensation, the consistency of the stool and the presence or absence of IBS. As a result of the heterogeneity of these and other factors in different studies, the degree of incontinence following fistulotomy described in the literature varies widely. However, examples of consistency exist. For example, recent studies at St Mark's hospital examining patients undergoing fistulotomy by a single surgeon have demonstrated a consistent level of impairment of continence (mostly minor, found in around one in three to one in four patients) in separate, mixed groups of fistulas with large contingents of high and complex tracts [8, 17]. In a recent study from the Oxford group Bokhari et al. found an incontinence rate of 16 % in those patients undergoing fistulotomy for simple fistulas (defined as those with a low risk for incontinence) [39].

In a study of mixed surgical procedures in which around a quarter underwent fistulotomy, Stremitzer et al. reported minor incontinence in 9 % and severe incontinence in 4 % in the fistulotomy group [40]. Toyonaga et al. found 20 % of patients undergoing fistulotomy for intersphincteric tracts developed some impairment of continence [10]. Chang et al. laid open 45 intersphincteric fistulas with a worsening of continence in 38 % of patients although the incontinence was mostly minor and less than a third noted any alteration to their lifestyle [11]. Westerterp et al. examined the post-operative continence of 60 patients undergoing fistulotomy for various height fistulas with long-term review (up to 4 years) [41]. Impairment occurred in 82, 24 and 44 % of patients with high, middle and low tracts, respectively. Satisfaction was 87 % across the group in spite of this and perhaps due to the fact that there were no recurrences. van Tets et al. found minor incontinence in 27 % of 267 patients undergoing fistulotomy for predominantly transsphincteric and intersphincteric fistulas although some extrasphincteric tracts were included and higher tracts were more likely to suffer incontinence [42].

Risk Factors for Incontinence

Several studies have tried to identify risk factors for postoperative incontinence after fistulotomy. Jordan et al. found that preoperative incontinence was the only factor significantly associated with post-operative impairment on multivariate analysis, although fistula complexity, height and recurrent tracts were also identified on univariate analysis [43]. In a more recent study, we found that time to referral was associated with a worsening of continence postoperatively, presumably because this identified patients who had undergone surgery previously, had more complex tracts and, perhaps, were more willing to accept a functional disadvantage in return for a cure [17]. However, Cavanaugh et al. found that incontinence was only associated with the amount of EAS divided in 110 patients who had undergone fistulotomy for transsphincteric (59 %) or intersphincteric fistulas [7]. Toyonaga et al. found on multivariate analysis of 148 patients undergoing fistulotomy for intersphincteric fistulas that low preoperative voluntary squeeze pressure and previous drainage surgery were associated with a greater impairment of continence [10], whereas Chang et al. found that the preoperative resting pressure was the only factor associated on multivariate analysis [11]. In 1994 van Tets et al. found that height and location of internal opening and the presence of secondary extensions were all associated with impairment of continence after fistulotomy [42]. Although there is inconsistency between studies, fistula complexity, indicated by duration of symptoms, previous surgery or complex anatomy, and preoperative impairment of continence have been found by several groups as factors associated with functional impairment after fistulotomy.

Impact of Incontinence and Recurrence on Quality of Life

Impairment of continence does not necessarily equate to poor quality of life. In the large series of fistulectomy and/or fistulotomy patients published by Rosa et al., 7 % of patients had a permanent impairment of continence but the satisfaction rate in the study was 97 % [25]. However, in the study by Cavanaugh described above, quality of life indicators were examined alongside the Faecal Incontinence Severity Index and a correlation was seen in which a greater degree of incontinence was associated with a deteriorating quality of life, especially with a very high incontinence score [7]. In another group of 21 patients with recurrent fistulas and a median of three previous operations who were cured by surgery (fistulectomy, cutting seton, advancement flap) during the study period, the gastrointestinal quality of life index (GIQLI) was used to assess quality of life. As one might expect, the GIQLI score improved after curative surgery. Incontinence decreased after surgery in the group as a whole, so its influence on quality of life is not clear in this study, but the significant improvement in quality of life after cure led the authors to conclude that cure should be sought despite the risk of (mostly minor) functional impairment.

In 1996 Garcia-Aguilar et al. reported a large series of patients undergoing sphincter dividing surgery with a recurrence rate of 8 % and impairment of continence in 46 % but dissatisfaction with the outcome of surgery in only 12% [6]. In order to investigate this, the Minnesota group then published a further analysis of factors associated with patient satisfaction (2000) in this group and found that the presence of recurrence was more likely to lead to dissatisfaction than the presence of incontinence [18]. In fact, flatus incontinence alone was not significantly associated with dissatisfaction at all, although more frequent and more severe incontinence episodes, and those which interfered with social activities, were increasingly associated with dissatisfaction. In opposition to this view, Ellis issued a questionnaire to patients and reported they preferred to avoid risk of impairment of continence and preferred sphincter preserving procedures. But as with all questionnaires/referendums, word choice significantly impacts on the result [2]. The degree of pain, success and impairment of continence, the latter described as 'worsening your ability to control gas and bowel movements', were presented as percentages in various scenarios. Patients were then asked to rank the scenarios and naturally patients opted for the choices with lowest risk and highest success. However, the most popular scenarios involved fibrin glue or fistula plug success rates of 70 % which have been reported by only a few authors, most finding a much higher rate of failure. The vague definition of impairment of continence falls exactly into the trap described above and allows the patient to assume atrocious bowel function when a minor functional impairment is the norm. Over all, it does seem that a minor functional impairment may be less likely to dissatisfy the patient than recurrence.

It is very difficult to assess the relative impacts on quality of life of recurrence and incontinence in an objective way and different patients will have different expectations and thresholds for satisfaction following surgery. Those with recurrent fistulas and a pre-existing continence impairment will likely have a different viewpoint to those with a short history of a primary fistula or those with a cultural emphasis on personal hygiene during religious practices, for example. Careful and detailed preoperative counselling helps the surgeon determine the patient's approach to this dilemma and choose the appropriate operative strategy.

Conclusions

Fistulotomy is the operation most likely to lead to fistula cure, whether the tract is high or low, recurrent or primary, complex or simple. The fear of functional impairment is in our view over-exaggerated. Because of this fear, many surgeons perhaps undertake too many sphincter preserving techniques, resulting in much recurrence and misery. Recurrence may be more likely to dissatisfy a patient than minor incontinence. Careful patient selection and preoperative counselling remain crucial when choosing fistulotomy. Fistula anatomy, bowel habit, the presence or absence of IBS and above all a proper understanding of the patient's wishes will all help decision making.

As a ball park figure, a consenting patient with normal bowel habit and without IBS could have 2 cm of cephalad anal sphincter left behind: two thirds would not notice continence disturbance, and one third would experience only inadvertent loss of flatus and occasional 'skid marks' on the underwear. In referral centres and with much experience of assessment that distance can be reduced to 1 cm and with some patients with a weekly bowel habit to 0.5 cm.

Summary

- Fistulotomy works and has a recurrence rate of approximately 5 %.
- All fistulotomy carries a one quarter to one third risk of mild mucus leakage/flatus incontinence, mostly related to internal sphincter division.
- Higher fistulas can also be laid open safely with equivalent results so long as 1–2 cm of good quality contractile sphincter remains cephalad to the fistulotomy and bowel function is normal and there is no IBS.
- The patient needs to understand the balance between cure (mostly excellent) and potential functional deficit (usually minor).

References

1. Jacob TJ, Perakath B, Keighley MR. Surgical intervention for anorectal fistula. Cochrane Database Syst Rev. 2010;5:CD006319.
2. Ellis CN. Sphincter-preserving fistula management: what patients want. Dis Colon Rectum. 2010;53(12):1652–5.
3. Jorge JM, Wexner SD. Etiology and management of fecal incontinence. Dis Colon Rectum. 1993;36(1):77–97.
4. Vaizey CJ, Carapeti E, Cahill JA, Kamm MA. Prospective comparison of faecal incontinence grading systems. Gut. 1999;44(1):77–80.
5. Milligan E, Morgan C. Surgical anatomy of the anal canal with special reference to anorectal fistulae. Lancet. 1934;ii:1150–6.
6. Garcia-Aguilar J, Belmonte C, Wong WD, Goldberg SM, Madoff RD. Anal fistula surgery. Factors associated with recurrence and incontinence. Dis Colon Rectum. 1996;39(7):723–9.
7. Cavanaugh M, Hyman N, Osler T. Fecal incontinence severity index after fistulotomy: a predictor of quality of life. Dis Colon Rectum. 2002;45(3):349–53.
8. Atkin GK, Martins J, Tozer P, Ranchod P, Phillips RK. For many high anal fistulas, lay open is still a good option. Tech Coloproctol. 2011;15(2):143–50.
9. Lunniss PJ, Kamm MA, Phillips RK. Factors affecting continence after surgery for anal fistula. Br J Surg. 1994;81(9):1382–5.
10. Toyonaga T, Matsushima M, Kiriu T, Sogawa N, Kanyama H, Matsumura N, et al. Factors affecting continence after fistulotomy for intersphincteric fistula-in-ano. Int J Colorectal Dis. 2007;22(9):1071–5.
11. Chang SC, Lin JK. Change in anal continence after surgery for intersphincteral anal fistula: a functional and manometric study. Int J Colorectal Dis. 2003;18(2):111–5.
12. Kennedy HL, Zegarra JP. Fistulotomy without external sphincter division for high anal fistulae. Br J Surg. 1990;77(8):898–901.
13. Bennett RC, Goligher JC. Results of internal sphincterotomy for anal fissure. Br Med J. 1962;2(5318):1500–3.
14. Khubchandani IT, Reed JF. Sequelae of internal sphincterotomy for chronic fissure in ano. Br J Surg. 1989;76(5):431–4.
15. Lindsey I, Jones OM, Smilgin-Humphreys MM, Cunningham C, Mortensen NJ. Patterns of fecal incontinence after anal surgery. Dis Colon Rectum. 2004;47(10):1643–9.
16. Zbar AP, Khaikin M. Should we care about the internal anal sphincter? Dis Colon Rectum. 2012;55(1):105–8.
17. Tozer P, Sala S, Cianci V, Kalmar K, Atkin GK, Rahbour G, et al. Fistulotomy in the tertiary setting can achieve high rates of fistula cure with an acceptable risk of deterioration in continence. J Gastrointest Surg. 2013. doi:10.1007/s11605-013-2198-1. Epub ahead of print.

Generic

18. Garcia-Aguilar J, Davey CS, Le CT, Lowry AC, Rothenberger DA. Patient satisfaction after surgical treatment for fistula-in-ano. Dis Colon Rectum. 2000;43(9):1206–12.
19. Sahakitrungruang C, Pattana-Arun J, Khomviali S, Tantiphlachiva K, Atittharnsakul P, Rojanasakul A. Marsupialization for simple fistula in ano: a randomized controlled trial. J Med Assoc Thai. 2011;94(6):699–703.
20. Pescatori M, Ayabaca SM, Cafaro D, Iannello A, Magrini S. Marsupialization of fistulotomy and fistulectomy wounds improves healing and decreases bleeding: a randomized controlled trial. Colorectal Dis. 2006;8(1):11–4.
21. Ho YH, Tan M, Leong AF, Seow-Choen F. Marsupialization of fistulotomy wounds improves healing: a randomized controlled trial. Br J Surg. 1998;85(1):105–7.
22. Lindsey I, Smilgin-Humphreys MM, Cunningham C, Mortensen NJ, George BD. A randomized, controlled trial of fibrin glue vs. conventional treatment for anal fistula. Dis Colon Rectum. 2002;45(12):1608–15.
23. Ho KS, Tsang C, Seow-Choen F, Ho YH, Tang CL, Heah SM, et al. Prospective randomised trial comparing ayurvedic cutting seton and fistulotomy for low fistula-in-ano. Tech Coloproctol. 2001;5(3):137–41.
24. van der Hagen SJ, Baeten CG, Soeters PB, van Gemert WG. Long-term outcome following mucosal advancement flap for high perianal fistulas and fistulotomy for low perianal fistulas: recurrent perianal fistulas: failure of treatment or recurrent patient disease? Int J Colorectal Dis. 2006;21(8):784–90.
25. Rosa G, Lolli P, Piccinelli D, Mazzola F, Bonomo S. Fistula in ano: anatomoclinical aspects, surgical therapy and results in 844 patients. Tech Coloproctol. 2006;10(3):215–21.
26. Hyman N, O'Brien S, Osler T. Outcomes after fistulotomy: results of a prospective, multicenter regional study. Dis Colon Rectum. 2009;52(12):2022–7.
27. van Koperen PJ, Wind J, Bemelman WA, Bakx R, Reitsma JB, Slors JF. Long-term functional outcome and risk factors for recurrence after surgical treatment for low and high perianal fistulas of cryptoglandular origin. Dis Colon Rectum. 2008;51(10):1475–81.
28. Parkash S, Lakshmiratan V, Gajendran V. Fistula-in-ano: treatment by fistulectomy, primary closure and reconstitution. Aust N Z J Surg. 1985;55(1):23–7.
29. Christiansen J, Ronholt C. Treatment of recurrent high anal fistula by total excision and primary sphincter reconstruction. Int J Colorectal Dis. 1995;10(4):207–9.
30. Jivapaisarnpong P. Core out fistulectomy, anal sphincter reconstruction and primary repair of internal opening in the treatment of complex anal fistula. J Med Assoc Thai. 2009;92(5):638–42.
31. Roig JV, Garcia-Armengol J, Jordan JC, Moro D, Garcia-Granero E, Alos R. Fistulectomy and sphincteric reconstruction for complex cryptoglandular fistulas. Colorectal Dis. 2010;12(7 Online):e145–52.
32. Arroyo A, Perez-Legaz J, Moya P, Armananzas L, Lacueva J, Perez-Vicente F, et al. Fistulotomy and sphincter reconstruction in the treatment of complex fistula-in-ano: long-term clinical and manometric results. Ann Surg. 2012;255(5):935–9.
33. Perez F, Arroyo A, Serrano P, Candela F, Sanchez A, Calpena R. Fistulotomy with primary sphincter reconstruction in the management of complex fistula-in-ano: prospective study of clinical and manometric results. J Am Coll Surg. 2005;200(6):897–903.
34. Malouf AJ, Norton CS, Engel AF, Nicholls RJ, Kamm MA. Long-term results of overlapping anterior anal-sphincter repair for obstetric trauma. Lancet. 2000;355(9200):260–5.
35. Kronborg O. To lay open or excise a fistula-in-ano: a randomized trial. Br J Surg. 1985;72(12):970.
36. Lewis A. Excision of fistula in ano. Int J Colorectal Dis. 1986;1(4):265–7.
37. Toyonaga T, Matsushima M, Tanaka Y, Suzuki K, Sogawa N, Kanyama H, et al. Non-sphincter splitting fistulectomy vs conventional fistulotomy for high trans-sphincteric fistula-in-ano: a prospective functional and manometric study. Int J Colorectal Dis. 2007;22(9):1097–102.
38. Jain BK, Vaibhaw K, Garg PK, Gupta S, Mohanty D. Comparison of a fistulectomy and a fistulotomy with marsupialization in the management of a simple anal fistula: a randomized, controlled pilot trial. J Kor Soc Coloproctol. 2012;28(2):78–82.
39. Bokhari S, Lindsey I. Incontinence following sphincter division for treatment of anal fistula. Colorectal Dis. 2010;12(7 Online):e135–9.

40. Stremitzer S, Strobl S, Kure V, Birsan T, Puhalla H, Herbst F, et al. Treatment of perianal sepsis and long-term outcome of recurrence and continence. Colorectal Dis. 2011;13(6):703–7.

41. Westerterp M, Volkers NA, Poolman RW, van Tets WF. Anal fistulotomy between Skylla and Charybdis. Colorectal Dis. 2003;5(6):549–51.

42. van Tets WF, Kuijpers HC. Continence disorders after anal fistulotomy. Dis Colon Rectum. 1994;37(12):1194–7.

43. Jordan J, Roig JV, Garcia-Armengol J, Garcia-Granero E, Solana A, Lledo S. Risk factors for recurrence and incontinence after anal fistula surgery. Colorectal Dis. 2010;12(3):254–60.

Fistulectomy with Primary Sphincter Reconstruction

10

Alexander Herold

Introduction

Even in the new millennium, high anal fistulas are still a challenge in colorectal surgery. In former years, the standard of care was complete fistulectomy with a high rate of continence disorders [1, 2]. Over the last 20–30 years, flap procedures have gained wide acceptance and were used in these cases. Also, many patients stayed with a long-term seton as definite treatment. The main problem of all surgical possibilities is a high recurrence rate with 30–50 % in flap procedures and 100 % of persistence in seton treatments. In recent years, we started to do a direct repair (primary reconstruction) in distal fistulas with excellent results and evolved our technique for proximal (high) anal fistulas.

Method

Primarily, patients present with a primary abscess or a chronic inflammation of a residual fistula tract. Therefore, it is necessary to reduce inflammation with wide abscess excisions or partial fistulectomies and to place a seton for 12 weeks. After complete resolution of the inflammation, patients were planned for fistulectomy with primary sphincter reconstruction.

Before surgery all patients received a complete bowel lavage and preoperative single-shot antibiotics, because to date no results are available as to whether no bowel cleaning might be equivalent or superior in accordance with other large bowel surgeries.

Primarily, the fistula situation is examined again to check suitability. Therefore, the tract is probed with a fine fistula probe. With a palpating finger, the amount of involved muscle can be calculated. The inner opening lies at the dentate line in the vast majority. Directly at the distal part of the inner opening incision starts to incise the anoderm to the anocutaneous line. From there the external opening is excised in an elliptical shape. After dissection of all subcutaneous tissues, the fistula tract is gently excised as far as the outer border of the external sphincter. Now all tissue except the muscle is excised or divided. The sphincter muscle then is incised straight forward till the fistula tract is reached. This lay-open allows a perfect view to the tracts and all surrounding tissues. No other techniques give better exposure. In many cases, you will not find a single tract, but residual cavities and holes especially in the deep part of the sphincter. With this technique, all these are visualized and can be excised. Starting from the distal external side the dorsal aspect of the granulous tract is completely excised including all cavities, leaving a healthy tissue behind. This gives the surgeon a perfect view of the fistula—much better than in all other techniques—enabling a complete excision of all granulation and scarred tissue. Due to inflammation and chronic sclerosis in most cases no separation of internal and external sphincter is possible, for reconstruction it is not necessary. To achieve good mobility and approximation, the sphincter muscle is mobilized from the anoderm and the external ischioanal fat. Mostly a few millimeters are therefore enough. Reconstruction starts at the most proximal part of the dissection, the first stitches are placed at a 45° angle to the fistula axis to get the uppermost tissue adapted. With every muscle stitch, you take a deep bite to both sides and adapt the muscle by suturing a firm knot. After two to three stitches of the muscle the upper part of the anoderm or distal part of the rectal mucosa around or above the dentate line is gently approximated, so that the anoderm as well is reconstructed. The retracter is no stepwise closed and the next part of the muscle is sutured followed by the anoderm of this section. Finally the complete sphincter complex is anatomically reconstructed, the distal wound of the ischioanal space is left open to allow lateral drainage (for the complete procedure, see Fig. 10.1a–g). The operation is finished with soft gauze dressing, no

A. Herold, M.D., Ph.D. (✉)
Deutsches End-und Dickdarm-Zentrum Mannheim,
Bismarckplatz 1, Mannheim 68165, Germany
e-mail: a.herold@enddarm-zentrum.de

H. Abcarian (ed.), *Anal Fistula: Principles and Management*, DOI 10.1007/978-1-4614-9014-2_10,
© Springer Science+Business Media New York 2014

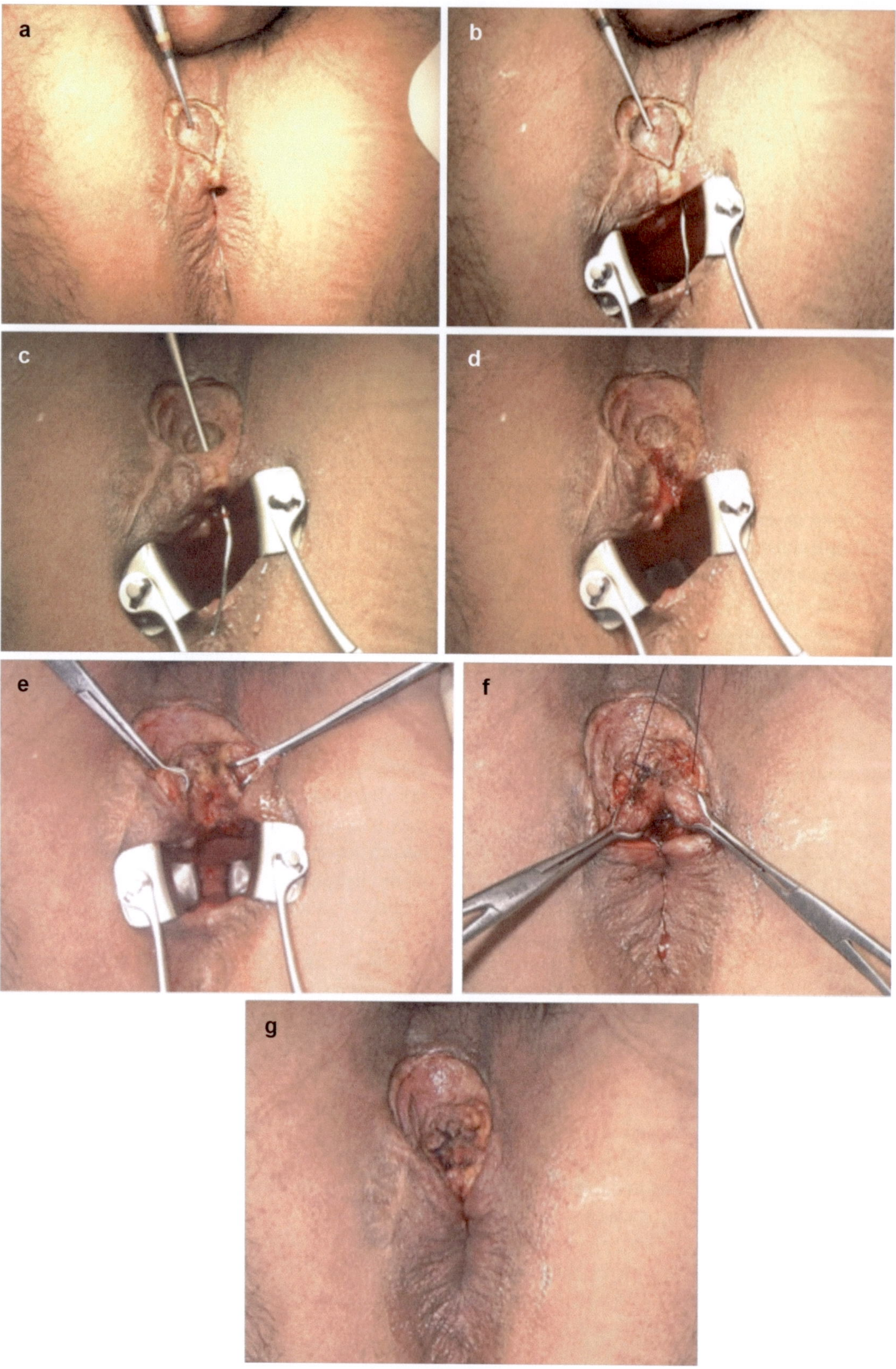

Fig. 10.1 Fistulectomy with primary sphincter reconstruction: individual steps of the technique. (**a**) Skin and anodermal incision. (**b**) Subcutaneous dissection. (**c**) Complete excision of fat and scar to the external sphincter. (**d**) Sphincter dissection, direct vision of the dorsal fistula aspect. (**e**) Mobilization of the sphincter. (**f**) Approximation of the muscle with single sutures. (**g**) Final aspect with complete reconstruction

Table 10.1 Published results

Authors	Year	n	Fistula type	Dehiscence (%)	Recurrence (%)	Incontinence (%)
Parkash et al. (Ind) [3]	1985	120	Distal	–	2.5	–
Lux and Athanasiadis (D) [4]	1991	46	Mixed	0	0	20 (1+2°)
Christiansen and Ronholt (DK) [5]	1995	14	Mixed	–	15	21 (1+2°)
Gemsenjäger (CH) [6]	1996	21	Mixed	5	5	5
Lewis (GB) [7]	1996	32	Mixed	–	9.5	
Roig et al. (E) [8]	1999	31	Mixed	4	10	24 (1+2°)
Perez et al. (E) [9]	2005	35	Mixed	–	6	12
Perez et al. (E) [10]	2006	16	Mixed	0	6	(Improved)
Bernal-Sprekelsen et al. (E) [11]	2008	8	Distal	–	12	25 (1°)
Ruppert (D), Personal communication	2010	153	Trans	6	21	12
Herold et al. (D) [12]	2009	148	Mixed	4	15	1.5 (3°)
Arroyo et al. (E) [13]	2012	70	Trans	0	8.5	17

Distal, lower third of the sphincter; Mixed, all types; Dehiscence, rupture of the muscle sutures; Recurrence, recurrence rate; Incontinence, grade of incontinence

intraanal plug is necessary. No special wound care is employed, the wound can be showered starting at the first day after the operation, the patient can walk, and physical exercises should be restrained for 4–6 weeks.

Results

Our experience with complete fistulectomy with primary sphincter reconstruction started already in 2004. Since then we have gained experience in up to 1,000 patients. In a retrospective study, we evaluated detailed results. In this study, 148 patients (51 females) with a mean age of 48 years were operated. In 43 % surgery was applied for recurrences following other fistula operations, 16 % were suprasphincteric and 84 % transsphincteric situations. No patient was operated with a covering stoma. The primary healing rate after a mean follow-up of 20 months (12–48 months) was 85 %. Adding revisionary surgery, this reaches 89 %. Recurrence and a number of previous operations had a significant influence on the outcome, whereas age, sex, smoking, other anal operations, and concomitant medication did not. In all patients new onset of incontinence was observed in 25 %, but the majority of these patients suffered from incontinence for flatus (16 %) and liquid stool (8 %). These results could be confirmed by others (Table 10.1). Overall recurrence rates are mostly around 10 % with acceptable low rates of incontinence.

Discussion

In this large cohort of patients we were able to demonstrate the practicability of an up-to-now rarely used procedure, and to achieve very promising initial results superior to results reported from advancement flaps, fibrin glue, and anal fistula plugs. By using this technique one normally is in fear of a rupture of the muscle sutures, but this appeared only in 0–8 % in the different studies—much rarer than expected. In our experience all of these insufficiencies could be repaired in a secondary operation, if performed in the first 4 postoperative weeks. So this fear—not present in other procedures, e.g., flap procedures—is not altogether neglectable, but has to be weighted against the benefit of a low recurrence rate and it can be solved in a second operation. A rupture of the mucosal or anodermal sutures occurred in 30–40 % without negative influence on the outcome, especially healing of the sphincter muscle. Today the recurrence rate in intermediate and high anal fistulas is still quite high, but this problem up to now is not solved by new procedures like plug operations or LIFT. Fistulectomy with primary sphincter reconstruction has a lower recurrence rate compared to those techniques. For those patients, wherein the majority several operations have been applied, and who are seeking for fistula cure, a minor continence disturbance is very acceptable. No patient in our group claimed his continence disorder and details were reported only after targeted questioning. So, in our daily practice, the patient's primary concern is recurrence and not incontinence.

Summary

Fistulectomy with primary sphincter reconstruction is a feasible procedure resulting in a low recurrence rate. Continence disorders are of minor concern for the patients.

References

1. Hull T, El-Gazzaz G, Gurland B, Church J, Zutshi M. Surgeons should not hesitate to perform episioproctotomy for rectovaginal fistula secondary to cryptoglandular or obstetrical origin. Dis Colon Rectum. 2011;54:54–9.

2. Ommer A, Herold A, Berg E, Fuerst A, Sailer M, Schiedeck T. Clinical practice guideline: cryptoglandular anal fistula. Dtsch Arztebl Int. 2011;108(42):707–13.

3. Parkash S, Lakshmiratan V, Gajendran V. Fistula-in-ano: treatment by fistulectomy, primary closure and reconstitution. Aust N Z J Surg. 1985;55(1):23–7.

4. Lux N, Athanasiadis S. [Functional results following fistulectomy with primary muscle suture in high anal fistula. A prospective clinical and manometric study]. Chirurg. 1991;62(1):36–41.

5. Christiansen J, Ronholt C. Treatment of recurrent high anal fistula by total excision and primary sphincter reconstruction. Int J Colorectal Dis. 1995;10:207–9.

6. Gemsenjäger E. [Results with a new therapy concept in anal fistula: suture of the anal sphincter]. Schweiz Med Wochenschr. 1996;126(47):2021–5.

7. Lewis A. Core out. In: Phillips RKS, Lunniss PJ, editors. Anal fistula: Surgical evaluation and management. London: Chapman & Hall; 1996. p. 81–86.

8. Roig JV, Garcia-Armengol J, Jordan J, Alos R, Solana A. Immediate reconstruction of the anal sphincter after fistulectomy in the management of complex anal fistulas. Colorectal Dis. 1999;1(3):137–40.

9. Perez F, Arroyo A, Serrano P, Candela F, Sanchez A, Calpena R. Fistulotomy with primary sphincter reconstruction in the management of complex fistula-in-ano: prospective study of clinical and manometric results. J Am Coll Surg. 2005;200(6):897–903.

10. Perez F, Arroyo A, Serrano P, Candela F, Perez MT, Calpena R. Prospective clinical and manometric study of fistulotomy with primary sphincter reconstruction in the management of recurrent complex fistula-in-ano. Int J Colorectal Dis. 2006;21:522–6.

11. Bernal-Sprekelsen J, Landente F, Morera F, Ripoll F, De Tursi L, Garcia-Granero M, Millan J. Treatment of anal fistulae followed by sphincteroplasty. Colorectal Dis. 2008;10 Suppl 2:51.

12. Herold A, Joos A, Hellmann U, Bussen D. Treatment of high anal fistula: is fistulectomy with primary sphincter repair an option? Colorectal Dis. 2009;11 Suppl 2:15.

13. Arroyo A, Pérez-Legaz J, Moya P, Armañanzas L, Lacueva J, Pérez-Vicente F, Candela F, Calpena R. Fistulotomy and sphincter reconstruction in the treatment of complex fistula-in-ano: long-term clinical and manometric results. Ann Surg. 2012;255(5):935–9.

José R. Cintron

Introduction

The management of fistula-in-ano remains a difficult and frustrating problem for surgeons and patients alike. Although fistulotomy is the gold standard to which other therapies must be compared, preservation of continence is also an important goal of any operation for fistula-in-ano. Extensive laying open of anorectal fistulas places the patient at varying risks of incontinence, as documented in a number of studies [1–6]. Additionally, a layopen fistulotomy leaves the patient with an open wound to care for which, in addition to pain, can be a process that takes weeks or even months to fully heal. For these reasons surgeons have searched for alternative methods of treating fistula-in-ano. Setons (cutting or loose), staged division of the sphincters, endorectal advancement flaps, dermal advancement flaps, and ligation of the intersphincteric fistula tract (LIFT procedure) have all been used as alternatives to primary fistulotomy with variable success rates; however, each of these procedures carries risks of pain, wound healing complications, and incontinence [7–18]. The ideal objectives in the treatment of a fistula would effectively heal the fistula with minimal pain, preserve sphincter function, and at the same time provide an early return to activities of daily living. These objectives led to less invasive approaches, specifically fibrin glue in the management of anorectal fistulae.

Biology and Scientific Rationale

Fibrin glue (also referred to as fibrin tissue adhesive and fibrin sealant and used interchangeably in this chapter) is a tissue adhesive that simulates the terminal steps of the natural clotting cascade (Fig. 11.1). Part of the scientific rationale for the success of fibrin glue is not just its ability to provide air and fluid tightness through the polymerization of fibrinogen within the fistula tract, but also its ability to provide a scaffold into which fibroblasts can infiltrate. Furthermore, Factor XIII, which is present and essential for fibrin cross-linking to occur, has been shown to have a physiological role by stimulating fibroblast proliferation. Other components, such as fibronectin, thrombin, glycoproteins, and fibrinogen itself, also play a role in or contribute to fibroblast migration, attachment, re-epithelialization, and neovascularization [19, 20].

During the provisional matrix that forms in the wound during early healing, fibrin becomes coated with vitronectin from the serum and fibronectin derived from both serum and aggregating platelets. Fibronectins are a class of glycoproteins that facilitate the attachment of migrating fibroblasts as well as other cell types to the fibrin lattice. Because of its influence on cellular attachment, fibronectin is a key modulator of the migration of various cell types in the wound. Additionally, the fibrin-fibronectin lattice binds various cytokines released at the time of injury and serves as a reservoir for these factors in the later stages of healing [19, 20]. The theory behind the treatment of fistulae with fibrin sealant is twofold. First, occlusion of the fistula tract with sealant immediately halts the ongoing contamination of the tract with stool, mucus, blood, and pus. Second, the proteins contained within the sealant stimulate native tissue in-growth and provide biologic scaffolding for the wound-healing process. The sealant is degraded as the fibrotic reaction progresses, and ultimately the sealant is entirely replaced by native tissues. Thus, no foreign body persists and the tract simply scars closed [21]. Fibrin gluing of anal fistulas is simple and repeatable. These factors make it a highly desirable treatment option. The use of fibrin sealant has grown in popularity over the last one and a half decades, although its appeal may be waning because of the variable results published over time.

J.R. Cintron, M.D., F.A.C.S., F.A.S.C.R.S. (✉)
Division of Colon and Rectal Surgery, John H. Stroger Hospital of Cook County, Chicago, 1900 West Polk St, Ste 402, Chicago, IL 60612, USA
e-mail: cintron2@gmail.com

H. Abcarian (ed.), *Anal Fistula: Principles and Management*, DOI 10.1007/978-1-4614-9014-2_11,
© Springer Science+Business Media New York 2014

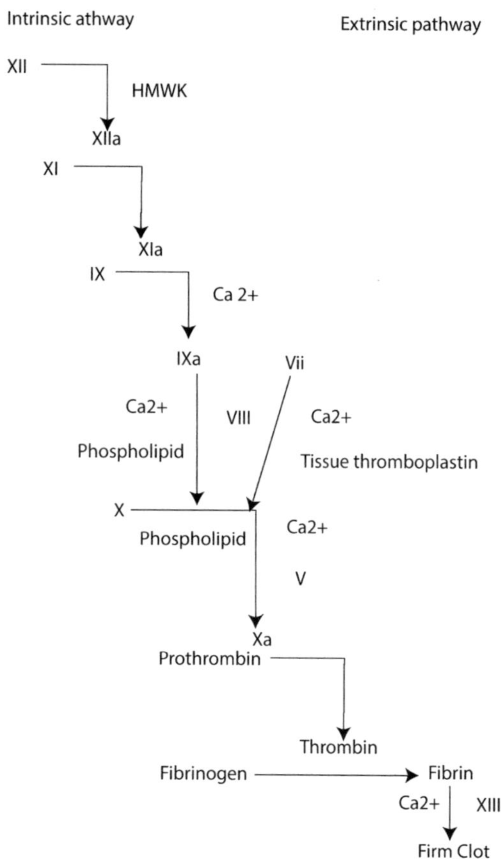

Fig. 11.1 Schematic of classic coagulation cascade

History

Fibrin tissue adhesive was first used successfully as a hemostatic agent in the early 1900s [19]. The efficacy of fibrin sealant was markedly improved through the addition of bovine thrombin to fibrinogen in 1944 [22]. Commercial plasma fractionation methods in the 1970s generated highly concentrated fibrinogen preparations that were made available in Europe in the late 1970s. Unfortunately, pooled fibrinogen concentrates were associated with an increased risk of viral transmission, especially hepatitis B and hepatitis C and later HIV. This led to license revocation in the United States by the Food and Drug Administration in 1978. Two decades later in 1998, the Food and Drug Administration relicensed the commercial preparation of fibrin sealant.

In the United States prior to 1998 fibrinogen was obtained primarily through autologous donation and "home-made" preparations. Implementation of viral inactivation procedures has made the use of commercial sealants quite safe and popular now and the preferred source of fibrin due to its ease of use and quick preparation, as evidenced by abundant clinical literature from throughout the world.

Autologous Fibrin Glue

The use of an autologous source to prepare fibrin glue minimizes the risk of disease transmission and provides a safe and simple method to treat anorectal fistulas. Abel et al. [23] published their results on the use of autologous fibrin glue in the treatment of rectovaginal and complex fistulas in ten patients and reported an overall success rate of 60 %. The authors combined autologous fibrinogen in cryoprecipitate (AFTA-C) with reconstituted bovine thrombin, thereby reproducing the final stage of the coagulation cascade. This process was reported to recover approximately 20–40 % of the fibrinogen in a unit of plasma that in total yielded approximately 10–35 mg/mL of fibrinogen concentrate. The fibrinogen concentrate is then combined with reconstituted thrombin (1,000 U/mL). Unfortunately, the process of autologous fibrinogen preparation through cryoprecipitation (AFTA-C) in the study by Abel et al. [23] took greater than 24 h to manufacture and required donation of a unit of blood. In addition, patients in the study by Abel et al. [23] underwent outpatient bowel preparation, received preoperative parenteral antibiotics, and stayed in the hospital taking nothing by mouth for 2 days postoperatively.

Autologous fibrin tissue adhesive made from a patient's own blood and based on ammonium sulfate precipitation (AFTA-A) is another method of producing autologous fibrin tissue adhesive. This tissue adhesive is biodegradable, is without side effects, and minimizes the risk of viral transmission. However, the bonding power of AFTA-A is significantly less than commercially produced fibrin tissue adhesives, hence limiting its effectiveness in cases where bonding power is essential such as in anorectal fistulas.

Another alternative method of producing autologous fibrin tissue adhesive uses a combination of ethanol and freezing to precipitate fibrinogen (AFTA-E). This method produces a biodegradable, autologous, and superior bonding power product than AFTA-A. AFTA-E is a third-generation autologous fibrin tissue adhesive developed after the first-generation (AFTA-C) and second-generation (AFTA-A) adhesives. The technical aspects of preparation of AFTA-E have been reported elsewhere [24]. Component one of AFTA-E is manufactured from 100 mL of a patient's blood. The fibrinogen is obtained via ethanol precipitation. Component two of the adhesive is prepared by combining a calcium chloride solution with thrombin and aminocaproic acid. The final thrombin concentration is 450 U/mL and the total preparation time for ATFA-E is 60 min. The results reported by Cintron et al. [25] using autologous fibrin glue parallel those of prior generation tissue adhesives [23]; however, several important differences should be pointed out. The use of a third-generation autologous fibrin tissue adhesive (AFTA-E) allows the manufacture of fibrin sealant within 1 h of a scheduled operation in contrast to 24 h. In addition, the fibrinolytic inhibitor, aminocaproic acid, keeps AFTA-E present in vivo for over 40 days at the reported concentration [26]. Furthermore, a sufficient quantity of fibrinogen (3–4 mL) is precipitated from 100 mL of blood, which when combined with an equal volume of bovine thrombin adequately fills the fistula tracts. Thus, large blood donations are avoided. All procedures were done on an ambulatory basis, and bowel preparation, parenteral antibiotics, and fistula tract decontamination were not performed unlike the studies by Abel et al. [23] and Hjortrup et al. [27], respectively.

Commercial Fibrin Sealant

By the 1970s, highly concentrated fibrinogen became widely available, as did Factor XIII and aprotinin, which served to stabilize the fibrin clot. In 1978, however, the United States Food and Drug Administration (FDA) prohibited the use of fibrinogen concentrates derived from pooled donors because of the risk of viral transmission of hepatitis (and later HIV). As a result, surgeons in the United States were left to use single-donor fibrinogen products and bovine aprotinin. By 1998, donor screening, reliable testing methods, and viral deactivation techniques made pooled fibrinogen products safe again. The FDA subsequently approved the use of commercially produced products for patients. Since that time, the use of fibrin sealant has been described for nearly every organ system. The combination of the two components of fibrin sealant reproduces the final stage of the native clotting cascade. The two essential components are fibrinogen and thrombin. The thrombin converts the fibrinogen into active fibrin. One of the commercial products most widely used is Tisseel® VH fibrin sealant (Baxter Healthcare, Deerfield, IL). The sealant is available as a two-component system. One component contains a solution of fibrinogen, Factor XIII, and bovine aprotinin. The second contains thrombin and calcium, which acts as a cofactor. The two components are maintained in separate syringes until a specially designed dual syringe applicator (Duploject®, Baxter Healthcare) (Fig. 11.2) delivers the products to the surgical site. The two components remain separated until they are mixed at the tip of the applicator device. The fibrin clot begins to organize within seconds of the two components mixing. As with autologous fibrin glue the fibrin matrix contained within the clot also serves as scaffolding for tissue in-growth into the healing wound. The fibrin as well as the fibronectin and glycoproteins that migrate into the clot stimulate activate fibroblasts, collagen deposition, re-epithelialization, and neovascularization of the wound. In this way the sealant facilitates the wound healing process. The body's native plasminogen system will destabilize the clot, and within 2 weeks, the entire synthetic clot is destabilized and replaced by host tissues [19, 20].

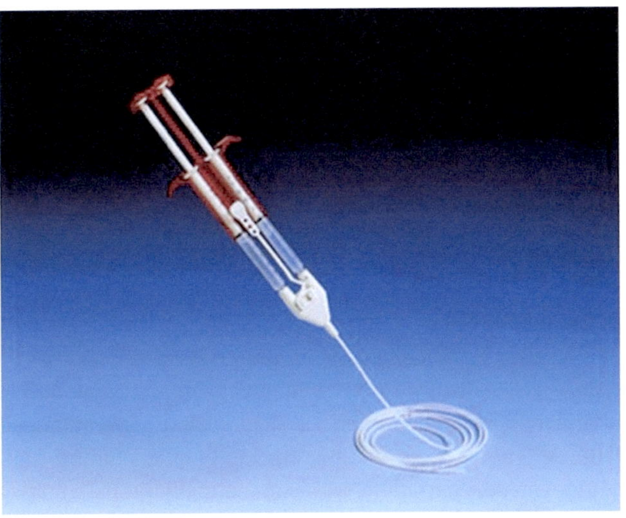

Fig. 11.2 Duploject® catheter system

Fibrin Sealant as a Carrier or Delivery Vehicle

Fibrin sealant has also been utilized to deliver cytokines, biomaterials, and most recently stem cells to the site of anal fistulas [28–30]. Singer et al. [29] reported on the use of fibrin sealant as a delivery vehicle for transforming growth factor beta (TGF-β) in an acute and chronic wound model in rats. Transforming growth factor is known to stimulate the inflammatory cascade and the wound healing process. They concluded that although fibrin sealant was an adequate delivery vehicle for TGF-β, unfortunately, it did not result in any significant changes in the healing of acute or chronic wounds in rats. Hammond et al. [28] assessed the safety, feasibility, and efficacy of cross-linked collagen in two different formats to heal anal fistulae. At operation patients were randomized to receive a solid collagen implant vs. collagen fibers suspended in fibrin glue. At the end of 29 months 80 % of the patients who underwent collagen-fibrin glue treatment were healed compared to 54 % who received the collagen implant alone. Garcia-Olmo and colleagues [31] reported on a randomized controlled multicenter Phase II study looking at fibrin glue vs. fibrin glue with adipose-derived stem cells in the treatment of 49 patients with complex perianal fistulas. After a 1-year follow-up there was a 16 % success rate in patients receiving fibrin glue alone compared to 71 % for patients who received fibrin glue in combination with adipose-derived stem cells. Herreros et al. [30] subsequently reported their results from a multicenter, randomized, single blind phase III trial utilizing autologous-expanded adipose-derived stem cells for the treatment of complex cryptoglandular perianal fistulas. Patients underwent surgical closure of the internal opening and then were randomized to receive either stem cells alone, stem cells with fibrin glue, or fibrin glue alone. The authors concluded that healing rates of approximately 40 % at 6 months were equivalent to fibrin glue alone and that when the three groups were compared no statistically significant differences were found. The utilization of fibrin sealant for these applications is still in its infancy and continues to evolve.

Technique

Although the operative procedure for fibrin glue injection of anal fistulas in the United States was performed with autologous fibrin sealant prior to 1998, most surgeons now utilize commercially prepared fibrin sealant when gluing anorectal fistulas. The reasons for this are multiple, including high fibrinogen concentrations with commercially prepared products, uniform production, advanced viral inactivation techniques, easy and quick preparation, no need for patient blood donation, greater quantities easily available, and consistent high bonding power. Operative procedures are typically performed as an outpatient. Preoperative mechanical bowel preparation is not required, other than an enema on the morning of surgery to evacuate the distal rectum. Oral and/or intravenous antibiotics are not necessary for this procedure. Patient positioning is at the discretion of the surgeon, provided that the primary and secondary openings of the fistula are easily accessible. The secondary or external opening is easily identified. Location of the primary or internal opening is essential in order to improve the success of the procedure. Occasionally hydrogen peroxide is utilized in order to inject the fistula tract in order to locate the primary opening. The tract should then be gently debrided without undue dilatation of the tract. Either an unfolded gauze sponge, a silk suture with a series of knots, a small curette, or a cytology brush works well (Fig. 11.3). Aggressive curettage or debridement should be avoided so as not to dilate the fistula tract. Dilation of the tract can lead to a greater quantity of sealant required to fill the fistula and to a higher risk of fibrin clot extrusion from the tract. After debridement the tract should be irrigated with saline or hydrogen peroxide to further cleanse the tract. Iodine irrigation of the tract should be avoided because iodine solutions can destabilize the fibrin clot. The fibrin sealant is prepared according to the manufacturer's instructions. A dual syringe applicator and dual lumen catheter is utilized containing the two components, which will mix together at the tip when injected. A variety of delivery systems are available. The author prefers a long, flexible catheter tip as seen in Fig. 11.2. Other delivery systems are available including malleable dual lumen catheters (Fig. 11.4). The dual lumen catheter is passed through the entirety of the fistula tract, at least up to the internal or primary opening and in most cases preferably through the internal opening. The catheter tip is first placed into the external orifice, through the tract, and into the anal canal towards the primary opening. This is usually accomplished by placing a tie/seton through the

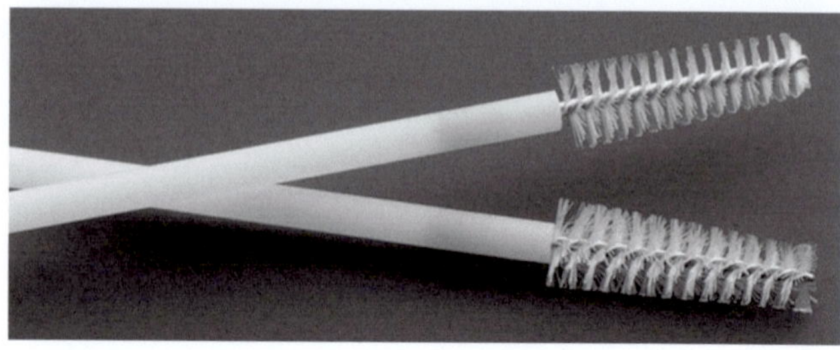

Fig. 11.3 Cytology brush used to debride fistula tract

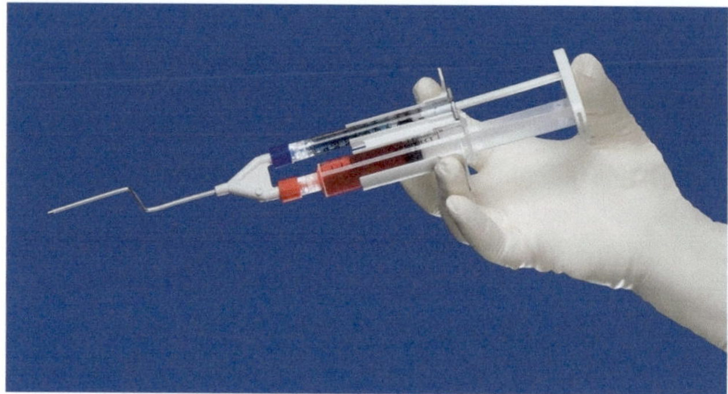

Fig. 11.4 First-generation Micromedics® malleable catheter system. With permission © Micromedics Inc., St. Paul, MN

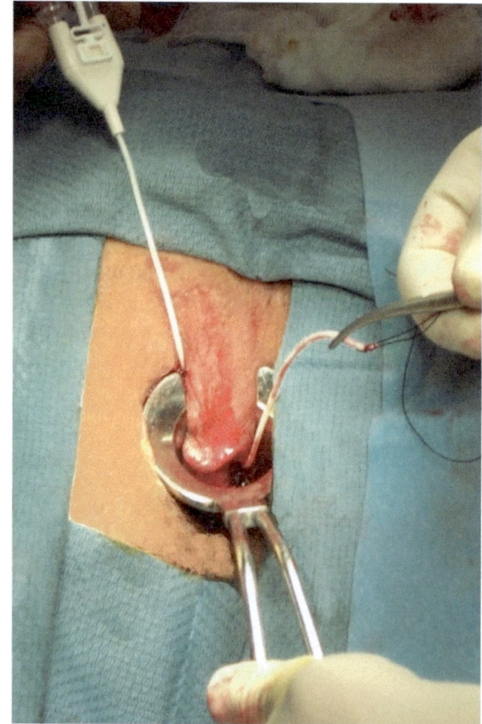

Fig. 11.5 Seton used to drag dual lumen flexible catheter through fistula tract

tract initially, which can then be secured to the catheter. The tie is then used to drag the dual lumen catheter with it and into the tract towards the primary opening (Fig. 11.5).

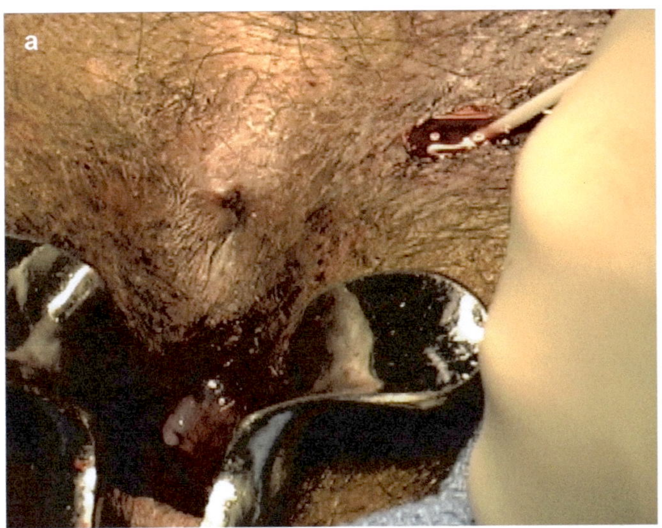
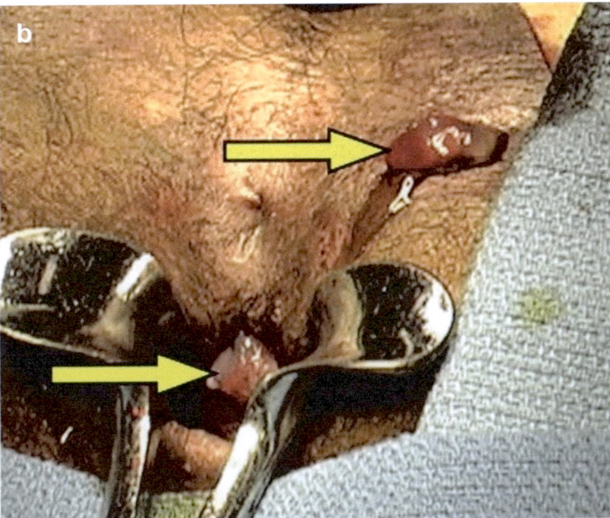

Fig. 11.6 (**a**) Dual lumen catheter trimmed and injection commenced occluding primary opening. (**b**) Completed injection demonstrating fibrin plugs present by arrows at primary and secondary fistula orifices (With permission Singer et al. [40])

The sealant is slowly injected at the internal opening and allowed to set (Fig. 11.6a). Once the clot stabilizes at the primary opening, the catheter is slowly withdrawn through the tract as sealant is being injected, thus obliterating the entire tract (Fig. 11.6b). The clot is allowed to solidify for 5–10 min. Figure 11.7a–c graphically demonstrates the injection process. The external orifice is then dressed with a non-adherent dressing. Patients are discharged home on the day of surgery, as there is minimal or no postoperative pain. Patients are instructed to avoid strenuous activity and are placed on a bowel regimen for approximately 2 weeks. Additionally, patients are instructed not to take Sitz or tub baths for 2 weeks, so as not to prematurely disrupt the fibrin clot. Showering is permitted. Complete obliteration of the tract and any of its side branches with sealant is the critical feature of the procedure. If an abscess is identified at the time of examination, it should be drained and a seton placed, and fibrin gluing deferred for a later date.

Complications Associated with Fibrin Sealant

One of the most common complications associated with the use of fibrin sealant for anorectal fistulas is the development of infection typically at the site of the external or secondary opening. This is reported in approximately 0–10 % of patients. It is important not to suture close the secondary opening at the time of gluing as this can lead to an increased incidence of infection. Other complications or side effects may be secondary to the components that constitute the product itself. These include but are not limited to hypersensitivity or allergic anaphylactoid reactions (bradycardia, tachycardia, hypotension, flushing, bronchospasm, wheezing,

dyspnea, nausea, urticaria, angioedema, pruritus, erythema, paresthesias) as well as infectious risks. Anaphylactic reactions to the antifibrinolytic protein aprotinin have been reported especially in patients who have had prior exposure to aprotinin [32, 33]. Additionally, as the commercial sealants are manufactured from human plasma, there is always the risk that the plasma may contain infectious agents such as known viruses (parvovirus), emerging viruses, or other pathogens that can potentially transmit disease including Creutzfeldt–Jakob disease (CJD) that are not eliminated by current inactivation procedures [33].

In autologous preparations or in preparations in which bovine thrombin is used, there have been some reports regarding excessive bleeding following the use of bovine thrombin particularly after reexposure to thrombin [34, 35]. Some patients have been reported to develop acquired coagulation factor inhibitors in response to bovine thrombin exposure. This does not seem to be the case when patients are reexposed to recombinant human thrombin which is utilized with greater frequency today [36]. The antibodies to bovine Factor V have been shown to elicit cross-reactivity with human Factor V, which potentially can decrease the amount of Factor V available, with subsequent inhibition of the clotting cascade [37]. This reaction is minimized via lower thrombin concentrations and through the use of Factor V-depleted bovine thrombin preparations [38].

Literature Review

Over the past one and a half decades there have been an increased amount of publications on the topic of fibrin glue in the management of anal fistulas that corresponds to the period after the FDA approved commercial sealants for use

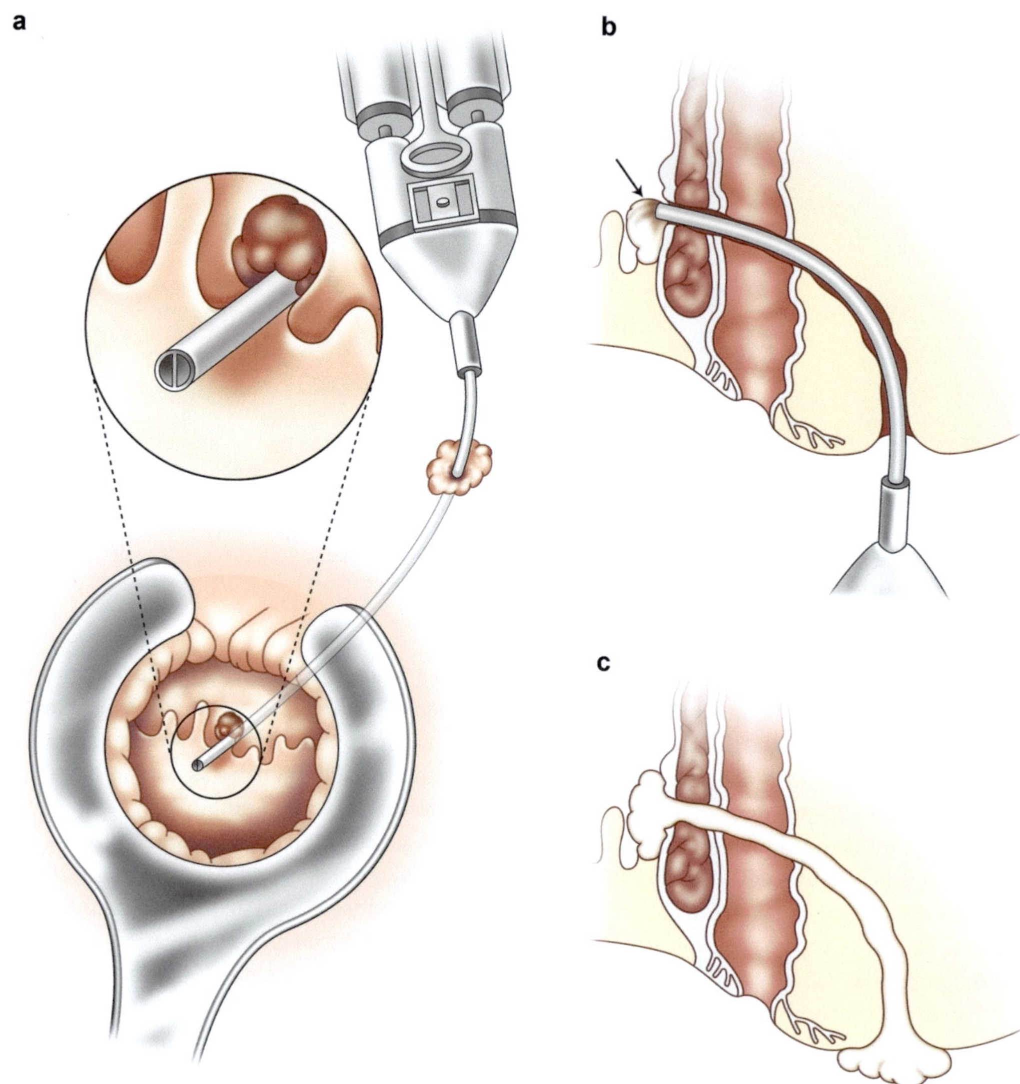

Fig. 11.7 (**a**) Dual lumen catheter system in place ready for fibrin sealant injection. (**b**) Fibrin sealant injection commenced with fibrin plug present at primary opening. (**c**) Fibrin sealant injection completed with entire tract sealed and plugs present at the primary and secondary openings (With permission Singer et al. [40])

in the United States, despite it being an off-label use for anal fistulas. The high variability regarding the design and methodology of reported studies makes comparison difficult. Few trials were initially prospective and randomized [39, 40], some were prospective and nonrandomized [23, 27, 41–48], while others were retrospective [49, 50]. The patients included in the majority of the trials were usually not standardized. They included patients who had acute and chronic fistulae, Crohn's disease, HIV-positive patients, postoperative patients, rectovaginal fistulae, and anastomotic fistulae. The commercial preparations of sealant are varied, and the intraoperative protocols differ in terms of preoperative preparation of the patient, management of the fistula in the operating room, and postoperative monitoring. The follow-up was relatively short in many of the trials, although several

trials have reported long-term data as can be seen in Table 11.1. As previously described, it is critical to obliterate the entirety of the fistula and any attached branches. For this reason, some authors chose to exclude patients in whom additional tracts were identified [27, 39, 43, 46] or deferred the injection until adequate drainage was achieved [25, 40, 41, 48, 49, 51]. Other investigators chose to include these patients and make attempts to fill all tracts and cavities with sealant [23, 42, 44]. Preoperative antibiotic use was also highly variable in these studies. Authors administered parenteral antibiotics [23, 43, 47], enteral antibiotics [44], or refrained from antibiotic use [39, 41]. There is evidence to suggest that antibiotics mixed within the fibrin sealant will be slowly released from the matrix over 24–48 h [52]. Several studies attempted to improve healing rates based on

Table 11.1 Summary of data over the last 2 decades

Authors	Year	N	Etiology	Success (%)	Type glue	Follow-up	Remarks
Hjortrup et al. [27]	1991	23	Crypto, postoperative	74	Commercial	12–26 m	First series including fistula-in-ano in 8 pts, nonrandomized
Abel et al. [23]	1993	10	Crypto, RVF, HIV, Crohn's	60	AFTA-C	3–12 m	Safe and effective, nonrandomized
Venkatash et al. [47]	1999	30	Crypto, RVF, HIV, Crohn's, urethro-vesicorectal	60	AFTA-C	9–57 m	Only recurrent pts enrolled, prospective
Aitola et al. [42]	1999	10	Crypto	0	Commercial	6 m	Pilot study
Cintron et al. [25]	1999	26	Crypto, Crohn's	85	AFTA-E	3.5 m	Third-generation autologous
Nelson et al. [7]	2000	10	Crypto	50	Commercial and dermal advancement flap	28 (4–63)	Dermal advancement flap and glue odds ratio for recurrence 4.3
Cintron et al. [41]	2000	26—A 53—C	Crypto, HIV, RVF, Crohn's	54 64	Autologous or commercial	12	Less efficacy in complex fistulae, failure seen 11 m
Patrlj et al. [46]	2000	69	Crypto	74	Commercial and cefotaxime	18–36	More effective in tracts ≥3.5 cm
El-Shobaky et al. [45]	2000	30	Crypto	87	Autologous	?	
Sentovich [53]	2001	20	Crypto, Crohn's	85	Autologous/commercial	10	
Lindsey et al. [39]	2002	19	Crypto, Crohn's	63	Commercial	3	Sealant better for complex fistulae Randomized, controlled
Chan et al. [44]	2002	10	Crypto	60	Commercial	6	Prospective nonrandomized
Tinay et al. [54]	2003	19	Crypto	78	Commercial	12	Prospective, nonrandomized
Sentovich et al. [48]	2003	48	Crypto, Crohn's,	69	Commercial	22 (6–46)	Better healing in shorter tracts, 89 % success if retreated, bowel preparation
Zmora et al. [49]	2003	24 (1°) 13 (flap and glue)	Crypto, Crohn's, postoperative	33-alone 54-flaps	Commercial	12.1 (1–36)	Retrospective, Sealant and flap yielded 54 % healing
Buchanan et al. [43]	2003	22	Crypto	14	Commercial	14	Prospective
Loungnarath et al. [50]	2004	42	Crypto, Crohn's postoperative	31	Commercial	26	Retrospective 3 pts lost to f/u
Jurczak et al. [55]	2004	31	Crypto	84	Commercial	9 (1–20)	
Gisbertz et al. [57]	2005	27	Crypto	33	Commercial	7	Complex fistulae excluded
Vitton et al. [58]	2005	14	Crohn's	57	Commercial	23 (12–26)	Similar success in Crohn's
Singer et al. [40]	2005	75	Crypto, HIV, Crohn's	35	Commercial ± Cefoxitin	27	Closure of internal opening and/or intra-adhesive cefoxitin not helpful
Zmora et al. [51]	2005	60	Complex crypto	53	Commercial (Quixil®) + ceftazidime	6	Prospective multicenter study + bowel preparation + IV cefonocid/flagyl antibiotics 1,000 U/mL thrombin
Dietz [59]	2006	39	Crypto, Crohn's, postoperative	31	Commercial	23	
Maralcan et al. [60]	2006	36	Crypto	83	Commercial	13.5 (10–17.5)	+Bowel preparation + I.V. antibiotics
Johnson et al. [61]	2006	10	Crypto	40	Commercial	3	Prospective cohort study
Ellis et al. [62]	2006	28	Advancement flap ± sealant	54	Commercial	22 (12–36)	Randomized controlled Worse result w/glue
Witte et al. [63]	2007	34	Crypto, IBD, HIV	55	Commercial	7	
Tyler et al. [64]	2007	89	Crypto, IBD, HIV	70	Commercial seton used		Success includes re-glued pts

(continued)

Table 11.1 (continued)

Authors	Year	N	Etiology	Success (%)	Type glue	Follow-up	Remarks
van Koperen et al. [65]	2008	26	Crypto	44 (1°) 59 (2°)	Commercial + Flap	13 (13–127)	Retrospective Outcome worse w/glue vs. flap alone
Adams et al. [66]	2008	36	Crypto	44	Commercial + closure 1° opening	40 (12–67)	Retrospective, long-term outcome
Hadzhiev [67]	2008	34	Crypto	74	Commercial	6	Retrospective, complex excluded, bowel preparation
Garcia-Olmo et al. [31]	2009	25 24	Crypto, Crohn's	16 71	Commercial [25] Commercial + adipose-derived stem cells [24]	12	Phase II multicenter randomized controlled
Chung et al. [68]	2009	23	Crypto	39	Commercial + closure 1° opening	3	Retrospective
Jurczak et al. [56]	2009	45	Crypto-complex	?	Commercial	67	
Damin et al. [69]	2009	32	Crypto	9	Commercial	12	Most failures w/in 3 m
de Parades et al. [70]	2010	30	Crypto-complex, Crohn's	50	Commercial Seton 8 weeks	11.7	Prospective nonrandomized Patients done under regional better outcome vs. general anesthesia
Grimaud et al. [71]	2010	36	Crohn's	38	Commercial	2	Multicenter, open label, randomized, controlled
Hammond et al. [28]	2011	16	Crypto	80	Commercial + collagen fibers	29	Prospective solid collagen implant vs. glue w/collagen fibers
Haim et al. [72]	2011	60	Crypto-complex	53 (32/60)– short 74 (17/23)– long	Commercial	78	Retrospective Recurrence 4.1 years postoperative 28 % lost to long-term f/u
Maralcan et al. [73]	2011	46	Crypto	87 (40/46) short-term 63 (29/46) long-term	Commercial	54	Prospective long-term study
de Oca et al. [74]	2012	28	Crypto	68	Commercial	20.6 (3–60)	Seton preoperative Recurrence 3–27 m
Herreros et al. [30]	2012	59 60	Crypto	37 52	Commercial + 1° closure vs. Commercial + adipose-derived stem cells	12	Phase III trial multicenter, randomized

AFTA-C autologous fibrin tissue adhesive-cryoprecipitate, *AFTA-E* autologous fibrin tissue adhesive-ethanol, *Crypto* cryptoglandular, *Pts* patients, *HIV* human immunodeficiency virus, *RVF* rectovaginal fistula, *f/u* follow-up, *IBD* inflammatory bowel disease

this laboratory data by including antibiotics within the sealant itself [40, 46]. Table 11.1 contains a summary of available data. Because of the variability in design, a formal systematic review or meta-analysis, although attempted, has not really provided useful information. Nonetheless, a review of the literature is warranted. The world literature review that follows primarily involves studies in which ten or greater patients had some form of fibrin glue treatment. Additionally, on occasion statistics may differ slightly as I thought it would be appropriate to not always dismiss patients who were lost to follow-up but include them on an intention to treat fashion.

In 1991 Hjortrup and colleagues [27] in Europe described the first cohort of patients successfully treated with a commercial sealant. This was a nonrandomized study of 23 patients of which only eight patients had fistula-in-ano, the remaining patients having postoperative persistent perineal sinuses. Although this series was small, it provided the first available data suggesting safety and efficacy for anal fistulas. Abel et al. [23] reported on a cohort of ten patients demonstrating safety and efficacy utilizing autologous fibrin glue. They reported a 60 % success with a mixed group of patients that included five patients who had rectovaginal fistulae, four of whom were successfully treated. Venkatesh and Ramanujam [47] reported results from 30 patients, all of whom had recurrent fistulae from various etiologies utilizing autologous fibrin glue. With a follow-up range from 9 to

57 months their overall success was 60 % in this complicated group, despite the variety of diagnoses and previous treatment failures. Aitola et al. [42] reported on their pilot study using commercial sealant with cryptoglandular fistulas over a 6-month follow-up. They reported zero success over the monitoring period. Cintron et al. [25] reported on a pilot study that enrolled 26 patients. The fistulas were of various etiologies and the fibrin adhesive was a third-generation autologous glue prepared via ethanol precipitation. Although reporting an 85 % success rate, follow-up was short at only 3.5 months. They subsequently published their long-term follow-up in a mixed cohort of patients utilizing autologous or commercial sealant in a prospective group of 79 patients [41]. Twenty-six patients were treated with autologous glue and 53 patients were treated with commercial sealant. Their follow-up was 12 months. There was a 54 % success rate in the autologous group and 64 % success in the commercial sealant group with an overall success at 61 %. More importantly, they recognized that recurrences occurred as late as 11 months in their study and urging even longer follow-up. Nelson and colleagues [7] published their results looking at derma island-flap anoplasty in a group of 65 patients. From that group commercial fibrin sealant was used in conjunction with a dermal island-flap anoplasty in ten patients with transphincteric fistulas. The anal fistulas were of cryptoglandular etiology and they reported a 50 % success rate over a 28-month follow-up on those patients who underwent concomitant fibrin glue injection. Of note, there was a higher failure rate when fibrin sealant was used in conjunction with dermal advancement flap with an odds ratio of 4.3. Although numbers were small, simultaneous use of fibrin glue was not advised. Patrlj et al. [46] enrolled 69 patients in a prospective study in which anal fistulae were treated with sealant that contained intra-adhesive cefotaxime. Their follow-up ranged from 18 to 36 months. They lavaged all fistula tracts with an antibiotic solution. Overall healing was 74 % and there was greater efficacy in patients whose fistula tract was ≥3.5 cm in length. This was the first study suggesting that intra-adhesive antibiotics may augment fistula healing. El-Shobaky et al. [45] presented at the Association of Coloproctology of Great Britain and Ireland their results with a series of 30 patients utilizing autologous fibrin glue in fistulas of cryptoglandular etiology. Although follow-up was not reported in their abstract, their patients enjoyed an 87 % success rate. Sentovich's [53] first report consisted of a cohort of 20 patients in 2001 utilizing autologous or commercial sealant with an 85 % success rate over a 10-month follow-up. His subsequent study in 2003 involved 48 patients utilizing commercial sealant only with a 69 % success rate with long-term follow-up of 22 months [48]. All patients were initially drained with setons and subsequently injected with sealant in a delayed fashion so as to insure adequate clearance of any perianal pus. Lindsey [39] described 19 patients in which a

commercial sealant was used to treat anal fistulae. This was the first randomized controlled trial published involving fibrin sealants with fistula-in-ano. They compared fibrin glue with conventional surgical treatments. Patients with rectovaginal fistulas or fistulas with side branches were excluded. They offered retreatment if initial injection failed. This strategy of reinjection brought initial healing rates of 42 % up to 63 % overall. This confirmed that retreatment is a reasonable option in patients failing their initial injection, although follow-up was short in their study. Additionally, they found sealant to be more efficacious in patients with complex fistulas compared to simple fistulas. Chan et al. [44] published their preliminary experience with commercial sealants for fistula-in-ano. They included ten patients in their study and also performed magnetic resonance imaging (MRI) monitoring. Overall success was 60 % over a 6-month follow-up. Additionally, they noted that MRI demonstrated a variable decrease in signal on STIR (Short Tau Inversion Recovery) images in those patients who had success. Tinay and El-Bakry [54] reported their results in 19 patients with a total of 21 fistulae from the Kingdom of Saudi Arabia. Three of their patients were lost to follow-up and 14 out of 18 had successful closure for an overall healing of 78 % with 1-year follow-up. Zmora and coworkers [49] performed a review of their experience with complex fistulae (high transsphincteric, suprasphincteric, high rectovaginal, and Crohn's fistulae) in 37 patients. Sealant alone afforded only a 33 % healing rate; however, when combined with a simultaneous endorectal advancement flap, healing was 54 %. The same author subsequently presented a prospective multicenter study enrolling 60 patients [51]. They utilized a concentrated commercial fibrin sealant with added ceftazidime. Additionally, the thrombin concentration was significantly enhanced. These patients had a 53 % success rate after 6-month follow-up. Buchanan et al. [43] from St. Marks presented their prospective trial with commercial fibrin sealant in conjunction with dynamic contrast-enhanced MRI combined with STIR imaging over a median 14-month follow-up. The majority of their patients consisted of transsphincteric fistulas. Despite the presence of healing of the secondary skin opening in 77 % of patients at 2 weeks, only 14 % remained healed at 16-month follow-up. This outcome was predicted with excellent accuracy when dynamic contrast-enhanced MRI with STIR was performed. Loungnarath and colleagues [50] in St. Louis published their retrospective study on a total of 42 patients utilizing commercial sealant with a median follow-up of 26 months. They found that durable healing was achieved in only 31 % of patients, but due to its low morbidity and simplicity should still be considered in patients with complex fistulas. Jurczak et al. [55] published their results with commercial sealant in 31 consecutive patients with a mean follow-up of 9 months. They achieved a healing rate of 84 %. Their long-term follow-up paper in 2009 with 45 patients demonstrates that all recurrences in their group occurred during the first 6 months and that durability of the procedure was present with a mean follow-up of 67 months [56]. Gisbertz et al. [57] reported on a pilot study in 27 patients. They excluded patients with complex fistulae. After a 6-month follow-up the overall success rate was 33 %. Patients with recurrent fistulae had a poorer outcome. Singer and colleagues [40] performed a randomized prospective study in the treatment of fistula-in-ano with commercial sealant. Seventy-five patients were randomized to sealant with cefoxitin, sealant with closure of the internal opening, or a combined arm. There were no significant differences between groups, with healing rates of 25 %, 44 %, and 35 %, respectively. Vitton and coworkers [58] published their results using commercial fibrin glue with modified aprotinin concentration in Crohn's disease fistulas in 14 patients. After 3 months there was a 71 % success rate. At the end of the follow-up period of almost 2 years the success rate was 57 %. In a varied cohort of patients Dietz [59] reported a 31 % success rate in 39 patients over a 2-year period utilizing a commercial sealant. Maralcan et al. [60] reported their results in a prospective study of 36 patients using commercial sealant. All their patients underwent preoperative mechanical bowel preparation and received intravenous antibiotics. After a mean follow-up of 54 weeks, they reported a 77.8 % success. Johnson et al. [61] reported on a trial comparing fibrin glue vs. anal fistula plug in a cohort of 25 patients. Of the 25 patients enrolled 10 were treated with a commercial fibrin sealant. There was a 40 % success rate after 3 months in the fibrin sealant group vs. 87 % in the anal fistula plug group. Ellis and Clark [62] reported a prospective randomized study comparing a flap procedure (mucosal advancement flap or anodermal advancement flap) to a flap procedure combined with fibrin glue obliteration of the fistula tract. With a median follow-up of 22 months, success was 80 % in those patients treated by advancement flap alone vs. 54 % in those treated by advancement flap in combination with fibrin glue injection. Witte et al. [63] reported their results with commercial sealant in complex and simple fistulas in 34 patients. They offered repeat injections to 8 of their 34 patients. Overall, closure after a median follow-up of 7 months was 55 % and success was similar in simple as well as complex fistulas. In a retrospective study, Tyler et al. [64] reported on 137 patients who underwent superficial fistulotomy vs. seton and glue, vs. seton and flap. The majority of these patients had a fistula of cryptoglandular etiology (116/137). The success rates were 100 %, 62 %, and 100 %, respectively. van Koperen and colleagues [65] published a retrospective study comparing advancement flap in conjunction with commercial sealant to advancement flap alone. Twenty-six patients underwent advancement flap combined with fibrin glue. After a median follow-up of 67 months the success rate in the group with fibrin glue was 44 % without any prior fistula surgery and 59 % with prior fistula surgery.

The patients who underwent flap without glue had 87 % and 77 % success rates, respectively. The authors concluded that using glue in combination with advancement flap led to worse outcomes. Adams et al. [66] retrospectively reviewed their results with commercial fibrin sealant in combination with suture closure of the primary opening in a cohort of 36 patients with cryptoglandular transsphincteric fistulas. Their overall success rate was 66 % at 3-month (short-term) follow-up (22/33). Of the patients that had successful closure at 3 months ($n=22$) and who were available for follow-up ($n=17$), 94 % (16/17) remained closed at 40-month follow-up. If you take the known long-term successes and consider intention to treat (16/36) then their overall long-term success was 44 %. Hadzhiev and colleagues [67] reported their retrospective review on 34 patients with non-complex fistulas of cryptoglandular etiology. Patients had an overall 74 % success after a 6-month follow-up; however, those patients with a history of recurrent fistula at the time of gluing had only a 50 % success rate. Chung et al. [68] retrospectively reviewed their treatment of patients with high transsphincteric fistulas. Of the 23 patients who underwent fibrin glue injection in combination with closure of the primary opening, their success rate after a 3-month follow-up was 39 %. Patients who underwent either anal fistula plug or advancement flap treatment had a better outcome in their study. Damin et al. [69] reported on 32 patients with cryptoglandular fistulas who underwent fibrin glue injection. Out of 32 patients who were glued only three healed for a 9 % success rate over a 12-month follow-up. de Parades et al. [70] prospectively studied 30 patients glued after an 8-week seton period. They included complex cryptoglandular fistulas and Crohn's fistulas. They reported a 50 % success rate over a 12-month follow-up. Additionally, for unclear reasons patients who underwent regional anesthesia had better outcomes than those patients done under general anesthesia. Grimaud et al. [71] published a multicenter open label randomized controlled trial in 36 patients with Crohn's fistulas involving the anus, low rectum, perineum, vulva, or vagina. Patients were randomized to commercial fibrin sealant injection ($n=36$) vs. observation ($n=41$) after removal of their setons. They reported a 38 % remission vs. 16 % remission in patients glued vs. those patients in the observation arm. Hammond et al. [28] reported their experience using fibrin glue in combination with suspended cross-linked collagen fibrils compared to a solid collagen implant alone in the treatment of anal fistulas of cryptoglandular etiology. Of 16 patients undergoing injection with fibrin glue and collagen fibrils, there was an 80 % success rate after a 29-month follow-up. Haim et al. [72] retrospectively reported on 60 patients who underwent fibrin sealant injection for complex fistulas of cryptoglandular etiology. Their short-term (6 months) success was 53 % and their long-term (6.5 years) success was 74 %. Most importantly, they reported a mean recurrence of

4.1 years postoperatively with recurrence as late as 6 years postoperatively. Maralcan et al. [73] prospectively reported their long-term results in 46 patients treated with fibrin sealant for cryptoglandular fistulas over a mean follow-up of 4.5 years. They reported a 63 % success rate over the long-term. Furthermore, patients with tracts greater than 4 cm and without side branches were more likely to have a positive outcome. de Oca et al. [74] reported their long-term results in 28 patients with cryptoglandular fistulas. They had a 68 % success rate after a mean follow-up of 20.6 months. Disease-free curves from their study demonstrated that the highest probability of recurrence occurred in the first 2 years after fibrin glue injection.

Meta-analysis and Cochrane

Cirocchi et al. [75] performed a meta-analysis of fibrin glue vs. surgery for the treatment of fistula-in-ano. Their aim was to evaluate recurrence and fecal incontinence rates in fibrin glue vs. surgical treatment (fistulotomy, cutting seton, non-cutting seton, mucosal advancement flap). The lack of homogeneity of results between studies did not allow the authors to perform any secondary outcome analysis. Of two randomized controlled trials (RCTs) and one non-randomized study, statistical analysis did not detect any significant difference for recurrence or anal incontinence between fibrin glue treatment and conventional surgical treatment. Jacob et al. [76] performed a Cochrane Review for surgical intervention of anorectal fistula. In their analysis there were no significant differences in recurrence rates or incontinence rates except in the case of advancement flaps. Although there was a low incontinence rate when glue was used in combination with a flap, this was offset by a higher recurrence rate when fibrin glue was used in combination with an advancement flap in comparison to advancement flap alone. Hence, favoring a flap-only technique.

Conclusion

Fistulotomy remains one of the most reliable methods of treating most fistulae; however, the incontinence rates make it prohibitive in many scenarios: high internal opening, anterior fistulae in women, prior anorectal surgery, and patients who either have disturbances of continence already or who have preexisting risk of incontinence (Crohn's, HIV+, elderly). Fibrin sealant injection carries essentially no risk of incontinence as there is no division of sphincter muscle. Additionally, there is very little postoperative pain, the procedure is easily repeatable, and most importantly it does not preclude any further surgical options later in the patient's treatment. In these respects, fibrin sealant is an ideal procedure for anal fistulae; however, the available data even in the

long-term suggest that the success rate is moderate at best. As previously explained, the data is highly variable, and the inconsistent trial design makes formal statistical analysis of the data difficult if not impossible. The operative procedure is technically simple; however, meticulous attention to the examination remains fundamental to its success. If there is any significant un-drained pus or unfilled side branches of the fistula, failure is likely to occur. Setons or drains should be used liberally, and injection delayed if pus is identified. The relationships between healing rates, fistula etiology, anatomy, tract length, antibiotic use, bowel preparation, and many other variables are not completely understood. Well-designed clinical trials may be required to properly evaluate these factors. Given its safety profile, ease of application, and repeatability, fibrin sealant injection should be in the armamentarium of the surgical specialist treating fistula-in-ano. Patients must be informed of its moderate success rate. Fistula-in-ano remains a complex disease that has evolved to include a variety of sphincter-preserving techniques [77]. Surgeons should become familiar with various surgical techniques including fibrin sealant injection in order that the treatment can be tailored to the patient.

Summary

1. Fibrin sealants simulate the terminal steps of the body's natural clotting cascade.
2. Fibrin sealants are safe, moderately effective, repeatable, and easy to use for the treatment of anal fistulas.
3. Fibrin sealants can be used as a carrier or delivery vehicle for other substances.
4. The outcomes of anal advancement flaps in the management of anal fistulas are worsened with the use of concomitant fibrin sealants.
5. The use of fibrin tissue adhesives continues to evolve and further randomized, prospective studies are needed.

References

1. Mazier WP. The treatment and care of anal fistulas: a study of 1,000 patients. Dis Colon Rectum. 1971;14(2):134–44.
2. Ramanujam PS, Prasad ML, Abcarian H, Tan AB. Perianal abscesses and fistulas. A study of 1023 patients. Dis Colon Rectum. 1984;27(9):593–7.
3. van Tets WF, Kuijpers HC. Continence disorders after anal fistulotomy. Dis Colon Rectum. 1994;37(12):1194–7.
4. Lunniss PJ, Kamm MA, Phillips RK. Factors affecting continence after surgery for anal fistula. Br J Surg. 1994;81(9):1382–5.
5. Pearl RK, Andrews JR, Orsay CP, Weisman RI, Prasad ML, Nelson RL, et al. Role of the seton in the management of anorectal fistulas. Dis Colon Rectum. 1993;36(6):573–7; discussion 577–9.
6. Garcia-Aguilar J, Belmonte C, Wong WD, Goldberg SM, Madoff RD. Anal fistula surgery. Factors associated with recurrence and incontinence. Dis Colon Rectum. 1996;39(7):723–9.

7. Nelson RL, Cintron J, Abcarian H. Dermal island-flap anoplasty for transsphincteric fistula-in-ano: assessment of treatment failures. Dis Colon Rectum. 2000;43(5):681–4.

8. Kodner IJ, Mazor A, Shemesh EI, Fry RD, Fleshman JW, Birnbaum EH. Endorectal advancement flap repair of rectovaginal and other complicated anorectal fistulas. Surgery. 1993;114(4):682–9; discussion 689–90.

9. Zimmerman DD, Briel JW, Gosselink MP, Schouten WR. Anocutaneous advancement flap repair of transsphincteric fistulas. Dis Colon Rectum. 2001;44(10):1474–80.

10. Jun SH, Choi GS. Anocutaneous advancement flap closure of high anal fistulas. Br J Surg. 1999;86(4):490–2.

11. Jones IT, Fazio VW, Jagelman DG. The use of transanal rectal advancement flaps in the management of fistulas involving the anorectum. Dis Colon Rectum. 1987;30(12):919–23.

12. Hamalainen KP, Sainio AP. Cutting seton for anal fistulas: high risk of minor control defects. Dis Colon Rectum. 1997;40(12):1443–6; discussion 1447.

13. Schouten WR, Zimmerman DD, Briel JW. Transanal advancement flap repair of transsphincteric fistulas. Dis Colon Rectum. 1999;42(11):1419–22; discussion 1422–3.

14. Williams JG, MacLeod CA, Rothenberger DA, Goldberg SM. Seton treatment of high anal fistulae. Br J Surg. 1991;78(10):1159–61.

15. Joo JS, Weiss EG, Nogueras JJ, Wexner SD. Endorectal advancement flap in perianal Crohn's disease. Am Surg. 1998;64(2):147–50.

16. Mizrahi N, Wexner SD, Zmora O, Da Silva G, Efron J, Weiss EG, et al. Endorectal advancement flap: are there predictors of failure? Dis Colon Rectum. 2002;45(12):1616–21.

17. Garcia-Aguilar J, Belmonte C, Wong WD, Lowry AC, Madoff RD. Open vs. closed sphincterotomy for chronic anal fissure: long-term results. Dis Colon Rectum. 1996;39(4):440–3.

18. Abcarian AM, Estrada JJ, Park J, Corning C, Chaudhry V, Cintron J, et al. Ligation of intersphincteric fistula tract: early results of a pilot study. Dis Colon Rectum. 2012;55(7):778–82.

19. Radosevich M, Goubran HI, Burnouf T. Fibrin sealant: scientific rationale, production methods, properties, and current clinical use. Vox Sang. 1997;72(3):133–43.

20. Romanos GE, Strub JR. Effect of Tissucol on connective tissue matrix during wound healing: an immunohistochemical study in rat skin. J Biomed Mater Res. 1998;39(3):462–8.

21. Singer M, Cintron J. New techniques in the treatment of common perianal diseases: stapled hemorrhoidopexy, botulinum toxin, and fibrin sealant. Surg Clin North Am. 2006;86(4):937–67.

22. Tidrick R, Warner E. Fibrin fixation of skin transplants. Surgery. 1944;15:90–5.

23. Abel ME, Chiu YS, Russell TR, Volpe PA. Autologous fibrin glue in the treatment of rectovaginal and complex fistulas. Dis Colon Rectum. 1993;36(5):447–9.

24. Park JJ, Cintron JR, Siedentop KH, Orsay CP, Pearl RK, Nelson RL, et al. Technical manual for manufacturing autologous fibrin tissue adhesive. Dis Colon Rectum. 1999;42(10):1334–8.

25. Cintron JR, Park JJ, Orsay CP, Pearl RK, Nelson RL, Abcarian H. Repair of fistulas-in-ano using autologous fibrin tissue adhesive. Dis Colon Rectum. 1999;42(5):607–13.

26. Siedentop KH, Chung SE, Park JJ, Sanchez B, Bhattacharya T, Marx G. Evaluation of pooled fibrin sealant for ear surgery. Am J Otol. 1997;18(5):660–4.

27. Hjortrup A, Moesgaard F, Kjaergard J. Fibrin adhesive in the treatment of perineal fistulas. Dis Colon Rectum. 1991;34(9):752–4.

28. Hammond TM, Porrett TR, Scott SM, Williams NS, Lunniss PJ. Management of idiopathic anal fistula using cross-linked collagen: a prospective phase 1 study. Colorectal Dis. 2011;13(1):94–104.

29. Singer M, Carillo T, Cintron J, Abcarian H. Evaluation of fibrin sealant as a delivery vehicle for TGF-B. Dis Colon Rectum. 2002;45:A46.

30. Herreros MD, Garcia-Arranz M, Guadalajara H, De-La-Quintana P, Garcia-Olmo D, FATT Collaborative Group. Autologous expanded adipose-derived stem cells for the treatment of complex cryptoglandular perianal fistulas: a phase III randomized clinical trial (FATT 1: fistula Advanced Therapy Trial 1) and long-term evaluation. Dis Colon Rectum. 2012;55(7):762–72.

31. Garcia-Olmo D, Herreros D, Pascual M, Pascual I, De-La-Quintana P, Trebol J, et al. Treatment of enterocutaneous fistula in Crohn's disease with adipose-derived stem cells: a comparison of protocols with and without cell expansion. Int J Colorectal Dis. 2009;24(1):27–30.

32. Shirai T, Shimota H, Chida K, Sano S, Takeuchi Y, Yasueda H. Anaphylaxis to aprotinin in fibrin sealant. Intern Med. 2005;44(10):1088–9.

33. Fibrin Sealant, TISSEEL, [package insert], Westlake Village, CA: Baxter Healthcare Corporation, Deerfield, IL; 1998.

34. Christie RJ, Carrington L, Alving B. Postoperative bleeding induced by topical bovine thrombin: report of two cases. Surgery. 1997;121(6):708–10.

35. Singla NK, Gasparis AP, Ballard JL, Baron JM, Butine MD, Pribble JP, et al. Immunogenicity and safety of re-exposure to recombinant human thrombin in surgical hemostasis. J Am Coll Surg. 2011;213(6):722–7.

36. Ofosu FA, Crean S, Reynolds MW. A safety review of topical bovine thrombin-induced generation of antibodies to bovine proteins. Clin Ther. 2009;31(4):679–91.

37. Lomax C, Traub O. Topical thrombins: benefits and risks. Pharmacotherapy. 2009;29(7 Pt 2):8S–12.

38. Bhandari M, Ofosu FA, Mackman N, Jackson C, Doria C, Humphries JE, et al. Safety and efficacy of thrombin-JMI: a multidisciplinary expert group consensus. Clin Appl Thromb Hemost. 2011;17(1):39–45.

39. Lindsey I, Smilgin-Humphreys MM, Cunningham C, Mortensen NJ, George BD. A randomized, controlled trial of fibrin glue vs. conventional treatment for anal fistula. Dis Colon Rectum. 2002;45(12):1608–15.

40. Singer M, Cintron J, Nelson R, Orsay C, Bastawrous A, Pearl R, et al. Treatment of fistulas-in-ano with fibrin sealant in combination with intra-adhesive antibiotics and/or surgical closure of the internal fistula opening. Dis Colon Rectum. 2005;48(4):799–808.

41. Cintron JR, Park JJ, Orsay CP, Pearl RK, Nelson RL, Sone JH, et al. Repair of fistulas-in-ano using fibrin adhesive: long-term followup. Dis Colon Rectum. 2000;43(7):944–9; discussion 949–50.

42. Aitola P, Hiltunen KM, Matikainen M. Fibrin glue in perianal fistulas—a pilot study. Ann Chir Gynaecol. 1999;88(2):136–8.

43. Buchanan GN, Bartram CI, Phillips RK, Gould SW, Halligan S, Rockall TA, et al. Efficacy of fibrin sealant in the management of complex anal fistula: a prospective trial. Dis Colon Rectum. 2003;46(9):1167–74.

44. Chan KM, Lau CW, Lai KK, Auyeung MC, Ho LS, Luk HT, et al. Preliminary results of using a commercial fibrin sealant in the treatment of fistula-in-ano. J R Coll Surg Edinb. 2002;47(1):407–10.

45. El-Shobaky M, Khafagy W, El-Awady W. Autologous fibrin glue in the treatment of fistula-in-ano. Colorectal Dis. 2000;2(Suppl):17.

46. Patrlj L, Kocman B, Martinac M, Jadrijevic S, Sosa T, Sebecic B, et al. Fibrin glue-antibiotic mixture in the treatment of anal fistulae: experience with 69 cases. Dig Surg. 2000;17(1):77–80.

47. Venkatesh KS, Ramanujam P. Fibrin glue application in the treatment of recurrent anorectal fistulas. Dis Colon Rectum. 1999;42(9):1136–9.

48. Sentovich SM. Fibrin glue for anal fistulas: long-term results. Dis Colon Rectum. 2003;46(4):498–502.

49. Zmora O, Mizrahi N, Rotholtz N, Pikarsky AJ, Weiss EG, Nogueras JJ, et al. Fibrin glue sealing in the treatment of perineal fistulas. Dis Colon Rectum. 2003;46(5):584–9.

50. Loungnarath R, Dietz DW, Mutch MG, Birnbaum EH, Kodner IJ, Fleshman JW. Fibrin glue treatment of complex anal fistulas has low success rate. Dis Colon Rectum. 2004;47(4):432–6.

51. Zmora O, Neufeld D, Ziv Y, Tulchinsky H, Scott D, Khaikin M, et al. Prospective, multicenter evaluation of highly concentrated fibrin glue in the treatment of complex cryptogenic perianal fistulas. Dis Colon Rectum. 2005;48(12):2167–72.

52. Kram HB, Bansal M, Timberlake O, Shoemaker WC. Antibacterial effects of fibrin glue-antibiotic mixtures. J Surg Res. 1991;50(2):175–8.

53. Sentovich SM. Fibrin glue for all anal fistulas. J Gastrointest Surg. 2001;5(2):158–61.

54. Tinay OE, El-Bakry AA. Treatment of chronic fistula-in-ano using commercial fibrin glue. Saudi Med J. 2003;24(10):1116–7.

55. Jurczak F, Laridon JY, Raffaitin P, Pousset JP. [Biological fibrin used in anal fistulas: 31 patients]. Ann Chir. 2004;129(5):286–9.

56. Jurczak F, Laridon JY, Raffaitin P, Redon Y, Pousset JP. Long-term follow-up of the treatment of high anal fistulas using fibrin glue. J Chir. 2009;146(4):382–6.

57. Gisbertz SS, Sosef MN, Festen S, Gerhards MF. Treatment of fistulas in ano with fibrin glue. Dig Surg. 2005;22(1–2):91–4.

58. Vitton V, Gasmi M, Barthet M, Desjeux A, Orsoni P, Grimaud JC. Long-term healing of Crohn's anal fistulas with fibrin glue injection. Aliment Pharmacol Ther. 2005;21(12):1453–7.

59. Dietz DW. Role of fibrin glue in the management of simple and complex fistula in ano. J Gastrointest Surg. 2006;10(5):631–2.

60. Maralcan G, Baskonus I, Aybasti N, Gokalp A. The use of fibrin glue in the treatment of fistula-in-ano: a prospective study. Surg Today. 2006;36(2):166–70.

61. Johnson EK, Gaw JU, Armstrong DN. Efficacy of anal fistula plug vs. fibrin glue in closure of anorectal fistulas. Dis Colon Rectum. 2006;49(3):371–6.

62. Ellis CN, Clark S. Fibrin glue as an adjunct to flap repair of anal fistulas: a randomized, controlled study. Dis Colon Rectum. 2006;49(11):1736–40.

63. Witte ME, Klaase JM, Gerritsen JJ, Kummer EW. Fibrin glue treatment for simple and complex anal fistulas. Hepatogastroenterology. 2007;54(76):1071–3.

64. Tyler KM, Aarons CB, Sentovich SM. Successful sphincter-sparing surgery for all anal fistulas. Dis Colon Rectum. 2007;50(10):1535–9.

65. van Koperen PJ, Wind J, Bemelman WA, Slors JF. Fibrin glue and transanal rectal advancement flap for high transsphincteric perianal fistulas; is there any advantage? Int J Colorectal Dis. 2008;23(7):697–701.

66. Adams T, Yang J, Kondylis LA, Kondylis PD. Long-term outlook after successful fibrin glue ablation of cryptoglandular transsphincteric fistula-in-ano. Dis Colon Rectum. 2008;51(10):1488–90.

67. Hadzhiev B. [Treatment of chronic anorectal fistulas by fibrin sealant]. Khirurgiia. 2008;3:41–5.

68. Chung W, Kazemi P, Ko D, Sun C, Brown CJ, Raval M, et al. Anal fistula plug and fibrin glue versus conventional treatment in repair of complex anal fistulas. Am J Surg. 2009;197(5):604–8.

69. Damin DC, Rosito MA, Contu PC, Tarta C. Fibrin glue in the management of complex anal fistula. Arq Gastroenterol. 2009;46(4):300–3.

70. de Parades V, Far HS, Etienney I, Zeitoun JD, Atienza P, Bauer P. Seton drainage and fibrin glue injection for complex anal fistulas. Colorectal Dis. 2010;12(5):459–63.

71. Grimaud JC, Munoz-Bongrand N, Siproudhis L, Abramowitz L, Senejoux A, Vitton V, et al. Fibrin glue is effective healing perianal fistulas in patients with Crohn's disease. Gastroenterology. 2010;138(7):2275–81.

72. Haim N, Neufeld D, Ziv Y, Tulchinsky H, Koller M, Khaikin M, et al. Long-term results of fibrin glue treatment for cryptogenic perianal fistulas: a multicenter study. Dis Colon Rectum. 2011;54(10):1279–83.

73. Maralcan G, Baskonus I, Gokalp A, Borazan E, Balk A. Long-term results in the treatment of fistula-in-ano with fibrin glue: a prospective study. J Korean Surg Soc. 2011;81(3):169–75.

74. de Oca J, Millan M, Jimenez A, Golda T, Biondo S. Long-term results of surgery plus fibrin sealant for anal fistula. Colorectal Dis. 2012;14(1):e12–5.

75. Cirocchi R, Santoro A, Trastulli S, Farinella E, Di Rocco G, Vendettuali D, et al. Meta-analysis of fibrin glue versus surgery for treatment of fistula-in-ano. Ann Ital Chir. 2010;81(5):349–56.

76. Jacob TJ, Perakath B, Keighley MR. Surgical intervention for anorectal fistula. Cochrane Database Syst Rev. 2010;5:006319.

77. Blumetti J, Abcarian A, Quinteros F, Chaudhry V, Prasad L, Abcarian H. Evolution of treatment of fistula in ano. World J Surg. 2012;36(5):1162–7.

Samuel Eisenstein and Alex Jenny Ky

Introduction

Sphincter-sparing procedures for the treatment of anal fistulae are the standard of care. Full resolution, however, may be challenging to achieve in patients with complex fistulae, defined as fistulae that involve greater than 30 % of the sphincter mechanism, fistulae in the setting of Crohn's disease or irradiation, in patients with a history of incontinence, and anterior fistulae in women [1, 2]. Historically cutting setons have been used in treating complex fistulae, however their efficacy has recently been called into question with up to a 60 % incontinence rate in some studies and significant pain caused by seton placement [3]. When simple fistulotomy is not an option, usually in the setting of a recurrent or complex fistulae, surgeons are turning to new biological agents as an option to achieve fistula closure while preserving continence.

Numerous biologic agents have been developed over the last 20 years for use in treating anal fistulae. Hjortrup et al. first described the use of fibrin glue to achieve closure of anal fistulae in 1991 [4]. Since then many other biologic agents have also been employed to this end, primarily in the form of plugs composed of either acellular biologic matrices or xenografted biologic tissue.

Surgical closure of a fistula consists primarily of two steps, closure of the internal opening and separation of the fistulous tract. Biologic agents have been used to achieve both of these ends and primarily work as a scaffolding to promote tissue ingrowth. Prior to placement of a biologic agent, the surgeon must first clear the acute septic episode and effective drainage must be achieved through either wide drainage or seton placement. At the time of the plug placement or glue injection the tract should be curetted to remove all granulation tissue and epithelialization. Interestingly, further obliteration of the fistula opening via endorectal advancement flap (ERAF) after either plug or fibrin glue placement has not been shown to improve results and therefore is not routinely recommended [5, 6].

While there are numerous biologic agents available for fistula therapy, the results thus far have been mixed and good results have not been reproducible. This is primarily because most studies to date have been too small to demonstrate significant results and few prospective studies have been performed. With time the data will likely improve, however the use of biologic agents in the treatment of anal fistulae is still in its infancy. Outlined here is a comprehensive list of the various agents which have been used for this purpose to date.

Injectable Glue

Fibrin Glue

Fibrin glue was the first biologic event described in the treatment of anal fistula in 1991 [4]. The glue, which is composed of fibrinogen and thrombin which when combined, form a fibrin clot, fills the fistula tract completely, adheres to local tissues, and acts as a scaffolding for ingrowth of healthy tissue. The procedure is noninvasive, only requiring removal of any granulation tissue or epithelialization prior to glue injection, and therefore has little impact on continence.

Initial reports were impressive, with a 75 % healing rate without loss of continence. More recent studies have been less promising, however, with cure rates between 40 and 54 % [7], with only one recent study, by Maralcan et al. in 2006 demonstrating a strong healing rate of 78 % [8]. Several recent meta-analyses of the literature have been published and demonstrate no advantage for the use of fibrin glue over conventional surgical therapies [7, 9]. However, because it is considered safe, with a minimal side-effect profile, and does not make future fistula repairs more difficult, fibrin glue can

S. Eisenstein, M.D. • A.J. Ky, B.A., M.D. (✉)
Department of Surgery, Mount Sinai School of Medicine,
5 East 98th St., Box 1259, New York, NY 10029, USA
e-mail: alex.ky@mountsinai.org

H. Abcarian (ed.), *Anal Fistula: Principles and Management*, DOI 10.1007/978-1-4614-9014-2_12,
© Springer Science+Business Media New York 2014

be considered as an adjunctive therapy to achieve closure in complex fistulae which may have failed previous attempts at closure.

Cryolife Bioglue

Bioglue is a combination of bovine serum albumin and glutaraldehyde which has been primarily used in achieving intraoperative hemostasis. It's use has been described in the treatment of anal fistulae, however, due to a low cure rate of 21 % at 60 months, an unacceptably high rate of acute sepsis necessitating repeat drainage, as well as demonstrably toxic serum levels of glutaraldehyde, it should not be used for this purpose [10–12].

Biologic Fistula Plugs

Numerous fistula plugs comprising a variety of biological agents have found their way to market over the last decade. Plugs are composed of a variety of acellular biologic materials and come in a variety of shapes and sizes. Placement usually involves identifying the fistula tract with a standard fistula probe followed by curettage. Once the probe has been placed through the tract, the plug can be tied to the probe with a silk tie and pulled through the tract. The plug should be trimmed at the level of the mucosa internally and sutured in place with an absorbable suture, usually in figure-of-8 fashion to prevent extrusion. The external end of the plug is also trimmed at the level of this skin for patient comfort and to prevent accidental removal of the plug. It is advised that some space be left at the external opening to allow for drainage of the tract, and for this reason the plug is not sewn in distally.

Ideally, the material from which the plug is composed should allow good tissue ingrowth as well as vascular ingrowth while being resistant to infection and extrusion. Plugs are an appealing therapeutic option because they do not require ligation of the fistula or division of the sphincters, both of which can lead to postoperative decrease in continence. Plug placement is also not particularly technically demanding, making their use more appealing than challenging procedures such as ERAF. To date, however, the data on their efficacy is mixed with closure rates ranging between 13 and 86 % [13, 14].

The reason for this lack of efficacy is not clear. Plug extrusion clearly accounts for a significant number of early postoperative failures with a 0–41 % extrusion rate reported in the literature [13, 15]. Extrusion is thought to be a technical failure from plug placement and rates are thought to decrease as one masters the learning curve. This however does not account for failure in patients who retained their plugs. Short tract length, less than 4 cm, was also shown to be a risk factor for plug failure in another study where longer tracts were shown to be three times as likely to achieve closure when compared to their shorter counterparts [16].

Ineffective clearance of the infectious process, failure to appropriately de-epithelialize the tract, and failure to optimize the patients' inherent ability to heal the fistula, such as diabetic control and smoking cessation, have all been implicated in further failures [17]. Several technical and postoperative considerations have been implicated in improving closure rates, including cleaning the tract with hydrogen peroxide, postoperative antibiotics, avoiding strenuous activities postoperatively, and the implementation of a clear liquid diet for several days, however none of these has been demonstrated to be effective in a study [18].

Cost is another consideration in plug placement. With most plugs costing around $1,000 significant expense can be added onto the procedure cost. Adamina et al. looked at the overall costs for patients receiving plugs vs. those receiving ERAF and found that when factoring in the need for reoperation and the length of stay, fistula plug placement saved the institution $1,588. This study was limited, however, by the fact that ERAF patients had a length of stay of 2.5 days vs. 1 day for plug patients since these procedures are both currently being done on an outpatient basis at most institutions. Results were also skewed by the poor cure rate of the ERAF group where 33 % achieved fistula closure vs. 50 % in the plug group. When hospital stay was controlled for the savings were $825, demonstrating a financial advantage for using fistula plugs [14].

Due to the expense and the overall scarcity of biologic materials, non-biologic absorbable plugs have been developed. These are less expensive and have demonstrated similar results in preliminary studies as their biologic counterparts, however little data is available to date on long-term outcomes and more research needs to be performed before they can be considered equivalent or better.

Xenograft

Xenograft materials are currently in use for a variety of applications, and have been a mainstay of treatment when mesh is required in contaminated surgical fields. These same materials have been repurposed for use in anal fistulae based on their ability to avoid vigorous host inflammatory reactions as well as maintain resistance to infection while being rapidly absorbed by host tissues after stimulating tissue ingrowth.

Xenograft tissues are readily available and less expensive than allografts. Their primary drawback is that since they are not human tissue, it is thought that their base components, collagen, elastin, and peptidoglycans may not be compatible with human tissue ingrowth and may lead to increased plug rejection. This has not been demonstrated to be the case with the materials currently available on the market, however.

Cook Surgisis Plug

The Cook Surgisis plug was released in 2006 and was the first commercially available fistula plug. This plug consists of a lyophilized porcine small bowel submucosal matrix. It consists of 90 % collagen (primarily types I, III, and V). It has been demonstrated to be resistant to infection and to be resistant to giant cell foreign body reactions, both of which could potentially lead to plug failure. The plug is completely degraded by host tissues over a period of 3 months [19, 20].

Initial studies demonstrated an 83 % cure rate at 12 months with minimal morbidity or impact on continence [21]. Despite promising initial results, further studies failed to demonstrate the same efficacy with cure rates ranging from 24 to 78 % at 6 months [13, 22–24]. However, because this plug has been on the market the longest time, it is the plug for which most data is available.

Multiple prospective, blinded studies have been carried out comparing the Surgisis plug to ERAF, and results have been disappointing. Van Kopernen et al. demonstrated in 60 patients a recurrence rate of 71 % in the plug arm with 52 % recurrence in patients receiving ERAF and there were no differences in preoperative or postoperative continence or soiling between the groups, nor were there any differences in quality of life [23]. These results however were not significant due to study size. Ortiz et al. however were forced to stop their trial early when 12 of the 15 patients accrued in the plug group recurred early while only demonstrating two recurrences in 16 patients treated with ERAF. These results were called into question, however, as it was felt that technical errors led to an unacceptably high extrusion rate which led to early plug failures [22].

Our own personal experience with the Surgisis plug has been mixed. We observed that over time the efficacy of plug closure decreased from 72.7 % closure rate at 8 weeks to 62.4 % at 12 weeks to 54.6 % at a median of 6.5 months with Crohn's disease patients doing significantly worse than non-Crohn's (26.6 % vs. 66.7 % closure rate long term). Also, interestingly, patients who received multiple plugs did significantly worse than those treated with a single plug (12.5 % vs. 63.9 %) indicating that multiple attempts at placement of a fistula plug is unlikely to prove effective [25]. Long-term follow-up of that same cohort demonstrated a 51 % closure rate at 24 months indicating that those fistulae that stayed closed at 6 months were likely to remain closed over the long term.

More recently, the Surgisis material has been employed in conjuncture with the LIFT procedure which has been termed the BioLIFT. In this procedure, a sheet of Surgisis is placed in the intersphincteric space following fistula tract ligation. Initial studies demonstrated a 94 % cure rate at 15 months with minimal postoperative morbidity [26]. Surgisis sheets have also been used as interposition material after rectovaginal fistula closure with success rates between 66 and 81% at 12 months [27, 28].

Covidien Permacol

Permacol is composed of cross-linked acellular dermal matrix (ADM) of porcine origin. It is approximately 95 % type I collagen with a small amount of elastin as well as type III collagen. It is manufactured in two constructs, a porous sheet and milled fibers in saline suspension [29, 30]. The fibrous suspension has been hypothesized to be more effective at filling irregular fistula tracts after injection, potentially improving cure rates. This hypothesis was tested, comparing Permacol strips sutured into fistula tracts to the milled fibers, suspended in fibrin glue, injected into the tracts. At a median of two and a half years the suspension group achieved an 80 % cure rate vs. 54 % in the Permacol sheet group, however these results were not statistically significant [31].

Other Xenografted Acellular Dermal Matrices

A variety of other porcine and bovine ADMs are being manufactured worldwide and there are several anecdotal reports of their use in the treatment of anal fistulae. One example of the work being done with these various ADMs come from a study from China where they examined the J-I type ADM which is manufactured similarly to the Surgisis plug. This prospective randomized trial demonstrated a significant improvement in fistula healing using this plug when compared to ERAF in 90 patients (82 % vs. 64 %) with no difference in incontinence or anal deformity rates between the two groups [32]. No individual ADM has yet to distinguish itself as superior to the rest and the vast majority of the available data is from individual case reports.

Allograft

Several types of allografts have been harvested from cadavers and employed as fistula plugs. Because they are composed of a variety of tissue types, including collagens, fibrin, elastin, and glycosaminoglycans [33, 34], it was initially thought that they would lead to improved fistula closure rates when compared to xenografted tissue. While this has not been demonstrated unequivocally, allografted tissues have demonstrated acceptable closure rates with minimal incontinence. These grafts all lack any cellular component which could potentially lead to rejection.

The primary drawback associated with allograft use stems from the scarcity of the product due to the manner in which is harvested. Cadaveric tissue is donated by the deceased leading to a much greater cost when compared to easily acquired xenograft sources. Interestingly, studies have also demonstrated no difference in biocompatibility between porcine and human ADMs [35].

Ruinuo Human Acellular Dermal Matrix

The ADM plug is an allogenic tissue graft derived from donated human skin. This plug consists of collagen, elastin, and glucosaminoglycans. Cones are formed from thin sheets of ADM, pulled through the fistula tract, and sutured into the internal sphincter.

One of the larger studies on any type of plug use comes from China and employs this ADM. Retrospective analysis of a prospective database demonstrated that 54.4 % of 114 patients achieved fistula closure at 6 months with only two reported cases on incontinence at this time. Factors associated with plug success included nonsmoking, longer duration of fistula, anterior location of fistula, short length of fistula, and procedure performed by an "expert" surgeon [36].

Recently, a variant of the LIFT procedure called the "LIFT-Plug" was also described using this ADM. The authors described closure of the internal opening of the fistula coupled with intrasphincteric ligation of the tract and placement of an ADM plug into the remaining external component of the tract. Healing rate for this procedure was reported at 95 % at a median of 14 months with a mean time to resolution of approximately 2 weeks, however it is unclear from this preliminary study whether this procedure is better than the LIFT alone as the authors did not compare the two [37].

Lifecell Alloderm

Alloderm is the most widely available ADM in the United States. No large studies have been performed to date employing Alloderm in closing complex anal fistulae, however several case reports have been published in which Alloderm sheets were used interpositionally in a layered closure in treating rectovaginal fistulae with good short-term results [38, 39]. Due to its similarity to other allograft ADMs, Alloderm should be used similarly when it is the only available ADM and an allograft is desired.

Considerations

Crohn's Disease

Managing perineal Crohn's disease can be very complicated, requiring multiple interventions, and often exhausting the armamentarium of a skilled colorectal surgeon. By definition all of these fistulae are complex and each proves a unique challenge in treating. Few studies have looked specifically at patients with Crohn's, however, a recent meta-analysis pooled similarly matched patients with and without Crohn's and demonstrated similar fistula closure rates in both groups with usage of the Surgisis plug (54.8 % vs. 54.3 %) with minimal impact on fecal continence between the groups [15]. This study was, however, limited by the number of Crohn's patients included, with only 42 of 530 total patients having Crohn's disease from 20 separate studies.

Head-to-Head Comparisons

Rarely have fistula plugs been compared head to head, but in one recent study, Buchberg et al. retrospectively analyzed their results from their use of both the Surgisis plug and the non-biologic, absorbable Gore Bio-A plug. They demonstrated that in their hands 6 of 11 patients treated with the Gore plug had successful closure of their fistulae while only 2 of 16 patients treated with the Surgisis plug achieved this outcome [40]. This ultimately demonstrates the limitations of the data demonstrated to this point as this study was very small, retrospective, and poor overall closure rates were demonstrated in both arms. More prospective head-to-head comparisons are needed to determine which plugs may be the most efficacious; however there has always been resistance by industry to put forth these studies.

Conclusions

Despite mixed results thus far, the use of biologic agents, such as fibrin glue or fistula plugs have demonstrated some success. While it is unlikely that one of the currently available plugs is vastly better than any other, further studies need to be performed, including head-to-head studies to identify superiority. This is a constantly evolving field and new plugs and new biologic agents are becoming available for use on a regular basis.

Despite the variability of the results, there is currently a place in the colorectal surgeon's armamentarium for these devices as they do offer another method to encourage fistula closure with minimal morbidity. That place is likely in the patient who has a complex fistula or who has failed multiple other attempts at fistula closure. This is a therapy in its infancy and many more studies, particularly prospective and randomized studies, need to be carried out to truly demonstrate the efficacy and long-term results achievable by each agent.

Summary

1. Numerous biologic agents have been employed in the closure of complex anal fistulae, including fibrin glue, allograft plugs, and xenograft plugs with mixed results.
2. To achieve effective fistula closure with the use of biologic agents, the fistula tract must first be drained with a seton. The procedure-involving placement of the plug must then include closure of the internal opening and ligation of the tract.
3. The ideal fistula plug should be composed of material, which allows good tissue and vascular ingrowth while being resistant to infection and extrusion.
4. While there is some promising data to date, most data is mixed. Prospective and head-to-head studies are necessary to determine optimal material selection for use in fistula plugs.
5. Fistula plugs are a viable option in recurrent and hard-to-treat complex anal fistulae.

References

1. Mizrahi N, Wexner SD, Zmora O, Da Silva G, Efron J, Weiss EG, et al. Endorectal advancement flap: are there predictors of failure? Dis Colon Rectum. 2002;45(12):1616–21.
2. Parks AG, Stitz RW. The treatment of high fistula-in-ano. Dis Colon Rectum. 1976;19(6):487–99.
3. Ritchie RD, Sackier JM, Hodde JP. Incontinence rates after cutting seton treatment for anal fistula. Colorectal Dis. 2009;11(6):564–71.
4. Hjortrup A, Moesgaard F, Kjaergard J. Fibrin adhesive in the treatment of perineal fistulas. Dis Colon Rectum. 1991;34(9):752–4.
5. Mitalas LE, van Onkelen RS, Gosselink MP, Zimmerman DD, Schouten WR. The anal fistula plug as an adjunct to transanal advancement flap repair. Dis Colon Rectum. 2010;53(12):1713.
6. van Koperen PJ, Wind J, Bemelman WA, Slors JF. Fibrin glue and transanal rectal advancement flap for high transsphincteric perianal fistulas; is there any advantage? Int J Colorectal Dis. 2008;23(7):697–701.
7. Cirocchi R, Santoro A, Trastulli S, Farinella E, Di Rocco G, Vendettuali D, et al. Meta-analysis of fibrin glue versus surgery for treatment of fistula-in-ano. Ann Ital Chir. 2010;81(5):349–56.
8. Maralcan G, Baskonus I, Aybasti N, Gokalp A. The use of fibrin glue in the treatment of fistula-in-ano: a prospective study. Surg Today. 2006;36(2):166–70.
9. Hammond TM, Grahn MF, Lunniss PJ. Fibrin glue in the management of anal fistulae. Colorectal Dis. 2004;6(5):308–19.
10. Abbas MA, Tejirian T. Bioglue for the treatment of anal fistula is associated with acute anal sepsis. Dis Colon Rectum. 2008;51(7):1155; author reply 1156.
11. Alexander SM, Mitalas LE, Gosselink MP, Oom DM, Zimmerman DD, Schouten WR. Obliteration of the fistulous tract with BioGlue adversely affects the outcome of transanal advancement flap repair. Tech Coloproctol. 2008;12(3):225–8.
12. de la Portilla F, Rada R, Vega J, Cisneros N, Maldonado VH, Sanchez-Gil JM. Long-term results change conclusions on BioGlue in the treatment of high transsphincteric anal fistulas. Dis Colon Rectum. 2010;53(8):1220–1.
13. Lewis R, Lunniss PJ, Hammond TM. Novel biological strategies in the management of anal fistula. Colorectal Dis. 2012;14(12):1445–55.
14. Adamina M, Hoch JS, Burnstein MJ. To plug or not to plug: a cost-effectiveness analysis for complex anal fistula. Surgery. 2010;147(1):72–8.
15. O'Riordan JM, Datta I, Johnston C, Baxter NN. A systematic review of the anal fistula plug for patients with Crohn's and non-Crohn's related fistula-in-ano. Dis Colon Rectum. 2012;55(3):351–8.
16. McGee MF, Champagne BJ, Stulberg JJ, Reynolds H, Marderstein E, Delaney CP. Tract length predicts successful closure with anal fistula plug in cryptoglandular fistulas. Dis Colon Rectum. 2010;53(8):1116–20.
17. Dudukgian H, Abcarian H. Why do we have so much trouble treating anal fistula? World J Gastroenterol. 2011;17(28):3292–6.
18. Schwandner T, Roblick MH, Kierer W, Brom A, Padberg W, Hirschburger M. Surgical treatment of complex anal fistulas with the anal fistula plug: a prospective, multicenter study. Dis Colon Rectum. 2009;52(9):1578–83.
19. Hodde J. Extracellular matrix as a bioactive material for soft tissue reconstruction. ANZ J Surg. 2006;76(12):1096–100.
20. Soiderer EE, Lantz GC, Kazacos EA, Hodde JP, Wiegand RE. Morphologic study of three collagen materials for body wall repair. J Surg Res. 2004;118(2):161–75.
21. Champagne BJ, O'Connor LM, Ferguson M, Orangio GR, Schertzer ME, Armstrong DN. Efficacy of anal fistula plug in closure of cryptoglandular fistulas: long-term follow-up. Dis Colon Rectum. 2006;49(12):1817–21.
22. Ortiz H, Marzo J, Ciga MA, Oteiza F, Armendariz P, de Miguel M. Randomized clinical trial of anal fistula plug versus endorectal advancement flap for the treatment of high cryptoglandular fistula in ano. Br J Surg. 2009;96(6):608–12.
23. van Koperen PJ, Bemelman WA, Gerhards MF, Janssen LW, van Tets WF, van Dalsen AD, et al. The anal fistula plug treatment compared with the mucosal advancement flap for cryptoglandular high transsphincteric perianal fistula: a double-blinded multicenter randomized trial. Dis Colon Rectum. 2011;54(4):387–93.
24. Ellis CN, Rostas JW, Greiner FG. Long-term outcomes with the use of bioprosthetic plugs for the management of complex anal fistulas. Dis Colon Rectum. 2010;53(5):798–802.
25. Ky AJ, Sylla P, Steinhagen R, Steinhagen E, Khaitov S, Ly EK. Collagen fistula plug for the treatment of anal fistulas. Dis Colon Rectum. 2008;51(6):838–43.
26. Ellis CN. Outcomes with the use of bioprosthetic grafts to reinforce the ligation of the intersphincteric fistula tract (BioLIFT procedure) for the management of complex anal fistulas. Dis Colon Rectum. 2010;53(10):1361–4.
27. Schwandner O, Fuerst A. Preliminary results on efficacy in closure of transsphincteric and rectovaginal fistulas associated with Crohn's disease using new biomaterials. Surg Innov. 2009;16(2):162–8.
28. Schwandner O, Fuerst A, Kunstreich K, Scherer R. Innovative technique for the closure of rectovaginal fistula using Surgisis mesh. Tech Coloproctol. 2009;13(2):135–40.
29. Hammond TM, Chin-Aleong J, Navsaria H, Williams NS. Human in vivo cellular response to a cross-linked acellular collagen implant. Br J Surg. 2008;95(4):438–46.
30. Shevchenko RV, Sibbons PD, Sharpe JR, James SE. Use of a novel porcine collagen paste as a dermal substitute in full-thickness wounds. Wound Repair Regen. 2008;16(2):198–207.

31. Hammond TM, Porrett TR, Scott SM, Williams NS, Lunniss PJ. Management of idiopathic anal fistula using cross-linked collagen: a prospective phase 1 study. Colorectal Dis. 2011;13(1):94–104.

32. Aba-bai-ke-re MM, Wen H, Huang HG, Chu H, Lu M, Chang ZS, et al. Randomized controlled trial of minimally invasive surgery using acellular dermal matrix for complex anorectal fistula. World J Gastroenterol. 2010;16(26):3279–86.

33. Bellows CF, Alder A, Helton WS. Abdominal wall reconstruction using biological tissue grafts: present status and future opportunities. Expert Rev Med Devices. 2006;3(5):657–75.

34. Han JG, Xu HM, Song WL, Jin ML, Gao JS, Wang ZJ, et al. Histologic analysis of acellular dermal matrix in the treatment of anal fistula in an animal model. J Am Coll Surg. 2009;208(6):1099–106.

35. Ge L, Zheng S, Wei H. Comparison of histological structure and biocompatibility between human acellular dermal matrix (ADM) and porcine ADM. Burns. 2009;35(1):46–50.

36. Han JG, Wang ZJ, Zhao BC, Zheng Y, Zhao B, Yi BQ, et al. Long-term outcomes of human acellular dermal matrix plug in closure of complex anal fistulas with a single tract. Dis Colon Rectum. 2011;54(11):1412–8.

37. Han JG, Yi BQ, Wang ZJ, Zheng Y, Cui JJ, Yu XQ, et al. Ligation of the intersphincteric fistula tract plus bioprosthetic anal fistula plug (LIFT-Plug): a new technique for fistula-in-ano. Colorectal Dis. 2012;15(5):582–6.

38. Shelton AA, Welton ML. Transperineal repair of persistent rectovaginal fistulas using an acellular cadaveric dermal graft (AlloDerm). Dis Colon Rectum. 2006;49(9):1454–7.

39. Miklos JR, Kohli N. Rectovaginal fistula repair utilizing a cadaveric dermal allograft. Int Urogynecol J Pelvic Floor Dysfunct. 1999;10(6):405–6.

40. Buchberg B, Masoomi H, Choi J, Bergman H, Mills S, Stamos MJ. A tale of two (anal fistula) plugs: is there a difference in short-term outcomes? Am Surg. 2010;76(10):1150–3.

Synthetic Fistula Plug

13

Alex Jenny Ky, Michael Polcino, and Alero T. Nanna

Introduction

The importance of understanding and treating anorectal fistulae is evidenced not only by the prevalence of this condition but also by the variety of approaches involved. There is currently neither a consensus nor a set of guidelines on the management of anorectal fistulae. Whether the fistula is simple or complex, it is paramount to maintain fecal continence and decrease recurrence. Historical approaches have included fistulotomy with or without marsupialization, seton placement, and endorectal advancement flaps, each with variable success rates. More recently, synthetic and biologic plugs have become available as adjuncts in fistula management. In this chapter, we discuss the available plugs, their chemical composition, and contraindications to and recommended techniques of application, including optimal disk placement. We also review several studies with a focus on success and recurrence rates when using the Surgisis or Gore Bio-A plug. Overall the Gore Bio-A appears to be an improvement over the Surgisis plug. However, further studies are required to clearly define its indications and application.

Anal fistula is one of the most frequently treated anorectal diseases, with an estimated 10–30% of all colorectal interventions performed to treat anal fistula [1]. Although being a common condition, there is not a single surgical technique to repair this disease due to the complex anatomic and physiologic aspects of this disease. Prior to focusing on synthetic anal fistula plugs, it is first necessary to focus on the classification of fistula and the history leading up to the development and incorporation of synthetic anal fistula plugs.

Anal fistulas can be classified into two main groups: simple and complex fistulas. Simple fistulas are generally low fistulas with single tracts and carry a low risk of incontinence when treated. In contrast, a complex fistula involves greater than 30–50 % of the sphincter muscle; anterior in woman; or the patient has a history of preexisting incontinence, Crohn's disease, or local irradiation [2].

When treating either type of fistula, maintaining fecal continence is essentially tantamount to healing the fistula itself. Garcia-Aguilar et al. published a report in 1996 of 75 patients who underwent surgery for anal fistulas between 1988 and 1992. Treatment included fistulotomy and marsupialization ($n=300$), seton placement ($n=63$), endorectal advancement flap ($n=3$), and other ($n=9$). Fistulas recurred in 31 patients (8 %) and 45 % reported some degree of postoperative incontinence [3].

The traditional treatment of complex anal fistulas often times involved advancement flaps. There is a wide variance of success rates. Jun and Choi reported an initial success rate of 95 % (38 of 40) patients who underwent anocutaneous flaps with zero reports of incontinence to either flatus or stool [4]. Conversely, Sonoda et al. reported the Cleveland Clinic experience. The study was a retrospective review of 105 patients. Sixty-two patients had anorectal fistulas while 37 patients had rectovaginal fistulas. The rate of primary healing was found to be 63.6 %. Greater body surface area, history of incision and drainage of a perianal abscess preceding advancement flap, previous placement of a seton drain, and short duration of fistula were associated with higher success rates. Conversely, Crohn's disease and rectovaginal fistulas were associated with lower success rates [5].

Since the 1940s, fibrin glue has been used as surgical sealant [6]. Fibrin glue began to come into favor as a treatment for anal fistulas in the 1990s. Venkatesh et al. published a series of 30 patients treated with autologous fibrin glue treated over a 4-year period. Success rate was 60 % [6]. Urinary tract-related fistulas, Crohn's disease-related fistulas, and fistulas related to AIDS failed to heal completely with fibrin glue application. Haim et al. looked at their long-term results [7]. The initial success rate was 53 % (32/60). Of the 32 patients who were initially treated successfully,

A.J. Ky, B.A., M.D. (✉) • M. Polcino, M.D. • A.T. Nanna, B.S., M.D.
Department of Surgery, Mount Sinai School of Medicine,
5 East 98th St, Box 1259, New York, NY 10029, USA
e-mail: alex.ky@mountsinai.org

H. Abcarian (ed.), *Anal Fistula: Principles and Management*, DOI 10.1007/978-1-4614-9014-2_13,
© Springer Science+Business Media New York 2014

23 were located and contacted at a mean follow-up of 6.5 years. Seventeen of 23 patients (74 %) remained disease-free. Despite the low rate of success, the application of fibrin glue has several advantages. These include easy application, no risk of damage to the sphincter complex, minimal patient discomfort, and the capacity to repeat application if the initial treatment fails [7].

Moving forward to the 2000s, anal fistula plugs began to come into practice in the mid 2000s. In 2005, the FDA approved Cook Medical's Surgisis Fistula Plug. It comprises porcine intestinal submucosa. It can be used in infected fields, host tissues colonize the graft, and it does not injure the sphincter complex [8]. Despite the scientific belief that this product would have excellent success rate, the results varied substantially. Success rates ranged from 13.9 to 87 % [9, 10]. This wide range of healing ultimately led to a consensus conference that was held in 2007. The results of the conference are presented here [8].

A consensus conference was held in Chicago on 27 May 2007 at the Illinois Airport Hilton Hotel to develop uniformity of opinion from surgeons with considerable experience in the use of the anal fistula plug. Of the 15 surgeons in attendance, 5 had performed 50 or more anal fistula plug procedures. Success rates with this approach have been reported to be as high as 85 %. Anecdotal communications have however suggested lower rates of success. Concerns have been expressed over plug extrusion and inadequacy of long-term follow-up. It was thought prudent to hold this conference because, despite a number of publications attesting to the safety and efficacy of the procedure, to date there has not been uniformity of opinion regarding indications and technique, nor has there been level I evidence of any actual benefit.

Plug Material, Mechanism, and Applications

Small intestinal submucosa (SIS) is a natural biomaterial harvested from porcine small intestine and fabricated into a biomedical product of various shapes and thicknesses [2]. As such it has been applied to a host of potential indications. These include reinforcement of soft tissue for incisional and inguinal herniorraphy; urethral sling placement in urogynaecology; staple line reinforcement; paraesophageal hernia repair and in the treatment of anal fistula. The fact that it has been demonstrably useful as a bioprosthetic material in infected fields makes its application in fistula surgery quite reasonable. The Surgisis AFP Anal Fistula Plug (the plug) has a biological configuration suitable for fistula disease. When SIS is implanted, host tissue cells and blood vessels colonize the "graft." In essence, SIS provides a scaffold or matrix to allow infiltration of the patient's connective tissue. The material is supplied in a sterile, peel-open package and is intended for one-time use.

Recommendations

All of the following recommendations and opinions of the Consensus Panel were unanimously agreed by those present unless otherwise indicated.

Inclusion/exclusion criteria indications for the use of the plug include:
Transsphincteric Fistula
This was considered to be the ideal indication for the use of the plug.
Anovaginal Fistula
While it was recognized that the shorter the tract the less likely the procedure would be successful, the plug was felt to be a reasonable alternative to other operations. Besides the financial cost of failure there appeared to be no disadvantage in attempting its use in this circumstance.
Intersphincteric Fistula
The Consensus Panel felt that the use of the plug for this indication was valid, if conventional fistulotomy posed a significant risk of incontinence. This would include those patients with inflammatory bowel disease and those who had previously undergone radiation therapy.
Extrasphincteric Fistula
While this was recognized to be an uncommon indication for fistula surgery, it was regarded as an indication for the fistula plug. Suturing the plug to the site of the internal opening was considered to be potentially technically difficult.

Contraindications for the Use of the Plug

Conventional, Uncomplicated Intersphincteric Fistula

Success approaches 100 % with minimal morbidity with standard fistulotomy. Thus, the cost/failure rate with the use of the plug cannot be justified. In addition, the following conditions were felt to be inappropriate because of the extremely low probability of success:

1. Pouch-vaginal fistula.
2. Rectovaginal fistula (because of the short length of the track).
3. Fistula with a persistent abscess cavity.
4. Fistula with any suggestion of infection. Examples included those with associated anorectal abscess formation, persistent cavity (as above), and a fistula with induration or purulent drainage.
5. Allergy to porcine products.

6. Inability of the surgeon to identify both the external and internal openings. This is an absolute contraindication for undertaking this procedure.

Preoperative Preparation

Some surgeons experienced in using the plug have prepared the bowel as for a major colon resection, with laxatives and antibiotics. The Consensus Panel questioned the value of attempts to delay defecation. They queried whether liquid stool was preferable to solid for prevention of extrusion of the plug. When the use of a small-volume preoperative enema was considered, there was no consensus: half of the Panel felt it would be useful. It was accepted that there was no evidence base for this consideration. Therefore, in the absence of data, the Panel concluded that bowel preparation and/or the use of a small-volume enema should be left to the individual surgeon's personal preference. The Panel did recommend a single preoperative dose of systemic antibiotics but felt that this should not be continued for longer.

Intraoperative Management

Anaesthetic

This was deemed to be a matter of the patient's or surgeon's preference.

Positioning the Patient

This was regarded as a matter of the surgeon's preference. The critical element, however, was to ensure adequate visualization of the internal opening to place the suture correctly.

Surgical Technique

Identifying the Internal and External Openings

The plug cannot be inserted unless there is clear delineation of the primary and secondary openings. Irrigation of the track with saline or peroxide was recommended.

Passing a Probe

Gentle passage of a probe was essential to confirm the position of the track and to facilitate insertion of the plug. The Panel unanimously affirmed that debridement, curettage, or brushing of the tract should not be performed. Such maneuvers would enlarge the fistula track.

Using a Seton

There was uniformity of opinion that a seton should always be employed temporarily until there was no evidence of acute inflammation, purulence, or excessive drainage. This would often take 6–12 weeks. However, the use of a seton prior to implantation was unnecessary if there was no acute inflammatory process.

Preparing the Plug

The AFP plug should be completely immersed in sterile saline for 2 min. Allowing immersion for >5 min risks fragmentation of the plug. Conversely, implantation of a nonhydrated plug is extremely painful.

Managing the Recessed Internal Opening

If there is epithelialization of the internal opening (dimpled or recessed), limited mobilization of the mucosal edges with debridement prior to suture placement should be considered.

Passing the Plug

The use of a suture or ligature was recommended to pull the narrow end of the plug from the internal opening through the track to the external opening until the plug is snug.

Trimming the Plug

Any excess plug should be trimmed at the level of the internal opening (the wide end) and sutured with 2-0 long-term, braided, absorbable material (e.g., Vicryl, Ethicon, Inc., Somerville, NJ, USA), incorporating the underlying internal anal sphincter. Monofilament material should not be used. There was no consensus, however, as to whether the plug should be buried under the mucosa. The excess external plug should be trimmed flush with the skin without fixation. The external opening may be enlarged if necessary to facilitate drainage.

Postoperative Care

The Panel had a stimulating discussion on various postoperative management alternatives. However, in the absence of evidence-based data, opinions revolved around what seemed reasonable and appropriate with more emphasis on the "art" rather than the "science" of surgery. There were nevertheless several unanimous conclusions.

1. Diet: No dietary restrictions.
2. Activity: No strenuous activity, exercise, or heavy lifting for 2 weeks. Abstinence from sexual intercourse for 2 weeks.
3. External dressing: For patient comfort only.
4. Topical antibiotics: Not indicated.

5. Cleansing: Showers with gentle cleaning.
6. Bowel management: Medications as necessary to prevent constipation or diarrhea.
7. Follow-up visits. Surgeon's preference: The tract should not be probed during these visits.

Outcome

Defining Failure

Early extrusion of the plug is either a technical error [the track being too large, the plug pulled too tightly, faulty fixation (i.e., to the mucosa rather than to the internal sphincter)] or infection. The Panel unanimously agreed that the overwhelming majority of fistulas which heal do so within 3 months, although some will take longer. The decision whether the operation should be considered a failure rests with the individual surgeon, but should not be taken for a minimum of 3 months.

Conclusions

The anal fistula plug was felt to be a reasonable alternative for the treatment of anal fistula. Members of the Panel were asked to state what they felt to be a reasonable rate of success and concluded that 50–60 % should be considered acceptable. To achieve the highest possibility of success, the Panel concluded that patient selection, avoidance of local infection, and meticulous technique were required. Besides the consideration of cost it was felt that the patient would not be adversely affected by insertion of the fistula plug because all other management options were still available. It was recognized, however, that even in patients with apparent healing the rate of subsequent recurrence was unknown. Prospective randomized trials comparing the anal fistula plug with other treatments such as seton fistulotomy were recommended. Finally it was unanimously agreed that the procedure should be undertaken only by trained surgeons familiar with anorectal anatomy and experienced in conventional anal fistula surgery and in the management of its complications.

Gore Bio-A Plug

In 2009, the synthetic Gore Bio-A plug was FDA approved. The Gore Bio-A is a synthetic plug as compared to Surgisis, which is a biologic plug. The Gore Bio-A fistula plug is a porous fibrous structure composed solely of a synthetic bioabsorbable polyglycolide–trimethylene carbonate copolymer (67 % polyglycolide, 33 % trimethylene carbonate). The copolymer has been found to be both biocompatible and

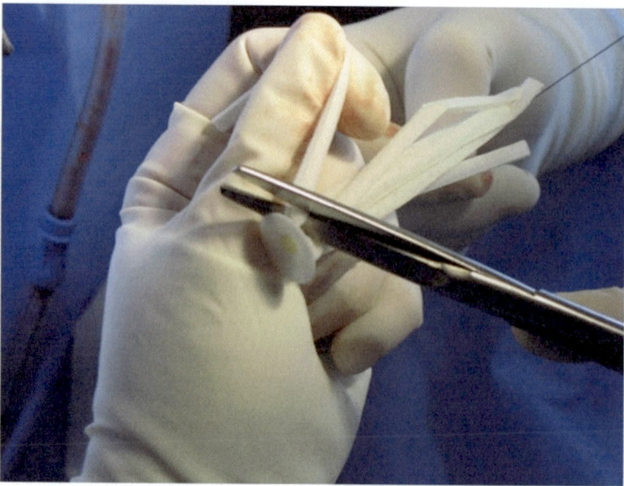

Fig. 13.1 Fistula plug placement. The fistula tract is identified and curetted. A silk tie is then placed through the tract. The tie is then affixed to the fistula plug so that it will be pulled through the internal orifice out the external. The plug is trimmed for optimal passage. The plug is gently brought through the fistulous tract. The plug is sutured into place and the internal orifice is closed with figure-of-8 absorbable suture. The external end of the plug is trimmed to skin level for patient comfort. Images courtesy of Dr. Alex Ky

nonantigenic because it is degraded via a combination of hydrolytic and enzymatic pathways. In vivo studies with this copolymer indicate that the bioabsorption process should be complete within 6 months [11]. The device consists of a disk 16 mm in diameter, attached to six tubes, each 9 cm in length. The size of the plug can be tailored by changing the number and length of the tubes so that it occupies the fistula tract until the bioabsorbable nature of the material allows the body to fill the defect with native tissue [12]. In comparison to the Surgisis plug, the disk was devised to decrease the incidence of dislodgement. The plug is depicted in Fig. 13.1.

The following technique is provided by Gore Medical (Flagstaff, AZ) and comprises the corporate recommendations for procedure [13].

Preparation

- Prepare the patient and surgical site using standard techniques appropriate for anal fistula repair.
- Remove the device from its sterile packaging using aseptic technique.
- Using sharp sterile scissors, trim the disk diameter to a size appropriate for the defect allowing for adequate fixation of the disk to the rectal mucosa. Care should be taken to avoid the creation of sharp edges or corners when trimming the disk.
- Individual tubes can be removed from the device to accommodate the diameter of the fistula tract. When removing

tubes, begin with the center-most tubes, carefully cutting the tube as close to the disk as possible (proximally adjacent) without compromising tube attachment.

- To facilitate introduction and deployment of the device in the fistula tract, it is recommended that a suture be used to gather the tubes and pull the device through the fistula tract. To do so, run a suture through the distal ends of the tubes. A bite depth of approximately 3 mm is recommended to ensure adequate suture retention strength.

Note: The use of a resorbable suture is recommended to minimize the potential that any permanent material is implanted.

- The GORE® BIO-A® Fistula Plug does not need to be hydrated prior to use. However, to facilitate passage of the tubes through the fistula tract, briefly immerse the entire device in sterile saline.

Device Placement

- Use standard techniques to define, clean, and prepare the fistula tract. If necessary, the tract may be defined with a curette to remove any granulation tissue.
- Insert a fistula probe or other suitable instrument through the fistula tract, entering through the external (secondary) opening and exiting via the internal (primary) opening.
- Grasp the suture attached to the distal end of the GORE® BIO-A® Fistula Plug.
- Gently draw the suture into the internal (primary) opening of the fistula tract. Continue to draw the suture through the fistula tract.
- Once the suture is visible at the external (secondary) opening, slowly draw the GORE® BIO-A® Fistula Plug into the defect until slight resistance is felt and the device disk is securely seated at the internal (primary) opening.

Note: Take care to ensure that disk lies flat and is well apposed to the rectal mucosa at the internal (primary) opening of the fistula tract.

- After the device is properly positioned in the fistula tract, one of the following fixation methods should be used to secure the disk at the internal (primary) opening.

Fixation Method I

– Using a suitable resorbable suture, secure the disk of the GORE® BIO-A® Fistula Plug to the adjacent tissue, obtaining adequate bites of rectal wall to prevent device migration and minimize the potential for leakage of bowel contents into the fistula tract.

Fixation Method II

– Using a suitable resorbable suture, close the rectal mucosa over the disk portion of the device to prevent device migration and minimize the potential for leakage of bowel

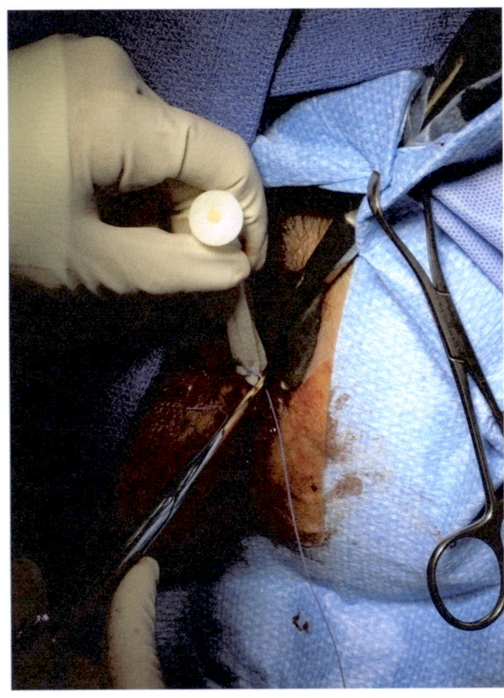

Fig. 13.2 The figure depicts fashioning disk and tube number to adequately close the fistula. Image courtesy of Dr. Alex Ky

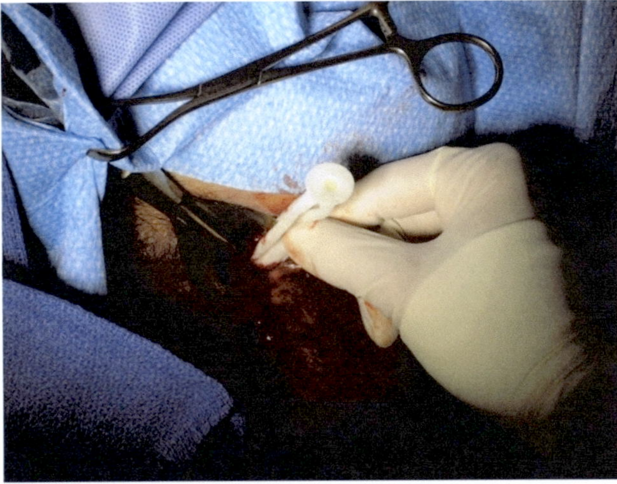

Fig. 13.3 The figure represents the fistula plug traversing the fistula from the internal to external opening. Images courtesy of Dr. Alex Ky

contents into the fistula tract. Figures 13.2, 13.3, 13.4, 13.5, 13.6, 13.7, and 13.8 depict the set-up and installation of the fistula plug.

Results

Buchberg et al. published a retrospective review of a prospectively maintained database between 2007 and 2009 comparing the Surgisis anal fistula plug to the Gore Bio-A

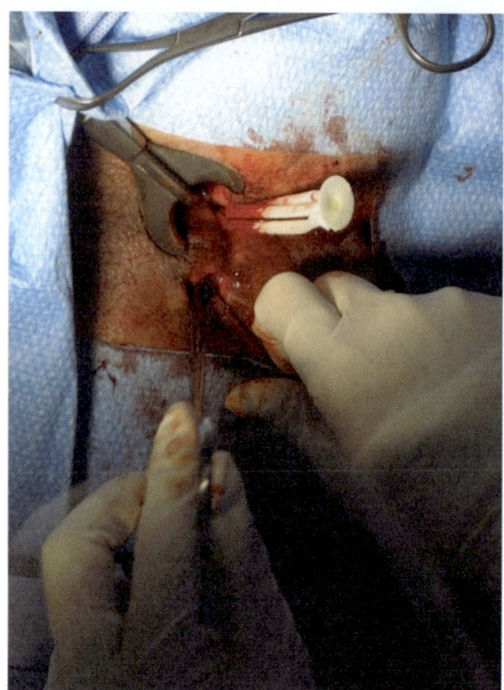

Fig. 13.4 The figure represents the fistula plug traversing the fistula from the internal to external opening. Images courtesy of Dr. Alex Ky

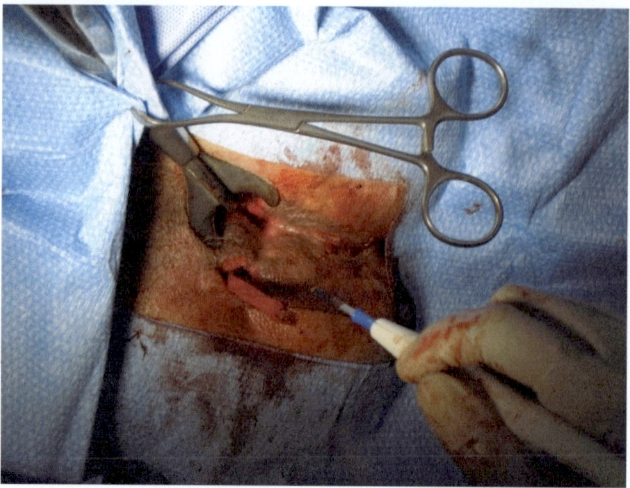

Fig. 13.6 The figure represents the fistula plug traversing the fistula from the internal to external opening. Images courtesy of Dr. Alex Ky

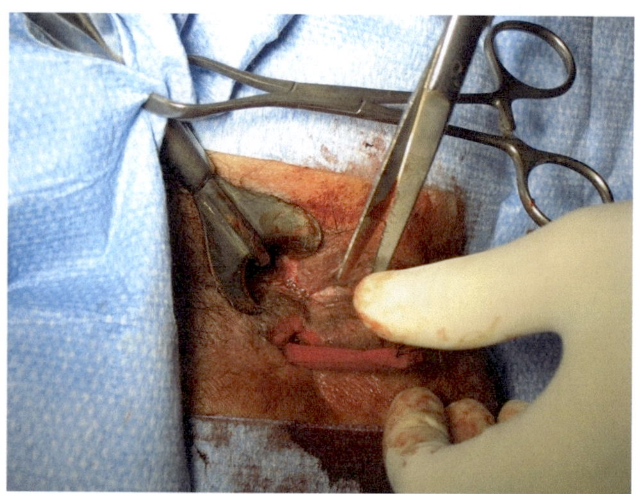

Fig. 13.7 The figure represents the fistula plug in its final position with the size of the external opening increased to allow for adequate drainage. Images courtesy of Dr. Alex Ky

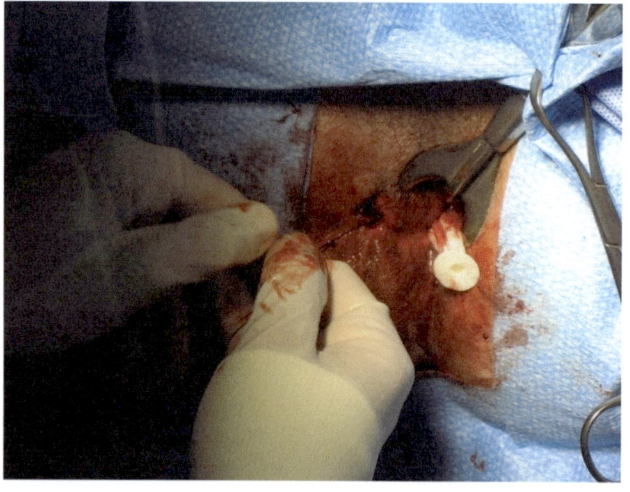

Fig. 13.5 The figure represents the fistula plug traversing the fistula from the internal to external opening. Images courtesy of Dr. Alex Ky

fistula plug [14]. There were a total of 27 plug insertions over a 28-month period in 16 patients. Twelve patients underwent 16 Cook plug insertions and 10 patients underwent 11 Gore plug insertions. Several patients who initially failed the Cook plug were subsequently receiving Gore plugs.

Successful closure (healing) was clinically defined as the absence of any discharge or swelling, with the internal opening closed by the time the anoscopy was performed and all external openings closed at the perineal examination at the last follow-up session. In regard to technique, the button was secured flush with the anal mucosa and secured with two to three 2-0 Vicryl sutures.

The overall procedural success rate in the Gore group was 54.5 % (6 of 11) vs. 12.5 % (2 of 16) in the Cook group. Of note, patients whose fistula plug was inserted after pretreatment of the fistula with a draining (loose) seton appeared to heal more often (55.6 %, 5/9) compared to those treated without a seton (28.6 %, 2/7).

De la Portilla et al. reported a series a total of 19 patients (18 men, 1 woman) with transsphincteric anal fistulas [12]. The median age was 49 (range, 33–65) years. Patients with known hypersensitivity to materials in the plug, those who had more than three external openings or Crohn's disease, and those who were under 18 years of age or were pregnant

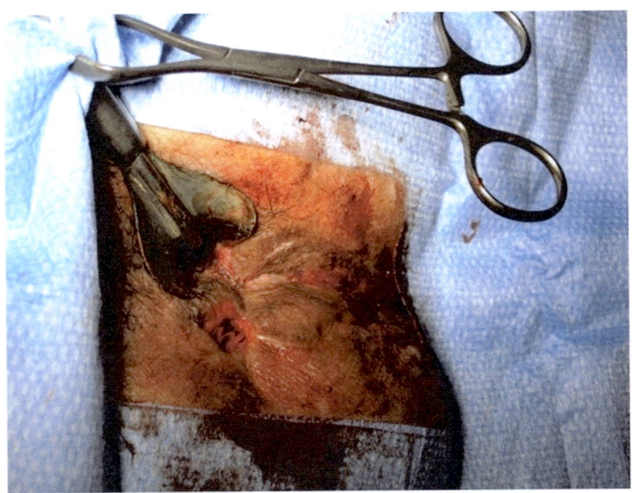

Fig. 13.8 The figure represents the fistula plug in its final position with the size of the external opening increased to allow for adequate drainage. Images courtesy of Dr. Alex Ky

were excluded form the study. The follow-up duration was 12 months and successful closure was clinically defined as the absence of any discharge or swelling, with the internal opening closed by the time the anoscopy was performed and all external openings closed at the perineal examination at the last follow-up session. In regard to technique, the disk was secured flush with the mucosa with interrupted absorbable sutures.

Concerning results, relapse occurred in 16 patients (with a perianal abscess in one patient). Successful closure was observed in only 3 out of 19 patients (15.8 %). The poor results from this study were attributed to the learning curve of the surgeons, the small number of patients, and the varied nature of the fistulas.

Ratto et al.'s study included 11 patients with a median age of 42 [15]. The fistulas were cryptoglandular in origin in all of the patients. There were five high anterior transsphincteric fistulas and six high posterior transsphincteric. The median duration of the procedure was 40 min. There were between 2 and 4 tubes inserted into the fistula tact. In regard to surgical technique, the submucosal pocket was closed with 3-0 Vicryl stitches. The disk was included in the suture to prevent plug migration and the protruding tubes were trimmed 2–3 mm beyond the surface of the perianal skin. The median follow-up was 5 months. All patients were evaluated by physical examination and endo-anal ultrasound. Success was defined as the absence of drainage, closure of the external opening, and the absence of perianal swelling or abscess formation. In regard to results, there was no early dislodgement, and closure occurred in 8 of 11 patients (72.7 %).

Ommer and colleagues recently published the initial results from Germany [16]. This series comprised 40 patients (30 male, 10 female, age 51 ± 12 years) who underwent closure of a high transsphincteric ($n=28$) or

Table 13.1 Summary of recent studies

Authors	Year	Number of patients	Crohn's patients	Healing rate (%)
Buchberg et al. [14]	2010	11	0	6/11 (54.5)
De la Portilla et al. [12]	2011	19	0	3/19 (15.7
Ratto et al. [15]	2012	11	0	8/11 (72.7)
Ommer et al. [16]	2012	40	4	23/40 (57.5)
Buchberg et al. [14]	2010	11	0	6/11 (54.5)
De la Portilla et al. [12]	2011	19	0	3/19 (15.7)
Ratto et al. [15]	2012	11	0	8/11 (72.7)
Ommer et al. [16]	2012	40	4	23/40 (57.5)

supra-sphincteric ($n=12$) fistula with Gore Bio-A Fistula Plug® in three surgical departments by five colorectal surgeons. Healing of the fistula was defined as complete closure of the internal opening and the external wound and no symptoms of inflammation. In describing the surgical technique, all arms of the plug were pulled tight and the head was fixated to the internal sphincter muscle using 2–3 sutures (PDS 2-0). The head was then covered with a mucosa-submucosa-flap (Vicryl 2-0).

The overall healing rate was 57.5 % (23/40). Six months after surgery the fistula had healed in 20 patients (50.0 %). Three additional fistulas healed after 7, 9, and 12 months. One patient developed an abscess which required surgical drainage and the plug had become dislodged in two patients during the first 2 weeks postoperatively. The healing rate varied significantly amongst the five surgeons with a range of 0–75%. In patients having only prior drainage of the abscess healing occurred in 63.6% (14/22) whereas in patients after one or more flap fistula reconstruction the healing rate decreased to 50% (9/18). No patient complained about any impairment of his or her preoperative continence status. Additionally, four Crohn's patients were treated with a success rate of 25 %. The following Table 13.1 is a summary of the recent studies.

Conclusion

The Gore Bio-A fistula plug is a new and evolving treatment modality for anal fistulas. There is a wide range of results in the data that has been published up to this point. This is due to the learning curve of the surgery, patient selection, and the small number of patients. One technical aspect that needs to be clarified is in regard to the fixation method of the disk. It is not clear whether it is optimal to secure the disk on top of the rectal mucosa or secure it beneath a flap. Intuitively, it seems that covering the disk with a mucosal flap would produce better results. This plug has also not been extensively studied in Crohn's patients. There are only four patients in the literature who have been treated with the Gore Bio-A plug.

Overall, the Gore Bio-A plug is a new technique that appears to be an improvement over the Surgisis plug and updated research will more clearly define the proper fixation method and surgical indications.

References

1. Parks AG, Gordon PH, Hardcastle JD. A classification of fistula-in-ano. Br J Surg. 1976;63:1–12.
2. Ellis CN. Bioprosthetic plugs for complex anal fistulas: an early experience. J Surg Educ. 2007;64:36–40.
3. Garcia-Aguilar J, Belmonte C, Wong WD, Goldberg SM, Madoff RD. Anal fistula surgery: factors associated with recurrence and incontinence. Dis Colon Rectum. 1996;39:723–9.
4. Jun SH, Choi GS. Anocutaneous advancement flap closure of high anal fistulas. Br J Surg. 1999;86(4):490–2.
5. Sonoda T, Hull T, Piedmonte MR, Fazio VW. Outcomes of primary repair of anorectal and rectovaginal fistulas using the endorectal advancement flap. Dis Colon Rectum. 2002;45:1622–8.
6. Venkatesh KS, Ramanujam P. Fibrin glue application in the treatment of recurrent anorectal fistulas. Dis Colon Rectum. 1999;42:1136–9.
7. Haim N, Neufeld D, Ziv Y, Tulchinsky H, et al. Long-term results of fibrin glue treatment for cryptogenic perianal fistulas: a multicenter study. Dis Colon Rectum. 2011;54(10):1279–83.
8. The Surgisis AFP. anal fistula plug: report of a consensus conference. Colorectal Dis. 2008;10:17–20.
9. Champagne BJ, O'Connor LM, Ferguson M, et al. Efficacy of anal fistula plug in closure of cryptoglandular fistulas: long-term follow-up. Dis Colon Rectum. 2006;49:1817–21.
10. Safar B, Jobanputra S, Cera S, et al. Anal fistula plug: Initial experience and outcomes meeting abstract. Dis Colon Rectum. 2007;50:725.
11. Katz AR, Mukherjee DP, Kaganov AL, Gordon S. A new synthetic monofilament absorbable suture made from poly-trimethylene carbonate. Surg Gynecol Obstet. 1985;161:213–22.
12. De la Portilla F, Rada R, Jiménez-Rodríguez R, et al. Evaluation of a new synthetic plug in the treatment of anal fistulas: results of a pilot study. Dis Colon Rectum. 2011;54(11):1419–22.
13. GORE® BIO-A® Fistula Plug instructions for use http://www.gore-medical.com/resources/dam/assets/AM0175-ML3_English.pdf. Accessed Nov 18, 2012.
14. Buchberg B, Masoomi H, Choi J, Bergman H, Mills S, Stamos MJ. A tale of two (anal fistula) plugs: is there a difference in short-term outcomes? Am Surg. 2010;76:1150–3.
15. Ratto C, Litta F. Parello et al. Gore Bio-A® Fistula Plug: a new sphincter-sparing procedure for complex anal fistula. Colorectal Dis. 2012;14(5):e264–9.
16. Ommer A, Herold A, Joos A, et al. Gore BioA Fistula Plug in the treatment of high anal fistulas—initial results from a German multicenter-study. Ger Med Sci. 2012;10:13. doi:10.3205/000164. Epub 2012 Sep 11.

Christine C. Jensen

Introduction

Treatment of anal fistula can be a delicate balance between maximizing the chances of successful healing and avoiding complications from the surgery itself, particularly incontinence from division of the anal sphincters. Many surgical procedures have been used in the treatment of anal fistula, with varying success. Endorectal advancement flap can be a useful tool in the armamentarium of the surgeon faced with an anal fistula, including in complex cases such as Crohn's disease or recurrent fistula.

First described by Noble in 1902 for rectovaginal fistulas [1], the application of this technique to anal fistulas was published soon after by Elting [2]. However, advancement flap did not gain wider popularity until much later. It was not until 1948 that Laird described modification of this to a partial-thickness flap [3], and widespread use of the technique did not follow for many decades. However, as the advantages of the operation became more apparent, endorectal advancement flap became one of the most widely used surgeries to treat fistula in ano.

The endorectal advancement flap has theoretical advantages over other strategies to treat anal fistula. By covering the internal opening of the fistula, it interrupts the course of the fistula, thus encouraging healing. The flap also avoids any full-thickness division of the anal sphincters, helping to preserve continence. The location of the flap on the high-pressure side of the fistula maintains the flap in place, rather than tending toward disruption of the flap by pressure transmitted through the fistula if the flap were to be located on the low-pressure side of the fistula. Thus, endorectal advancement flaps have great potential to effect cure in the treatment of anal fistulas.

C.C. Jensen, M.D., M.P.H. (✉)
Department of Surgery, University of Minnesota,
1055 Westgate Drive, Ste 190, St. Paul, MN 55114, USA
e-mail: cjensen@crsal.org

Technique

The patient needs no special preparation, although some surgeons may prefer enemas to clear the rectum of stool. Perioperative antibiotics are not necessary although they are used by many surgeons. The patient is placed under either regional or general anesthesia and positioned in the prone jackknife position. The buttocks are spread and taped to provide exposure. Careful attention to positioning, such that the patient's hips are at the break point in the bed, greatly facilitates good visualization during the course of the operation, and a headlight is indispensable. Although posterior fistulas can be more difficult to address in this position than anterior or lateral fistulas, the prone jackknife position is still preferable to lithotomy as it provides better exposure.

A Pratt or Hill-Ferguson retractor is used to visualize the internal opening and the fistula tract is probed to delineate the anatomy. The fistula should be characterized by type (intersphincteric, transsphincteric, extrasphincteric, or suprasphincteric), the amount of muscle involved, and the location of the internal opening. Careful attention should be paid to identifying any additional tracts, as undrained tracts will contribute to failure of the flap. Beginning distal to the internal opening, a partial-thickness flap is raised incorporating mucosa, submucosa, and some muscle fibers (Fig. 14.1). As the flap is developed, the width should gradually increase so that the base is at least twice the width of the apex of the flap to ensure adequate blood supply to the flap. Dissection of the flap continues cephalad until the flap reaches easily past the internal opening without excessive tension. At this point many surgeons perform a partial fistulectomy, coring out the fistula tract beginning at the external opening until the sphincter muscles are reached. If a fistulectomy is not performed, the fistula tract should be curetted to remove granulation tissue and debris.

The internal opening should be closed using interrupted absorbable sutures such as 2-0 polyglactin. The tip of the flap, containing the internal opening, is excised. The flap is then

H. Abcarian (ed.), *Anal Fistula: Principles and Management*, DOI 10.1007/978-1-4614-9014-2_14,
© Springer Science+Business Media New York 2014

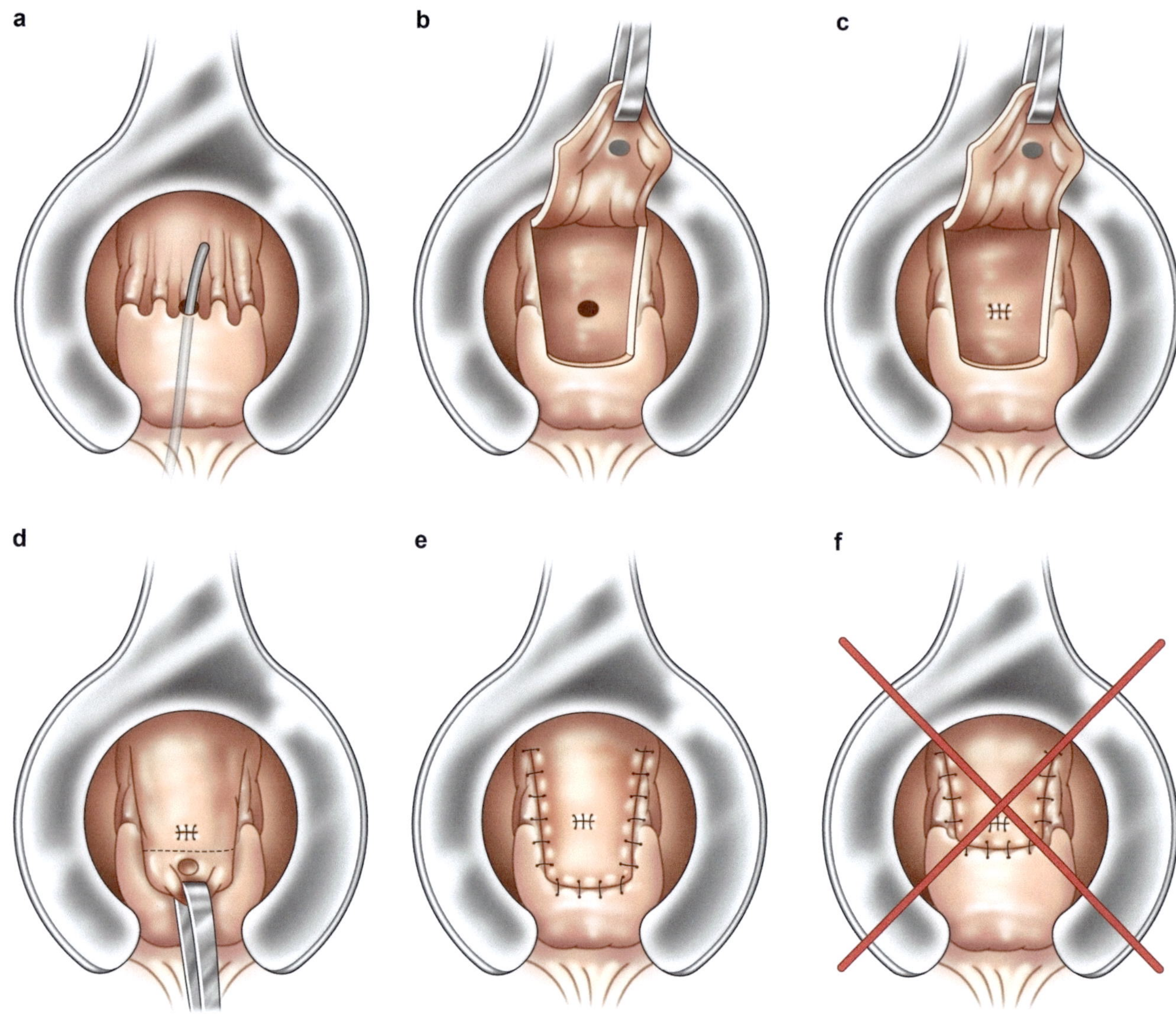

Fig. 14.1 Rectal advancement flap. (**a**) Fistula in ano, with internal opening at the dentate line. (**b**) Elevation of partial-thickness flap, exposing internal opening. (**c**) Closure of internal opening. (**d**) Advancement of flap with excision of portion containing internal opening. (**e**) Completed flap covering internal opening. Note this advances mucosa distal to dentate line. (**f**) Incorrectly illustrated flap, showing internal opening above dentate line and flap advancing only to dentate line

sewn into place using interrupted absorbable sutures, again such as 2-0 polyglactin. While doing this, the sutures should be spaced more closely together on the flap than on the rectal defect so that the flap is gradually advanced to cover the internal opening without excessive tension. When properly performed, the flap should extend distal to the dentate line if the internal opening was at the dentate line (Fig. 14.1, panel e). However, many publications regarding endorectal advancement flap erroneously illustrate the internal opening above the dentate line with the finished flap extending to the dentate line (Fig. 14.1, panel f); when properly performed an advancement flap for a fistula with the internal opening at the dentate line results in a slight degree of ectropion. The area is then inspected for hemostasis; rectal packing is not necessary.

Many publications report an inpatient stay after surgery of up to 3–4 or even 6 days [4–9], but the patient can be discharged the same day in the majority of cases. Pain medication, sitz baths, and bulk laxatives should be prescribed; no restricted diet or other laxatives are necessary.

Results

Healing of Fistula

The reported success rates for primary healing of cryptoglandular fistulas after endorectal advancement flap vary widely from 59 to 97 % (Table 14.1), but are generally in the

Table 14.1 Results of endorectal flap repair of cryptoglandular fistulas. Primary success rate is the percentage healed after first attempt at repair with advancement flap; ultimate success rate is percentage healed after additional intervention for initial failures

Authors	Number of patients	Fistula type	Primary success rate (%)	Ultimate success rate (%)	Comments
Christoforidis et al. [19][a]	43	TS	63	–	14 patients had fistulectomy and 7 had fibrin glue in addition to flap
Chung et al. [57][a]	96	TS	60	–	Mucosal rather than partial-thickness flaps
Dubsky et al. [41]	54	High TS or SS	76	–	
Golub et al. [20]	164	115 (70 %) TS, SS, ES 15 (9 %) IS 34 (21 %) not recorded	97	–	Success rate based on long-term follow-up in 61 patients; 10 patients had fistulas in the immediate postoperative period requiring additional intervention but were not considered recurrences
Koehler et al. [52][a]	15 mucosal 18 partial- or full-thickness	Dorsal horseshoe	73	88	Ultimate success rate includes patients who had anocutaneous flaps ($n=8$) or suture closure of internal opening ($n=11$)
Mitalas et al. [34][b]	162	TS	59	–	
Mitalas et al. [16][b]	80	TS	68	–	
Mitalas et al. [31][b]	54	TS	63	–	
Mitalas et al. [18][b]	26	TS	69	90	All of these patients were having repeat flap surgery, with a success rate of 69 %; in combination with the first surgery this leads to an ultimate success rate of 90 %
Mitalas et al. [39][b]	278	TS	64	–	
Ortiz and Marzo [49]	103	91 (88 %) TS 12 (12 %) SS	93	–	All patients also had fistulectomy
Ortiz et al. [17][a]	91	High TS or SS	82	–	
Ortiz et al. [14][a]	16	TS	88	–	
Perez et al. [8][a]	30	High TS or SS	93	–	
Schouten et al. [36]	44	TS	75	–	
van Koperen et al. [42][a]	54	TS	83	–	
Wang et al. [56][a]	26	TS	64	–	

TS transsphincteric, *SS* suprasphincteric, *ES* extrasphincteric, *IS* intersphincteric
[a]Study included other interventions (e.g., anal fistula plug, fibrin glue) but reported results are only for patients who had endorectal flap
[b]These studies include many of the same patients

70–80 % range. Some of this variation in success rates may be due to the duration of follow-up and the means of defining and detecting recurrence. The mean time to recurrence has been found to range widely from a median of 8 weeks to 9 months [10–12]. Some studies show the majority of recurrences occurring within the first year [13], or even all recurrences occurring within the first 3 months [14], while other studies have shown recurrences up to 55 months after surgery [7, 15].

Studies designed specifically to examine the length of follow-up needed to capture all recurrences demonstrate that the majority of recurrences occur early. Mitalas et al. [16] attempted to define the duration of follow-up required by following 80 patients who had an endorectal advancement flap for a median of 92 months. They found a median healing time of 3.6 months and one patient presenting with a recurrence at 28 months. However, in this study the long-term follow-up was performed by having patients fill out a questionnaire rather than by an office visit with examination, so some recurrent fistulas may not have been detected. Ortiz

et al. [17] conducted follow-up of 91 patients with examinations monthly until the wound healed and annually after healing. Their results, over a median follow-up of 42 months, did not differ significantly from those of Mitalas, showing a mean time to recurrence of 5 months and no recurrences after 1 year. Thus, it appears the majority of recurrences will become clinically apparent within the first year, but a small minority of patients may experience late recurrence after initial healing.

Healing Rates After Repeat Flap

If endorectal advancement flap fails and the patient has a recurrence, repeat flap is an option for treatment. Mitalas et al. performed a second advancement flap in 26 patients with transsphincteric cryptoglandular fistulas who had recurrence after an initial rectal advancement flap [18]. The healing rate after the second flap was 69 %. In combination with the patients with successful fistula healing after the first flap, endorectal advancement flap was successful in 90 % of patients after a maximum of two attempts. In addition, patients undergoing repeat flap had no change in fecal incontinence scores, suggesting that repeat flap carries a low risk of incontinence.

Complications

Endorectal advancement flap is generally associated with a low risk of complications; many case series do not report complications. The most common complication appears to be bleeding. In a case series of 189 patients with mucosal flaps by Aguilar et al. [4], there were two cases of delayed bleeding; bleeding was also reported in 2 of 43 patients by Christoforidis et al. [19], 1 of 167 patients by Golub et al. [20], 1 of 48 patients by Muhlmann et al. [12], and 1 of 31 patients by Joo et al. [6].

There are also reports of urinary retention [21], including a 7.8 % rate of postoperative urinary retention by Golub et al. [20]. For this reason it is reasonable to ensure patients can void before they are discharged from the recovery area, in order to avoid emergency room visits for urinary retention. In the Aguilar study [4] there were two cases of anal stenosis; however, 80 % of these patients also had a hemorrhoidectomy, so it is unclear whether these complications arose as a result of the advancement flap or the hemorrhoidectomy.

Effect of Other Factors on Healing Rates

Patient Characteristics

In general there is no effect of age on healing rates in multiple studies [22–27]. In studies that have shown a difference in healing rates with age, increased age is associated with a higher likelihood of healing. Gustafsson et al. found a trend toward a higher likelihood of healing with age greater than 50 [28]. Similarly, healing rates were 45.7 % for age less than 40, 67.9 % for those aged 40–60, and 100 % for those older than 60 in a paper by Sonoda et al. [29]. One confounding factor may be the prevalence of Crohn's; in the Sonoda paper a higher proportion of the younger patients had Crohn's disease while the older patients were more likely to have cryptoglandular fistulas. However, some of the studies demonstrating no effect of age on healing rates included significant numbers of patients with Crohn's disease [22, 26]. Thus, it is unclear whether the decreased healing at younger ages found in some studies is due to a differential prevalence of Crohn's among the study patients at different ages.

The majority of studies have found that gender does not affect fistula healing rates [28], including in multiple logistic regression analyses after controlling for other factors [24, 25, 27]. However, one study did find a significantly greater proportion of men had primary healing of their fistula [30]. Seventeen of 24 males vs. 6 of 18 women in this study had primary healing of their fistula after closure of the internal opening was performed; in the majority of cases this closure was done with a partial-thickness endorectal advancement flap.

The data on the effect of obesity on healing rates is mixed. Schwandner et al. found that obesity, defined as a body mass index (BMI) greater than 30 kg/m^2, was associated with a decreased success rate for full-thickness flaps [23]. In this study, the recurrence rate was 14 % for non-obese patients vs. 28 % for obese patients, and this association continued after adjustment for other factors. Among the patients with recurrence of their fistula, there was also a higher need for reoperation for abscess among obese patients vs. non-obese patients. However, other studies have found no difference in recurrence with obesity [24, 26, 28], or even increased healing with greater body surface area [29]. Many studies have found no effect of smoking on flap success [23, 25, 28, 31].

However, smoking is associated with a higher recurrence rate in other studies [22, 24, 27], which may be plausible due to the possibility of decreased blood flow to the rectal mucosa as a result of smoking [31]. All of these studies performed multivariate analyses which demonstrated that smoking was independently associated with fistula recurrence after endorectal advancement flap. Ellis and Clark [27] found a 51 % recurrence rate for smokers vs. 19 % for nonsmokers undergoing endorectal advancement flap. Similarly, Zimmerman et al. [24] found a 40 % recurrence rate among smokers vs. a 21 % recurrence rate among nonsmokers; in this study the healing rate was significantly less if the patient smoked more than ten cigarettes per day. It may therefore be prudent to encourage patients to quit smoking prior to endorectal advancement flap.

The use of systemic medications in Crohn's disease also has the potential to affect success rates. Steroid use has not been found to affect healing rates in some studies [10, 22], with other studies showing a trend toward an increased likelihood of failure with steroid use [26, 29]. This may be due to steroid use serving as a proxy for a greater severity of Crohn's disease, which would predispose patients to recurrence or persistence of their fistulas. In contrast, there is evidence that biologic immunomodulators may contribute to the success of endorectal advancement flaps in patients with Crohn's disease. In a case series of 19 patients with Crohn's disease who were treated with preoperative infliximab, eight healed and did not require surgery. The remaining 11 underwent endorectal advancement flaps with an 82 % success rate [32]. Similarly, in a retrospective review of 218 patients with Crohn's undergoing a variety of surgical interventions for anal fistulas, there was improvement or healing in 71.3 % of those receiving biologic immunomodulators vs. 35.9 % of those not receiving biologics, although the overall healing rate was low at 26.5 % for surgery alone and 36.6 % for surgery plus biologic immunomodulators [33]. Biologics thus show some promise as an adjunct to endorectal advancement flaps in patients with Crohn's disease.

Fistula Characteristics

Although there have been some studies that show no difference in recurrence rates based on etiology of the fistula [7], the preponderance of evidence suggests that fistulas associated with Crohn's disease tend to have a higher recurrence rate than fistulas of other etiologies [5, 10, 22, 29]. For example, Sonoda et al. [29] found a healing rate of 50 % for Crohn's fistulas vs. 77 % for cryptoglandular fistulas, and Mizrahi et al. found rates of 43 and 67 %, respectively [10]. There is some evidence that the activity of Crohn's disease, not just the presence of Crohn's, can affect recurrence rate also. A success rate of 25 % has been found in the presence of small bowel Crohn's, vs. 87 % in the absence of small bowel Crohn's [6]. In contrast, though, Crohn's activity was not found to affect the healing rate after rectovaginal fistula repair (done in most cases with a mucosal advancement flap although a significant minority of patients had other procedures performed) [26]. Patients with Crohn's disease should therefore be counseled that they may experience a higher rate of recurrence after endorectal advancement flap than patients with fistulas due to cryptoglandular or other causes.

Location of the fistula does not appear to affect healing rates, with anterior, posterior, and lateral fistulas having similar healing rates [23, 24, 34]. Data are mixed as to whether different types of fistulas have differential healing rates. Mizrahi et al. found no difference in healing rates between anorectal, rectovaginal, pouch-perineal, and rectourethral fistulas in a case series of 106 flaps in 94 patients [10], although there were necessarily small numbers of some of these types of fistulas. A number of studies have compared rectovaginal fistulas to other fistulas, with a higher healing rate [6, 35], lower healing rate [5], and no difference [27] all having been found.

Data are similarly mixed as to the effect of fistula complexity on healing rates. "Complex" fistulas (horseshoe, suprasphincteric, or anovaginal fistulas or those with other extensions) have not been found to have lower healing rates than more straightforward fistulas [28, 30]. Fistulas with a horseshoe component have been found to have higher [34], lower [13], and similar [24] healing rates when compared to fistulas without a horseshoe component. The healing rate for rectovaginal fistulas was not found to vary by the location of the fistula (high vs. low) or size of the fistula opening by Pinto et al. [22]. Referral to a tertiary institution may also serve as a proxy for fistula complexity, but has not been found to affect success rates in the studies that have examined this factor [23, 25]. Thus, surprisingly, the majority of studies show no effect of complexity on healing rates.

Prior surgical attempts to repair the fistula are another factor that may serve as a proxy for fistula complexity. Schouten et al. found a success rate of 87 % for transsphincteric cryptoglandular fistulas treated with endorectal advancement flaps if there had been only one or no prior attempts at repair vs. a success rate of 50 % if there had been two or more attempts at repair [36]. Lowry et al. found similar results for among a group of patients treated for rectovaginal fistulas with endorectal advancement flaps (of note, 31 % of these patients had concomitant overlapping sphincteroplasties). Success rates were 88% among those with no prior repairs, 85 % with one repair, 55 % with two repairs, and 100 % with three repairs, with the relative risk of failure for those with two prior attempts vs. none being 3.71 [37]. Additional studies have found a decreased success rate [7, 27] or trend toward this [38] with prior attempts at repair. However, many other studies have found no difference in the recurrence rate in the presence of prior attempts at repair [6, 10, 25, 28] or any relationship to the number of prior attempts at repair [23, 24, 26]. Thus, while patients with a history of multiple prior attempts at repair should be cautioned about the risk of failure, there is evidence that they can expect a success rate which may not be markedly different than patients who have not had prior attempts at repair.

Operative Technique

A seton is often placed prior to surgery to allow maturation of the fistula tract prior to endorectal advancement flap. There is some evidence that this may contribute to a greater likelihood of healing. A greater success rate for endorectal flap after seton placement [29], or a trend toward this, [26] has been found in some case series but not in others [24, 25, 39]. However, in all of these studies the choice of a preoperative seton was not random, suggesting that these were likely placed in situations where the surgeon anticipated a lower likelihood of healing. The finding of no difference or an increase in healing in these presumably more difficult fistulas suggests that setons are of benefit. Seton placement for a minimum of 6 weeks prior to flap should therefore be strongly considered.

Reports vary widely on the use of antibiotics and constipating medications. While the majority of centers administer a dose of perioperative antibiotics, some centers also continue antibiotics postoperatively for variable durations. Some centers limit patients to a clear liquid diet for a period of time and/or place them on constipating medications, while others have no particular restrictions. Studies in general do not show a benefit of postoperative antibiotics [7, 29] or a postoperative regimen including clear liquid diet, immobilization, and antibiotics [39]. Only one report demonstrates increased healing with postoperative antibiotics [30]. Not all of the patients in this study had flaps performed, and all had fistulectomy performed in addition, so the generalizability to patients undergoing endorectal advancement flap is limited. In terms of postoperative bowel regimen to promote constipation, no difference in healing rates has been found between a constipating regimen and no regimen [7, 10]. Thus, perioperative antibiotics may be used, but postoperative antibiotics and a restricted bowel regimen are not necessary.

Partial-thickness flaps are likely more successful than full-thickness flaps. In a review of the literature incorporating a total of 1,654 patients, Soltani and Kaiser examined the effect of flap type on healing rates [40]. They found that partial-thickness flaps were used more often in the studies reporting above-average success rates, while full-thickness flaps were associated with below-average success rates except in one study [41]. Mucosal flaps were represented equally in studies reporting above- and below-average success rates. Partial-thickness flaps, incorporating mucosa, submucosa, and some muscle fibers, should be preferred.

The presence of a diverting stoma has not been found to have an effect on fistula healing after endorectal advancement flap [10, 26, 29]. However, all of these studies were case series in which the choice of whether to perform a stoma was nonrandom. Most likely the patients selected to have a stoma had fistulas that were thought to have a low likelihood of healing, and as such it is unclear whether the stomas performed in these cases contributed to a higher healing rate than would otherwise have been found for these difficult fistulas. Diverting stoma may be a good option in selected cases.

Modifications to the Endorectal Advancement Flap

A number of modifications to the endorectal advancement flap technique have been attempted, but generally have not led to increased success rates. Perhaps the most enthusiasm surrounded the injection of fibrin glue into the fistula tract in addition to performing the flap. Although one study found no effect of glue injection on healing, there were only 12 patients who had glue injected. Instead, there is good evidence to suggest that fibrin glue decreases the chance of successful healing. Both a case–control study [42] and a randomized controlled trial [43] have demonstrated a decreased success rate with glue. In the case–control study, 26 patients who had fibrin glue and advancement flap were matched to 54 who had advancement flap only. The recurrence rate was 17 % for advancement flap alone vs. 46 % for flap and fibrin glue. Similarly, in the randomized controlled trial there was a recurrence rate of 20 % for flap alone vs. 46 % for flap and fibrin glue (but these patients had either mucosal advancement flaps or anodermal flaps rather than partial-thickness rectal flaps). Fibrin glue should not be used in conjunction

with advancement flap. Sileri et al. performed a similar injection with porcine dermal collagen matrix, achieving success in 10 of 11 patients [44], but experience with this material is limited.

Gustafsson and Graf did a randomized controlled trial comparing flap alone to flap with a gentamicin-collagen sponge implanted underneath and found no difference in healing rates between the two groups [28]. Similarly, van Onkelen et al. found a healing rate of only 51 % when performing the LIFT (ligation of intersphincteric fistula tract) procedure in addition to endorectal advancement flap [45]. Thus, there are no modifications to the endorectal advancement flap that have been found to consistently improve outcomes over flap alone.

Continence

Although endorectal advancement flaps do not divide full-thickness muscle, there are a number of reasons why they may negatively affect continence. A partial-thickness flap does take some muscle fibers, including some of the internal sphincter fibers if the flap extends distal to the dentate line as it does in most cases. If the internal opening is at the dentate line, flaps also cause the rectal mucosa to extend past the dentate line, creating some degree of ectropion. Finally, the amount of stretch that must be put on the sphincter muscles intraoperatively could cause some temporary or even permanent incontinence.

Clinical Results

Studies have come to a wide range of conclusions regarding continence after endorectal advancement flap. Encouraging findings regarding continence have been found by a number of studies, which have found no change in continence after flap [46, 47] or only transient changes in continence [15]. Similarly, when the Rockwood Fecal Incontinence Severity Index was measured preoperatively and postoperatively after initial and even repeat flaps, no change in scores was found [18]. Some studies even report improved continence after flap, perhaps because there is no longer drainage through the fistula tract [5, 35]. However, in one of these studies, which exclusively included patients with rectovaginal as opposed to anoperineal fistulas, some of the patients had sphincteroplasties in addition to advancement flaps, which may partially explain the improvement in continence [35].

The preponderance of studies indicates a decrement in continence in a minority of patients. Van der Hagen et al. found a decrease in continence postoperatively in 10 % of patients [48], and Mizrahi et al. similarly found 9% of patients to have a decrease in continence [10]. The reported postoperative prevalence of mild soiling or incontinence to flatus ranges from 8 to 15 % postoperatively [4, 11, 20, 49], although it is unclear what the preoperative prevalence of incontinence was in these populations.

When continence has been assessed more formally using incontinence scoring systems, there continues to be evidence for a moderate decrement in continence in a subset of patients. Ortiz et al. measured the Cleveland Clinic Florida Fecal Incontinence (CCF-FI) score preoperatively and postoperatively, and found that the proportion reporting a score of zero (perfect continence) decreased significantly from 89 % preoperatively to 77 % postoperatively [17]. When Christoforidis et al. used the CCF-FI score to assess continence after advancement flap, 48 % reported perfect continence, while 35 % reported scores of 3 or 4, representing occasional incontinence to flatus with rare incontinence to liquid stool. Seventeen percent reported scores of 7–12, representing frequent liquid or occasional solid incontinence, but this group comprised four patients, two of whom were incontinent preoperatively and one of whom could not recall what his continence status was preoperatively [19].

There are also studies that would support a substantial negative effect of endorectal advancement flaps on continence. Postoperatively, Joy and Williams found 50 % of patients were incontinent to flatus, 21 % to liquid, and no patients to solids (patients who were incontinent to flatus and liquid were counted in both groups) [50]. One report found a 43 % prevalence of postoperative soiling [25] and another a 38 % incidence of soiling or incontinence to flatus among patients who had reported normal continence preoperatively [36]. At 1 year after surgery, 31 % of patients reported a slight decrease and 11 % a major decrease in continence in another study, although some of these patients had additional surgery with division of the internal sphincter before their 1-year follow-up [30].

Thus, the data on postoperative continence are mixed, but most studies seem to support a decrement in continence in a subset of patients. This is supported by a meta-analysis by Soltani and Kaiser which found a prevalence of incontinence after advancement flap of 13.2 % in cryptoglandular disease and 9.4 % in Crohn's (although it was not specified whether this was incontinence to flatus, liquid, and/or solid stool) [40]. Most likely a minority of patients will experience impaired continence postoperatively, although in many cases this will be soiling or incontinence to gas rather than incontinence to solid stool. Informing patients of this risk is an important part of the preoperative counseling process.

Manometric Results

Several studies have used anal manometry to quantify any changes associated with endorectal advancement flap, and the findings have been mixed. Some have found no difference in resting or squeeze pressures when comparing preop-erative to postoperative values, although one of these studies included only nine patients [11, 47]. Many other studies have found manometric changes after endorectal advancement flap. Among 56 patients treated with advancement flap for mid to high transsphincteric fistulas, Uribe et al. found a significant decrease in resting pressure from a mean of 83.6 mmHg preoperatively to 45.6 mmHg postoperatively and in squeeze pressure from a mean of 208.8–169.5 mmHg, respectively [9]. Other studies, although also examining patients who had other procedures to treat anal fistulas, found decreases in resting [30, 51–53] and squeeze pressures [30, 52, 53] among the patients who had endorectal advancement flaps. These findings suggest that the incontinence reported by some patients after advancement flap is not due solely to ectropion causing fecal seepage, but results from decreases in the resting and squeeze pressures. Whether these decreases in resting and squeeze pressures are due to taking some internal sphincter fibers, stretching of the sphincter muscles during surgery or some other cause remains to be seen.

Risk Factors for Incontinence

Knowledge of factors associated with an increased risk of incontinence after endorectal advancement flap would be useful in counseling patients who may be at particularly high risk of incontinence. However, few studies have identified risk factors for incontinence. Schouten et al. found no difference in risk of incontinence based on age, sex, or the number of prior repairs [36]. Mizrahi et al. found an increased risk in the presence of prior attempts at repair [10]. Abbas et al. found an increased risk of incontinence with older age and high transsphincteric fistulas, but the majority of the patients in this study had fistulotomies, with only 10.6 % of patients having advancement flaps [13]. Although there is little data with which to counsel patients, the patients at higher risk for incontinence after advancement flap are likely those who are at higher risk with any procedure—those with baseline disturbances in continence, prior repairs, women, and older individuals.

Comparison with Other Surgeries for Fistula

Anal Fistula Plug

A number of studies have compared endorectal advancement flap to anal fistula plug, as both operations do not involve full-thickness division of the anal sphincter muscles. Two randomized controlled trials comparing plugs and advancement flaps have been conducted. In the first, by Ortiz et al., 43 patients with high transsphincteric fistulas of cryptoglandular origin were randomized to plug or flap and followed for up to 1 year [14]. This study was closed prematurely due to a significantly higher rate of recurrence in the plug arm, with recurrences in 12 of 15 plug patients vs. 2 of 16 flap patients (relative risk for recurrence for plug vs. flap, 6.40, $p < 0.001$). Van Koperen et al. similarly performed a randomized controlled trial of plug vs. advancement flap in high transsphincteric cryptoglandular fistulas [54]. This study found a 71 % recurrence in the plug arm vs. 52 % in the flap arm, which was not significant. However, this study was likely underpowered, as their power calculation assumed a 40 % difference in recurrence rate between the two arms. Conversely, a randomized controlled trial of acellular dermal matrix used in a manner similar to a plug found recurrence of only 4.5 % with acellular dermal matrix vs. 28.9 % with flap [55].

There are also a number of case series comparing success rates with plugs vs. flaps. Some have shown greater success rates with flap than plug [13, 19, 56], often despite longer follow-up in the flap group which would tend to predispose to a higher recurrence rate in the group with longer follow-up [19, 56]. Other studies demonstrated no difference in success rates between the two operations [12, 57]. However, in one of these studies the flaps were mucosal, rather than the more commonly performed partial-thickness flap, so it is unclear whether this would have affected the observed success rate [57]. Thus, the preponderance of evidence would suggest that the endorectal advancement flap has a higher success rate than the anal fistula plug, as many studies demonstrate this, and some of the studies demonstrating no difference in success rates between the two methods have methodologic concerns. In addition, there is an absence of any studies demonstrating the flap is inferior to the plug.

Fistulotomy

A number of retrospective reviews have compared fistulotomy and endorectal advancement flap. A higher recurrence rate has been found with flap as compared to fistulotomy [25, 48, 51], although one study found no difference in recurrence rate [13]. However, the problem with comparing these two methods, as acknowledged by many of the authors of these studies, is that endorectal advancement flap is generally used in situations where a fistulotomy would be associated with an unacceptably high risk of incontinence, either due to the high location of the fistula or due to preexisting impaired continence. Therefore, it is of little use to compare these two methods, particularly in retrospective reviews, as patients who underwent a flap were likely not candidates for fistulotomy. One randomized controlled trial comparing endorectal advancement flap vs. fistulotomy with concomitant sphincter repair has been conducted [8]. This study showed a 7.4 % recurrence rate in the flap group vs. 7.1 % in the fistulotomy group, with no difference in continence between the two groups. However, as the majority of surgeons do not perform sphincter repair at the time of fistulotomy or perform fistulotomy for high fistulas, this comparison cannot be generalized. Fistulotomies are appropriate for low fistulas in the absence of impaired continence, while endorectal advancement flaps are used for situations where fistulotomy is not an option.

Fibrin Glue

Two retrospective reviews by Chung et al. have examined the success rates with fibrin glue instillation vs. endorectal advancement flap. In one, fistula plug and endorectal flap were found to have superior healing rates compared to seton and fibrin glue [57]. In another study among 51 patients with inflammatory bowel disease, a 20 % success rate was found with the flap and 0 % success with glue; however, this study included only five patients with flaps and two with fibrin glue, so conclusions regarding the relative efficacy of these two procedures cannot be drawn from this study [58]. Flap may thus be more effective than glue, but there is very limited evidence upon which to base a conclusion.

Seton

While a seton is rarely used as a primary strategy to effect fistula healing, there are some studies that have compared endorectal advancement flap to setons. One found a high healing rate for flaps, loose setons, and cutting setons with no difference between groups [50], while another study that compared anal fistula plug, fibrin glue, endorectal advancement flap, and setons found plugs and flaps to be superior to glue and setons [57].

Special Situations

Endorectal advancement flap can also be useful in situations where the fistula may be especially complex or difficult to heal, such as rectovaginal fistulas, rectourethral fistulas, and Crohn's-associated fistulas.

Rectovaginal Fistula

Rectovaginal fistulas can pose particular challenges to the surgeon. Endorectal advancement flaps can play a role in the treatment of rectovaginal fistulas, whether alone or in conjunction with sphincteroplasty. For a discussion of the treatment of rectovaginal fistula in the setting of Crohn's disease, please see the later section on this topic; this section will deal exclusively with rectovaginal fistulas not due to Crohn's disease.

A wide range of results have been reported for endorectal advancement flap alone for rectovaginal fistulas associated with cryptoglandular disease or obstetric injury. Hoexter et al. reported no recurrences over a mean follow-up of 4 years in a group of 15 patients treated with advancement flaps for low rectovaginal fistulas [59], as did Hilsabeck in a group of nine patients followed for as long as 20 years [60]. Success rates were lower in a report by Russell and Gallagher, with healing in all six flaps performed for fistulas arising from obstetric injury, but just 12 of 15 flaps performed for fistulas arising from cryptoglandular disease [61]. Watson and Phillips also reported a lower initial success rate, with success in 7 of 12 patients with fistulas arising from a mix of obstetric injury and cryptoglandular disease [62]. Tsang reported an even lower success rate of just 41 % among 27 flaps performed for fistulas arising from obstetric injury [38]. In terms of functional results, flaps improve continence in this group because there is no longer gas and stool passing into the vagina. Among the 19 patients with anovaginal fistulas who had an endorectal advancement flap in the study by Mazier et al., only one was incontinent to flatus postoperatively, while preoperatively 14 were incontinent to flatus, four to liquid stool, and one to solid stool [63].

Advancement flap can also be performed in conjunction with sphincteroplasty to treat fistulas due to obstetric injury, and this may be associated with a greater success rate in healing the fistula than flap alone. A number of studies have reported success rates among groups of patients with rectovaginal fistulas in which a significant portion of the patients underwent sphincteroplasty in addition to flap. Success rates have ranged from 74 to 95 % [37, 64–66]. In a series where all 20 patients had mucosal flaps in addition to sphincteroplasties, Khanduja et al. reported that drainage of stool and flatus stopped in all, and 14 had perfect continence while six reported their continence was improved [67].

Rectourethral Fistula

There are some reports of using endorectal advancement flaps for rectourethral fistulas. Parks and Motson described this in 1983 using a full-thickness flap in five patients with rectoprostatic fistulas [68]. All of these were done under the protection of a sigmoid colostomy, and all healed. Garofalo et al. treated 23 patients for rectourethral fistula, 12 of whom were treated with endorectal advancement flap [69]. They achieved initial success in 8 of the 12 patients, and two of the failures healed after repeat flap. Most of these patients had stomas, and the authors advocated for both fecal and urinary diversion prior to flap repair. Advancement flap may

Table 14.2 Results of endorectal advancement flap in Crohn's-associated rectovaginal fistulas

Authors	Number of patients	Success rate (%)
El-Gazzaz et al. [26]	47	43
Hull and Fazio [74]	24	67
Penninckx et al. [73]	11	55
MacRae et al. [75]	8	0
Athanasiadis et al. [53]	7	29
O'Leary et al. [76]	6	50
Morrison et al. [77]	2	100

thus be an option for rectourethral fistulas, and avoids some of the morbidity associated with procedures such as gracilis muscle flaps.

Crohn's Disease

Advancement flap is an attractive option in Crohn's disease because full-thickness sphincter division is avoided, which is of particularly great importance in these patients as they will be at greater risk for future fistulas. However, results have not been particularly promising. Among the nine patients with Crohn's disease who underwent flaps, five recurred in one study [70]. In a larger study of 32 patients with Crohn's undergoing a total of 36 flaps, four did not heal in the immediate postoperative period and the same fistula recurred after healing in an additional 11 patients [71]. The risk of recurrence of the operated fistula (as opposed to a new fistula in another location) was 46 % at 2 years, despite 18 of the 36 flaps being done under the protection of a diverting stoma. Thus, endorectal advancement flap may result in healing in some patients with Crohn's disease, but the risk of recurrence is high.

Rectovaginal Fistula Associated with Crohn's Disease

As difficult as it is to treat fistulas in the setting of Crohn's disease, rectovaginal fistulas in the setting of Crohn's disease present even greater challenges, and as a result there is rather extensive literature on the subject. The majority of studies, however, include only a small number of patients with Crohn's-associated rectovaginal fistulas undergoing flap procedures. Reported success rates after initial flap tend to be quite low (Table 14.2). Rectovaginal fistulas associated with Crohn's disease tend to have higher recurrence rates than those due to other etiologies [22, 72]. Among those with Crohn's, the number of sites involved with Crohn's has also been found to be associated with outcome [73], although another study found no association between Crohn's activity and failure [26]. Thus, endorectal advancement flap can certainly be used in an attempt to heal rectovaginal fistulas associated with Crohn's disease, but success rates are low. It may be that increased success rates are seen as the use of biologic immunomodulators becomes more prevalent.

Conclusion

Endorectal advancement flaps are a useful technique in the treatment of anal fistula. Advancement flaps are associated with a success rate that compares favorably to other surgeries for anal fistula. Flaps are associated with only a small risk of a decrement in continence, as they avoid full-thickness division of the anal sphincters. They can also be used in special situations such as Crohn's disease and rectovaginal fistulas. Surgeons treating anal fistulas should be well-versed in the technique of endorectal advancement flap.

Summary

- Endorectal advancement flap for anal fistula is successful in many patients and is a valuable tool for treating anal fistulas.
- Endorectal advancement flap avoids division of the anal sphincter muscles, but may still have deleterious effects on continence.
- Complex fistulas such as those arising from Crohn's disease or persisting after prior attempts at repair can be successfully addressed with endorectal advancement flaps.
- In general, modifications of the endorectal flap technique have not led to increased success rates.

References

1. Noble G. A new operation for complete laceration of the perineum designed for the purpose of eliminating danger of infection from the rectum. Trans Am Gynecol Soc. 1902;27:357–63.
2. Elting AWX. The treatment of fistula in ano: with especial reference to the whitehead operation. Ann Surg. 1912;56(5):744–52.
3. Laird DR. Procedures used in treatment of complicated fistulas. Am J Surg. 1948;76(6):701–8.
4. Aguilar PS, Plasencia G, Hardy Jr TG, Hartmann RF, Stewart WR. Mucosal advancement in the treatment of anal fistula. Dis Colon Rectum. 1985;28(7):496–8.
5. Jarrar A, Church J. Advancement flap repair: a good option for complex anorectal fistulas. Dis Colon Rectum. 2011;54(12): 1537–41.
6. Joo JS, Weiss EG, Nogueras JJ, Wexner SD. Endorectal advancement flap in perianal Crohn's disease. Am Surg. 1998;64(2): 147–50.
7. Ozuner G, Hull TL, Cartmill J, Fazio VW. Long-term analysis of the use of transanal rectal advancement flaps for complicated anorectal/vaginal fistulas. Dis Colon Rectum. 1996;39(1):10–4.
8. Perez F, Arroyo A, Serrano P, Sanchez A, Candela F, Perez MT, et al. Randomized clinical and manometric study of advancement flap versus fistulotomy with sphincter reconstruction in the management of complex fistula-in-ano. Am J Surg. 2006;192(1): 34–40.
9. Uribe N, Millan M, Minguez M, Ballester C, Asencio F, Sanchiz V, et al. Clinical and manometric results of endorectal advancement flaps for complex anal fistula. Int J Colorectal Dis. 2007;22(3):259–64.
10. Mizrahi N, Wexner SD, Zmora O, Da Silva G, Efron J, Weiss EG, et al. Endorectal advancement flap: are there predictors of failure? Dis Colon Rectum. 2002;45(12):1616–21.
11. Kreis ME, Jehle EC, Ohlemann M, Becker HD, Starlinger MJ. Functional results after transanal rectal advancement flap repair of trans-sphincteric fistula. Br J Surg. 1998;85(2):240–2.
12. Muhlmann MD, Hayes JL, Merrie AE, Parry BR, Bissett IP. Complex anal fistulas: plug or flap? ANZ J Surg. 2011;81(10): 720–4.
13. Abbas MA, Jackson CH, Haigh PI. Predictors of outcome for anal fistula surgery. Arch Surg. 2011;146(9):1011–6.
14. Ortiz H, Marzo J, Ciga MA, Oteiza F, Armendariz P, de Miguel M. Randomized clinical trial of anal fistula plug versus endorectal advancement flap for the treatment of high cryptoglandular fistula in ano. Br J Surg. 2009;96(6):608–12.
15. Abbas MA, Lemus-Rangel R, Hamadani A. Long-term outcome of endorectal advancement flap for complex anorectal fistulae. Am Surg. 2008;74(10):921–4.
16. Mitalas LE, Gosselink MP, Oom DM, Zimmerman DD, Schouten WR. Required length of follow-up after transanal advancement flap repair of high transsphincteric fistulas. Colorectal Dis Offic J Assoc Coloproctol Great Brit Ireland. 2009;11(7):726–8.
17. Ortiz H, Marzo M, de Miguel M, Ciga MA, Oteiza F, Armendariz P. Length of follow-up after fistulotomy and fistulectomy associated with endorectal advancement flap repair for fistula in ano. Br J Surg. 2008;95(4):484–7.
18. Mitalas LE, Gosselink MP, Zimmerman DD, Schouten WR. Repeat transanal advancement flap repair: impact on the overall healing rate of high transsphincteric fistulas and on fecal continence. Dis Colon Rectum. 2007;50(10):1508–11.
19. Christoforidis D, Pieh MC, Madoff RD, Mellgren AF. Treatment of transsphincteric anal fistulas by endorectal advancement flap or collagen fistula plug: a comparative study. Dis Colon Rectum. 2009;52(1):18–22.
20. Golub RW, Wise Jr WE, Kerner BA, Khanduja KS, Aguilar PS, Golub RW, Wise Jr WE, Kerner BA, Khanduja KS, Aguilar PS. Endorectal mucosal advancement flap: the preferred method for complex cryptoglandular fistula-in-ano. J Gastrointest Surg Offic J Soc Surg Aliment Tract. 1997;1(5):487–91.
21. Hyman N. Endoanal advancement flap repair for complex anorectal fistulas. Am J Surg. 1999;178(4):337–40.
22. Pinto RA, Peterson TV, Shawki S, Davila GW, Wexner SD. Are there predictors of outcome following rectovaginal fistula repair? Dis Colon Rectum. 2010;53(9):1240–7.
23. Schwandner O. Obesity is a negative predictor of success after surgery for complex anal fistula. BMC Gastroenterol. 2011;11:61.
24. Zimmerman DD, Delemarre JB, Gosselink MP, Hop WC, Briel JW, Schouten WR. Smoking affects the outcome of transanal mucosal advancement flap repair of trans-sphincteric fistulas. Br J Surg. 2003;90(3):351–4.
25. van Koperen PJ, Wind J, Bemelman WA, Bakx R, Reitsma JB, Slors JF. Long-term functional outcome and risk factors for recurrence after surgical treatment for low and high perianal fistulas of cryptoglandular origin. Dis Colon Rectum. 2008;51(10):1475–81.
26. El-Gazzaz G, Hull T, Mignanelli E, Hammel J, Gurland B, Zutshi M. Analysis of function and predictors of failure in women under-

going repair of Crohn's related rectovaginal fistula. J Gastrointest Surg Offic J Soc Surg Aliment Tract. 2010;14(5):824–9.

27. Ellis CN, Clark S. Effect of tobacco smoking on advancement flap repair of complex anal fistulas. Dis Colon Rectum. 2007;50(4):459–63.

28. Gustafsson UM, Graf W. Randomized clinical trial of local gentamicin-collagen treatment in advancement flap repair for anal fistula. Br J Surg. 2006;93(10):1202–7.

29. Sonoda T, Hull T, Piedmonte MR, Fazio VW. Outcomes of primary repair of anorectal and rectovaginal fistulas using the endorectal advancement flap. Dis Colon Rectum. 2002;45(12):1622–8.

30. Gustafsson UM, Graf W. Excision of anal fistula with closure of the internal opening: functional and manometric results. Dis Colon Rectum. 2002;45(12):1672–8.

31. Mitalas LE, Schouten SB, Gosselink MP, Oom DM, Zimmerman DD, Schouten WR. Does rectal mucosal blood flow affect the outcome of transanal advancement flap repair? Dis Colon Rectum. 2009;52(8):1395–9.

32. Kraemer M, Kirschmeier A, Marth T. Perioperative adjuvant therapy with infliximab in complicated anal Crohn's disease. Int J Colorectal Dis. 2008;23(10):965–9.

33. El-Gazzaz G, Hull T, Church JM. Biological immunomodulators improve the healing rate in surgically treated perianal Crohn's fistulas. Colorectal Dis offic J Assoc Coloproctol Great Brit Ireland. 2012;14(10):1217–23.

34. Mitalas LE, Dwarkasing RS, Verhaaren R, Zimmerman DD, Schouten WR. Is the outcome of transanal advancement flap repair affected by the complexity of high transsphincteric fistulas? Dis Colon Rectum. 2011;54(7):857–62.

35. Kodner IJ, Mazor A, Shemesh EI, Fry RD, Fleshman JW, Birnbaum EH. Endorectal advancement flap repair of rectovaginal and other complicated anorectal fistulas. Surgery. 1993;114(4):682–9. discussion 9–90.

36. Schouten WR, Zimmerman DD, Briel JW. Transanal advancement flap repair of transsphincteric fistulas. Dis Colon Rectum. 1999;42(11):1419–22. discussion 22–3.

37. Lowry AC, Thorson AG, Rothenberger DA, Goldberg SM. Repair of simple rectovaginal fistulas. Influence of previous repairs. Dis Colon Rectum. 1988;31(9):676–8.

38. Tsang CB, Madoff RD, Wong WD, Rothenberger DA, Finne CO, Singer D, et al. Anal sphincter integrity and function influences outcome in rectovaginal fistula repair. Dis Colon Rectum. 1998;41(9):1141–6.

39. Mitalas LE, van Wijk JJ, Gosselink MP, Doornebosch P, Zimmerman DD, Schouten WR. Seton drainage prior to transanal advancement flap repair: useful or not? Int J Colorectal Dis. 2010;25(12):1499–502.

40. Soltani A, Kaiser AM. Endorectal advancement flap for cryptoglandular or Crohn's fistula-in-ano. Dis Colon Rectum. 2010;53(4):486–95.

41. Dubsky PC, Stift A, Friedl J, Teleky B, Herbst F. Endorectal advancement flaps in the treatment of high anal fistula of cryptoglandular origin: full-thickness vs. mucosal-rectum flaps. Dis Colon Rectum. 2008;51(6):852–7.

42. van Koperen PJ, Wind J, Bemelman WA, Slors JF. Fibrin glue and transanal rectal advancement flap for high transsphincteric perianal fistulas; is there any advantage? Int J Colorectal Dis. 2008;23(7):697–701.

43. Ellis CN, Clark S. Fibrin glue as an adjunct to flap repair of anal fistulas: a randomized, controlled study. Dis Colon Rectum. 2006;49(11):1736–40.

44. Sileri P, Franceschilli L, Del Vecchio BG, Stolfi VM, Angelucci GP, Gaspari AL. Porcine dermal collagen matrix injection may enhance flap repair surgery for complex anal fistula. Int J Colorectal Dis. 2011;26(3):345–9.

45. van Onkelen RS, Gosselink MP, Schouten WR. Is it possible to improve the outcome of transanal advancement flap repair for high transsphincteric fistulas by additional ligation of the intersphincteric fistula tract? Dis Colon Rectum. 2012;55(2):163–6.

46. Miller GV, Finan PJ. Flap advancement and core fistulectomy for complex rectal fistula. Br J Surg. 1998;85(1):108–10.

47. Lewis WG, Finan PJ, Holdsworth PJ, Sagar PM, Stephenson BM. Clinical results and manometric studies after rectal flap advancement for infra-levator trans-sphincteric fistula-in-ano. Int J Colorectal Dis. 1995;10(4):189–92.

48. van der Hagen SJ, Baeten CG, Soeters PB, van Gemert WG. Long-term outcome following mucosal advancement flap for high perianal fistulas and fistulotomy for low perianal fistulas: recurrent perianal fistulas: failure of treatment or recurrent patient disease? Int J Colorectal Dis. 2006;21(8):784–90.

49. Ortiz H, Marzo J. Endorectal flap advancement repair and fistulectomy for high trans-sphincteric and suprasphincteric fistulas. Br J Surg. 2000;87(12):1680–3.

50. Joy HA, Williams JG. The outcome of surgery for complex anal fistula. Colorectal Dis Offic J Assoc Coloproctol Great Brit Ireland. 2002;4(4):254–61.

51. Roig JV, Jordan J, Garcia-Armengol J, Esclapez P, Solana A. Changes in anorectal morphologic and functional parameters after fistula-in-ano surgery. Dis Colon Rectum. 2009;52(8):1462–9.

52. Koehler A, Risse-Schaaf A, Athanasiadis S. Treatment for horseshoe fistulas-in-ano with primary closure of the internal fistula opening: a clinical and manometric study. Dis Colon Rectum. 2004;47(11):1874–82.

53. Athanasiadis S, Yazigi R, Kohler A, Helmes C. Recovery rates and functional results after repair for rectovaginal fistula in Crohn's disease: a comparison of different techniques. Int J Colorectal Dis. 2007;22(9):1051–60.

54. van Koperen PJ, Bemelman WA, Gerhards MF, Janssen LW, van Tets WF, van Dalsen AD, et al. The anal fistula plug treatment compared with the mucosal advancement flap for cryptoglandular high transsphincteric perianal fistula: a double-blinded multicenter randomized trial. Dis Colon Rectum. 2011;54(4):387–93.

55. A ba-bai-ke-re MM, Wen H, Huang HG, Chu H, Lu M, Chang ZS, et al. Randomized controlled trial of minimally invasive surgery using acellular dermal matrix for complex anorectal fistula. World J Gastroenterol. 2010;16(26):3279–86.

56. Wang JY, Garcia-Aguilar J, Sternberg JA, Abel ME, Varma MG. Treatment of transsphincteric anal fistulas: are fistula plugs an acceptable alternative? Dis Colon Rectum. 2009;52(4):692–7.

57. Chung W, Kazemi P, Ko D, Sun C, Brown CJ, Raval M, et al. Anal fistula plug and fibrin glue versus conventional treatment in repair of complex anal fistulas. Am J Surg. 2009;197(5):604–8.

58. Chung W, Ko D, Sun C, Raval MJ, Brown CJ, Phang PT. Outcomes of anal fistula surgery in patients with inflammatory bowel disease. Am J Surg. 2010;199(5):609–13.

59. Hoexter B, Labow SB, Moseson MD. Transanal rectovaginal fistula repair. Dis Colon Rectum. 1985;28(8):572–5.

60. Hilsabeck JR. Transanal advancement of the anterior rectal wall for vaginal fistulas involving the lower rectum. Dis Colon Rectum. 1980;23(4):236–41.

61. Russell TR, Gallagher DM. Low rectovaginal fistulas. Approach and treatment. Am Journal Surg. 1977;134(1):13–8.

62. Watson SJ, Phillips RK. Non-inflammatory rectovaginal fistula. Br J Surg. 1995;82(12):1641–3.

63. Mazier WP, Senagore AJ, Schiesel EC. Operative repair of anovaginal and rectovaginal fistulas. Dis Colon Rectum. 1995;38(1):4–6.

64. Rothenberger DA, Christenson CE, Balcos EG, Schottler JL, Nemer FD, Nivatvongs S, et al. Endorectal advancement flap for

treatment of simple rectovaginal fistula. Dis Colon Rectum. 1982;25(4):297–300.

65. Baig MK, Zhao RH, Yuen CH, Nogueras JJ, Singh JJ, Weiss EG, et al. Simple rectovaginal fistulas. Int J Colorectal Dis. 2000;15(5–6):323–7.

66. Wise Jr WE, Aguilar PS, Padmanabhan A, Meesig DM, Arnold MW, Stewart WR. Surgical treatment of low rectovaginal fistulas. Dis Colon Rectum. 1991;34(3):271–4.

67. Khanduja KS, Padmanabhan A, Kerner BA, Wise WE, Aguilar PS. Reconstruction of rectovaginal fistula with sphincter disruption by combining rectal mucosal advancement flap and anal sphinctero-plasty. Dis Colon Rectum. 1999;42(11):1432–7.

68. Parks AG, Motson RW. Peranal repair of rectoprostatic fistula. Br J Surg. 1983;70(12):725–6.

69. Garofalo TE, Delaney CP, Jones SM, Remzi FH, Fazio VW. Rectal advancement flap repair of rectourethral fistula: a 20-year experience. Dis Colon Rectum. 2003;46(6):762–9.

70. van Koperen PJ, Safiruddin F, Bemelman WA, Slors JF. Outcome of surgical treatment for fistula in ano in Crohn's disease. Br J Surg. 2009;96(6):675–9.

71. Makowiec F, Jehle EC, Becker HD, Starlinger M. Clinical course after transanal advancement flap repair of perianal fistula in patients with Crohn's disease. Br J Surg. 1995;82(5):603–6.

72. Halverson AL, Hull TL, Fazio VW, Church J, Hammel J, Floruta C. Repair of recurrent rectovaginal fistulas. Surgery. 2001;130(4):753–7. discussion 7–8.

73. Penninckx F, Moneghini D, D'Hoore A, Wyndaele J, Coremans G, Rutgeerts P. Success and failure after repair of rectovaginal fistula in Crohn's disease: analysis of prognostic factors. Colorectal Dis Offic1 J Assoc Coloproctol Great Brit Ireland. 2001;3(6):406–11.

74. Hull TL, Fazio VW. Surgical approaches to low anovaginal fistula in Crohn's disease. Am J Surg. 1997;173(2):95–8.

75. MacRae HM, McLeod RS, Cohen Z, Stern H, Reznick R. Treatment of rectovaginal fistulas that has failed previous repair attempts. Dis Colon Rectum. 1995;38(9):921–5.

76. O'Leary DP, Milroy CE, Durdey P. Definitive repair of anovaginal fistula in Crohn's disease. Ann R Coll Surg Engl. 1998;80(4):250–2.

77. Morrison JG, Gathright Jr JB, Ray JE, Ferrari BT, Hicks TC, Timmcke AE. Results of operation for rectovaginal fistula in Crohn's disease. Dis Colon Rectum. 1989;32(6):497–9.

Dermal Advancement Flap

Christine C. Jensen

Introduction

Because of the challenging nature of anal fistulas, a number of procedures have been developed to treat fistulas. All of these procedures have their benefits and drawbacks; dermal advancement flap is no exception. Dermal flaps can be a useful tool in treating fistulas, and may have particular benefits in certain situations. The technique of dermal advancement flap is presented here, along with a review of the relevant literature including healing rates and effects on continence.

Technique

The patient undergoes no specific preparation other than perhaps some enemas to clear the rectum, and does not need perioperative antibiotics. Many surgeons, however, prefer to perform the procedure with the addition of bowel preparation and perioperative antibiotics. A general or regional anesthetic is induced, and the patient is positioned in prone jackknife position. Proper positioning is crucial, with the patient's hips on a hip roll at the break in the bed and the bed in maximum flexion. The buttocks are taped apart. A headlight is necessary to assist with visualization of the anal canal.

After the patient is prepped and draped, an elliptical incision is made incorporating the internal opening of the fistula (Fig. 15.1, panel a). The ellipse is slightly more narrow at the end with the internal opening of the fistula than at the distal end. The ellipse can also incorporate the external opening of the fistula, so that the fistula tract remains beneath the skin being used for the flap. The internal opening is then excised, including a small portion of the internal sphincter surrounding

the internal opening (Fig. 15.1, panel b). Once the flap is adequately mobilized and can reach without tension, the flap is advanced into the anal canal such that it covers the internal opening. It is then sewn into place with absorbable suture, such as 3-0 polyglactin. Because the flap has been advanced into the anal canal, there remains an open area of exposed subcutaneous fat in the perianal area, which is left open to heal by secondary intention (Fig. 15.1, panel c). Note that the fistula tract is not excised, and passes beneath the dermal flap.

Although some studies report a postoperative hospitalization of a few days [1–4], patients can usually be discharged the same day with narcotic pain medication and instructions for sitz baths. Postoperative antibiotics are not necessary. A bulking agent may be helpful to avoid postoperative constipation. Particularly for male patients, it is helpful to keep them in the recovery area until they have demonstrated the ability to void as urinary retention can occur.

Modifications of the dermal flap include the V-Y flap and the "house" flap (Fig. 15.2). As in the standard flap procedure, the internal opening is excised and the flap advanced into the anal canal. In both of these modifications, however, the open area in the perianal skin resulting from advancement of the flap is able to be closed due to the geometry of the flap.

Results

Healing of Fistula

Dermal flap has a good success rate for healing anal fistulas, with most healing rates reported to be in the 70–80 % range (Table 15.1). In fact, the healing rate may be even greater than this, as many of the studies demonstrating lower success rates had small numbers of patients. In the three largest studies, each including at least 40 patients and together comprising 170 patients, the healing rate was at least 80 % in each study [5–7]. When the three studies are aggregated, the combined success rate is 88 %. Thus, the healing rate for dermal flap is

C.C. Jensen, M.D., M.P.H. (✉)
Department of Surgery, University of Minnesota,
1055 Westgate Drive, Ste 190, St. Paul, MN, 55114, USA
e-mail: cjensen@crsal.org

H. Abcarian (ed.), *Anal Fistula: Principles and Management*, DOI 10.1007/978-1-4614-9014-2_15,
© Springer Science+Business Media New York 2014

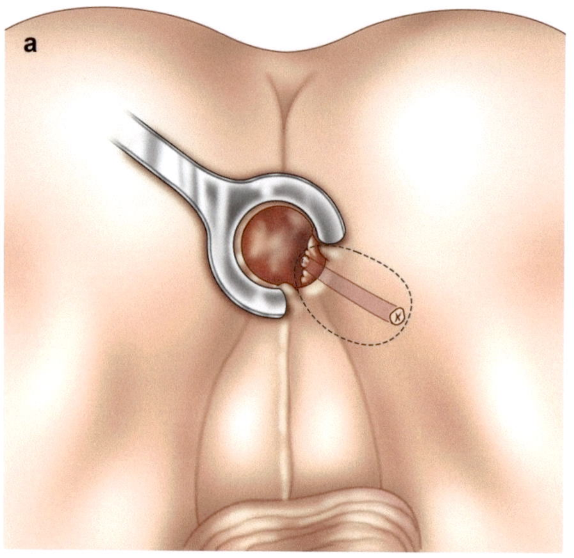

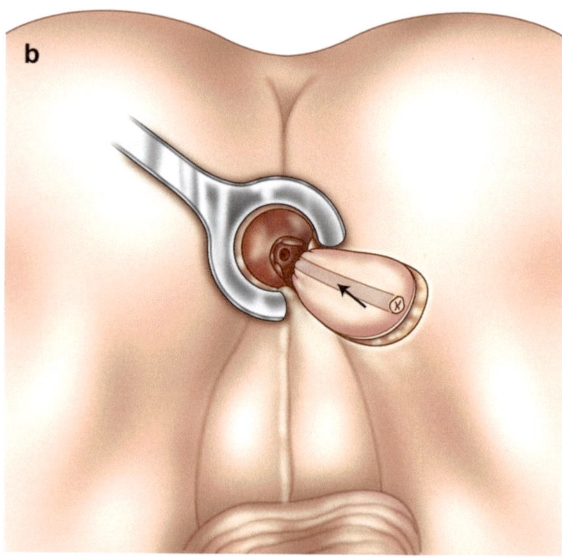

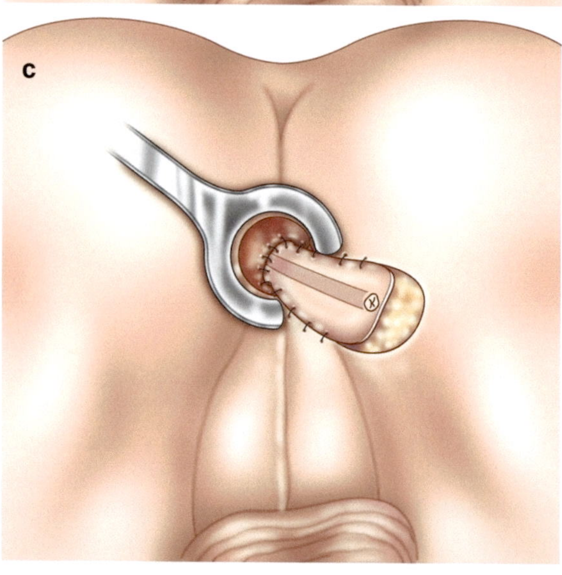

Fig. 15.1 Dermal flap for treatment of anal fistula. (**a**) Flap is marked out, incorporating both the internal and external fistula openings. (**b**) Originating crypt is excised and flap is advanced. (**c**) Flap is sewn into place, leaving open area of subcutaneous fat to heal by secondary intention

quite high, particularly if it is performed by surgeons who use dermal flaps frequently to treat anal fistula.

Because of the amount of dissection required, the wounds from dermal flap repair may take several weeks to heal. Overall, it appears most operative sites will heal in approximately 6 weeks [3, 7–9]. However, average healing times of as little as 2–3 weeks [5], or as long as 3 months [10], have been reported. Patients should therefore be counseled that it may be several weeks before complete healing is achieved.

The observed recurrence rate may depend partially on the duration for which the patient is followed. Among ten women with anovaginal fistulas associated with Crohn's disease and repaired with dermal flaps, Hesterberg et al. observed recurrences at 4, 8, and 13 months [11]. In the large case series by Nelson et al., the latest recurrence was at 20 months [6]. Thus, success rates may vary depending on the length of follow-up, as recurrences can occur even more than 1 year after operation.

Complications

Complications associated with dermal flap are generally minor. The most commonly reported complication is minor separation of the external portion of the flap. Reported rates of this complication range from 5 % [7] to 50 % [9], with other reports falling between these two extremes [1, 8]. However, if the dermal flap is performed in the manner described earlier in this chapter, leaving a portion of the wound in the perianal skin open, this complication is rare. It seems this complication is more likely to occur when the skin is completely closed, as with a V-Y or house flap, likely due to excessive tension on the wound.

Another reported complication is urinary retention. Urinary retention was reported in 6 of 65 patients by Sungurtekin et al. [7] and 8 of 29 patients by Sentovich et al. [4], although the vast majority of flaps in the Sentovich study were performed for indications other than anal fistula. Other reported complications include persistent external fistula tract after healing of the internal opening [6] and infectious complications (*Clostridium difficile* infection, urinary tract infection, cellulitis) [4]. In a randomized controlled trial, Ho and Ho found no difference in complication rates or postoperative pain between dermal flaps and fistulotomy or seton placement, although this study only included 20 patients [3]. Thus, dermal flap is associated with a low rate of complications, particularly if a portion of the external wound is left open to prevent dehiscence of the wound.

Effect of Other Factors on Healing Rates

Characteristics of the fistula can have an effect on whether the fistula heals, or whether it recurs after initial healing.

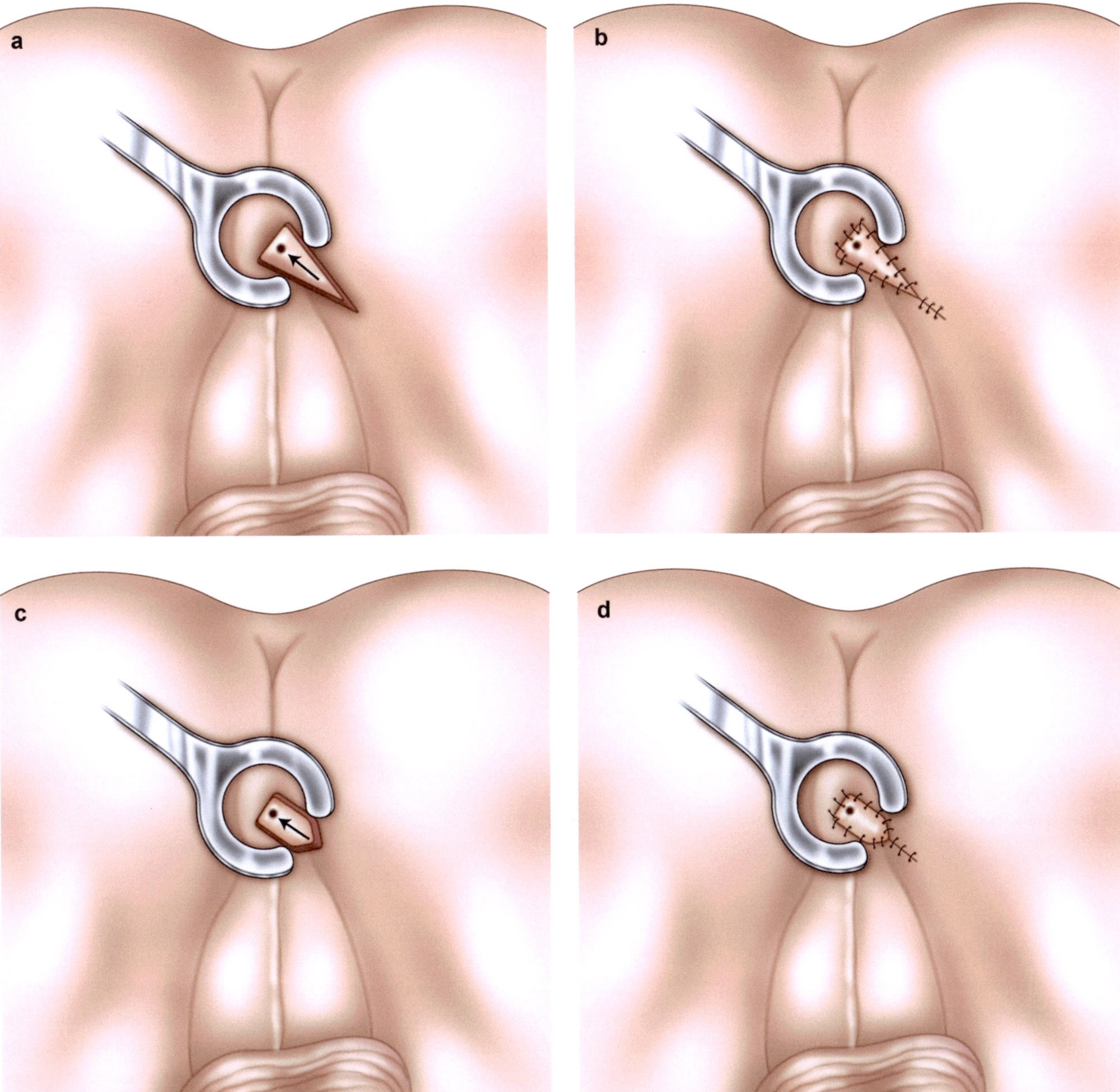

Fig. 15.2 Variations of dermal flap. (**a**) Mobilized tissue for V-Y flap. (**b**) Completed V-Y flap. (**c**) Mobilized tissue for house flap. (**d**) Completed house flap

Fistulas that have failed prior attempts at repair may be less likely to heal with a dermal flap. This was found by both Zimmerman et al. [10] and Ellis and Clark [12], with Nelson et al. also finding a trend toward greater recurrence in patients who had failed prior repairs [6]. Although type of fistula seems as if it would affect healing rates, this has not been demonstrated [12]; Nelson et al. did find that rectovaginal fistulas arising from obstetric injury were associated with a lower healing rate but this was due to a single patient requiring four operations to heal a rectovaginal fistula [6].

Similarly, patient characteristics may affect healing rates. There may be a slightly higher success rate in women [10].

Age has not been found to affect recurrence rates [10, 12]. Ellis and Clark also reported a higher recurrence rate with smoking, but less than a third of these patients had dermal flaps [12]. The majority had endorectal advancement flaps, so it is unclear whether this association would hold if only dermal flaps were examined.

Modifications to the dermal flap technique have not been demonstrated to improve the healing rate. Nelson et al. found that injection of fibrin glue into the fistula tract in conjunction with dermal flap actually increased recurrence rates [6]. Ellis also found increased recurrence with fibrin glue injection in a randomized controlled trial, although dermal flaps represented

Table 15.1 Results of dermal flap repair of anal fistulas

Authors	Number of patients	Fistula type	Primary success rate (%)	Ultimate success rate (%)	Comments
Alver et al. [1][a]	4	3 TS 1 RVF	75	100	RVF did not heal
Amin et al. [15]	18	10 TS 4 IS 4 SS	72	83	
Athanasiadis et al. [2][a]	14	RVF	85	–	All patients had Crohn's disease
Chew and Adams [14]	6	TS	100	–	Internal sphincter was incorporated into flap
Del Pino et al. [18]	11	TS	73	–	Recurrence in 2 of 3 patients with Crohn's
Ellis and Clark [13][a]	22	"Complex"	75	–	Success rate is for dermal flap without fibrin glue
Ellis and Clark [12][a]	27	25 TS 2 RVF	78	–	
Hesterberg et al. [11]	10	RVF	70	90	All patients had Crohn's disease
Ho and Ho [3][a]	10	TS	100	–	
Hossack et al. [9]	16	SS	94	–	
Jun and Choi [5]	40	35 TS 5 SS	98	–	
Koehler et al. [17][a]	8	Dorsal horseshoe	75	–	
Nelson et al. [6]	65	Mixed	80	–	
Robertson et al. [8]	20	Not stated	70	–	Six patients had Crohn's disease
Sentovich et al. [4][a]	1	"Perineal"	0	–	
Sungurtekin et al. [7]	65	49 TS 15 SS 1 RVF	91	–	
Zimmerman et al. [10]	26	TS	46	–	

Primary success rate is the percentage healed after first attempt at repair with advancement flap; ultimate success rate is percentage healed after additional intervention for initial failures

TS transsphincteric, *SS* suprasphincteric, *ES* extrasphincteric, *IS* intersphincteric

[a]Study included other interventions (e.g., endorectal flap) or other pathology (e.g., anal stenosis) but reported results are only for patients who had dermal flap for fistula

only 38 % of the flaps in this study, with the remainder being endorectal advancement flaps [13]. Chew described including a segment of internal sphincter with the flap and reported healing in all patients; however, this report only included six patients [14]. Thus, modifications to the dermal flap have not improved the success rate of the procedure.

Continence

Clinical Results

Although dermal flap does not involve division of anal sphincter musculature, it may still be associated with a decrement in continence. This may be due to stretching of the sphincter muscles by the retractor during operation, which would potentially have only a temporary effect on continence. Advancement of the dermal flap into the anal canal could also affect closure of the anus, preventing tight sealing and leading to seepage.

Data are mixed in terms of the effect of continence observed after dermal flap. Some studies have shown no effect on continence, although in some studies the means of assessing continence are not well detailed [7, 15, 16]. Robertson and Mangione found only 1 of 20 patients had deterioration in continence, which was the new onset of minor incontinence to flatus [8]. However, two studies that used questionnaires to assess pre- and postoperative continence show a more mixed result in terms of the effect of dermal flap on continence. Using the St. Mark's hospital incontinence score, Hossack et al. found that continence improved in 69 % of patients and mean incontinence scores decreased, likely due to cessation of drainage from the fistula [9]. Three of the 16 patients in this study had deterioration in continence, which was a decrease in control over flatus. However, all three also reported a decrease in soiling. One of these three patients reported increased urgency and the need to continue pad use as a result. Of note, the authors mention that some of the patients had a decrease in the ability to control flatus in the immediate postoperative period but ultimately reported improved continence. This may be due to stretching of the sphincters during surgery, and therefore patients who report decreased continence in the immediate postoperative period should be counseled that this may resolve.

The second study that used pre- and postoperative questionnaires provided less reassuring results regarding continence. Zimmerman et al. evaluated 26 patients having dermal flap repair of transsphincteric fistulas, 23 of whom completed a continence questionnaire [10]. Twenty-two percent had improvement in continence, but 30 % had a deterioration. Of 11 patients with perfect continence preoperatively, two had soiling and incontinence to flatus, and two had loss of full bowel movements postoperatively. Of those with some degree of preoperative incontinence, two had deterioration in continence. Perhaps some of the high prevalence of deterioration in continence may be due to the presence of prior attempts at repair, as 20 of the 26 patients in this study had prior attempts at repair. If these attempts involved division of part of the anal sphincters, the addition of the dermal flap may have been enough to make the incontinence clinically apparent. Thus, the effect of dermal flap on continence may vary significantly between patients, and patients should be cautioned as to the potential for increased symptoms of incontinence as a risk associated with dermal flap.

Manometric Results

Only one study has examined manometric results after dermal advancement flap. Koehler et al. treated 42 patients with dorsal horseshoe cryptoglandular fistulas with one of four methods of closing the internal opening: mucosal flap, partial- or full-thickness endorectal advancement flap, dermal flap, or direct (suture) closure [17]. Only eight of these patients underwent dermal flap. They reported new incontinence in 12 patients, but it is not possible to determine from the data presented how many of these were within the group treated with dermal flaps. Mean resting pressures decreased from 137 cm H_2O preoperatively to 101 cm H_2O postoperatively among patients who had a dermal flap, and mean squeeze pressures from 297 to 229 cm H_2O. No procedure was found to be better than another in terms of the change in resting and squeeze pressures. Since no sphincter muscle is divided during creation of the dermal flap, it may be that these decreases in sphincter pressure are due to stretching of the sphincter muscles by the retractor during the operation and may therefore be temporary. Thus, dermal flap is likely associated with some decrease in resting and squeeze pressures, but this decrease is similar to that observed with other procedures.

Comparison with Other Surgeries for Fistula

Several studies have compared the recurrence rates associated with dermal flap to other surgeries for fistula, and in general these studies have found no difference in recurrence rates between the various operations. Ho and Ho did a randomized controlled trial comparing dermal flap to "conventional treatment," which was fistulotomy or seton placement, and found no difference in success rates [3]. Similarly, Koehler et al. found no difference between mucosa–submucosa endorectal flap, partial- or full-thickness endorectal flap, internal opening closure, and dermal flap in healing of horseshoe fistulas [17]. In a meta-analysis among women with rectovaginal fistulas associated with Crohn's disease, Penninckx et al. found no difference in healing rates for endorectal advancement flap, vaginal flap, dermal flap, or perineoproctotomy [16]. However, only one study was included in the meta-analysis that included patients with dermal advancement flap. In contrast, Athanasiadis et al. found dermal flaps had an 85 % success rate in this population as compared to 29 % for rectal flaps [2]. However, all of these studies include relatively small numbers of patients undergoing each surgery, so their ability to detect a difference in success rates between methods is questionable.

Special Situations

Crohn's Disease

Dermal flap may be ideally suited to patients with Crohn's disease. Provided there is not extensive perianal disease with scarring from prior fistulas, dermal flap can bring unaffected tissue into the area in an attempt to heal the fistula. Many patients with Crohn's disease may also have anal stenosis, and dermal flap can be used to treat both problems at one operation. Unfortunately, there are few reports of the use of dermal flap in Crohn's disease. The largest number is in Nelson's report of 65 patients treated with dermal flap, of which 17 had Crohn's disease and successful healing was achieved in 15 [6]. Robertson and Mangione achieved healing in three of six patients with Crohn's, but pursued a very conservative regimen in these patients including either proximal diversion or total parenteral nutrition for 6 weeks after repair [8]. Among the 11 patients treated with dermal flap by Del Pino et al., three had Crohn's disease but only one healed [18]. Thus, dermal flap can be used successfully in Crohn's disease, but there are few reports on its efficacy.

Rectovaginal Fistulas Associated with Crohn's Disease

An even more difficult situation is rectovaginal or anovaginal fistula associated with Crohn's disease. Two studies have examined the use of dermal flaps in this situation. Athanasiadis et al. treated 37 women with Crohn's rectovaginal fistulas with a total of 56 procedures, 14 of which were dermal flaps [2]. They achieved an 85 % success rate over a period of follow-up ranging from 10 months to 18 years. Of note, the majority of these patients had diverting ileostomies, and the numbers of patients with dermal flaps were too small to evaluate whether the presence of an ileostomy contributed significantly to healing in these patients.

Hesterberg et al. performed dermal flaps in ten women with Crohn's anovaginal fistulas [11]. Seven of these had proctitis and therefore had diverting stomas. All patients healed initially, and three recurrences were observed during a median follow-up of 18 months. One healed after repeat flap, one healed after fibrin injection, and one patient had a seton in place at the time of the report. Of note, five of these patients had anal stenosis and four were reported to be improved after surgery. This demonstrates the utility of dermal flaps in Crohn's disease where anal stenosis can be a frequent problem, and can be addressed at the same time as the fistula by using a dermal flap. Thus, there appears to be a role for dermal flap in the treatment of anovaginal or rectovaginal fistulas related to Crohn's disease.

Conclusion

Dermal flap should be considered as an option when treating a patient with an anal fistula. Dermal flaps are associated with a good success rate, particularly when performed by a surgeon with experience performing dermal flaps. Dermal flaps can be particularly useful in the presence of coexisting anal pathology such as anal stenosis or Crohn's disease. Although dermal flap does not divide the anal sphincters, it can be associated with a decrement in continence in some patients, although other patients will experience improved continence. Surgeons should be familiar with dermal flaps as an option in order to allow most appropriate procedure to be selected to treat the patient with an anal fistula.

Summary

- Dermal advancement flap is an important procedure for the treatment of anal fistulas and is associated with a good success rate in healing the fistula.
- Dermal advancement flap avoids division of the anal sphincter muscles, but may still have deleterious effects on continence.
- Dermal advancement flap can be particularly useful in the presence of other anorectal pathology, such as anal stenosis or Crohn's disease.
- While dermal advancement flap is not used as frequently as other procedures for anal fistula, surgeons should be familiar with this technique.

References

1. Alver O, Ersoy YE, Aydemir I, Erguney S, Teksoz S, Apaydin B, et al. Use of "house" advancement flap in anorectal diseases. World J Surg. 2008;32(10):2281–6.
2. Athanasiadis S, Yazigi R, Kohler A, Helmes C. Recovery rates and functional results after repair for rectovaginal fistula in Crohn's disease: a comparison of different techniques. Int J Colorectal Dis. 2007;22(9):1051–60.
3. Ho KS, Ho YH. Controlled, randomized trial of island flap anoplasty for treatment of trans-sphincteric fistula-in-ano: early results. Tech Coloproctol. 2005;9(2):166–8.
4. Sentovich SM, Falk PM, Christensen MA, Thorson AG, Blatchford GJ, Pitsch RM. Operative results of house advancement anoplasty. Br J Surg. 1996;83(9):1242–4.
5. Jun SH, Choi GS. Anocutaneous advancement flap closure of high anal fistulas. Br J Surg. 1999;86(4):490–2.
6. Nelson RL, Cintron J, Abcarian H. Dermal island-flap anoplasty for transsphincteric fistula-in-ano: assessment of treatment failures. Dis Colon Rectum. 2000;43(5):681–4.
7. Sungurtekin U, Sungurtekin H, Kabay B, Tekin K, Aytekin F, Erdem E, et al. Anocutaneous V-Y advancement flap for the treatment of complex perianal fistula. Dis Colon Rectum. 2004; 47(12):2178–83.
8. Robertson WG, Mangione JS. Cutaneous advancement flap closure: alternative method for treatment of complicated anal fistulas. Dis Colon Rectum. 1998;41(7):884–6; discussion 6–7.
9. Hossack T, Solomon MJ, Young JM. Ano-cutaneous flap repair for complex and recurrent supra-sphincteric anal fistula. Colorectal Dis. 2005;7(2):187–92.
10. Zimmerman DD, Briel JW, Gosselink MP, Schouten WR. Anocutaneous advancement flap repair of transsphincteric fistulas. Dis Colon Rectum. 2001;44(10):1474–80.
11. Hesterberg R, Schmidt WU, Muller F, Roher HD. Treatment of anovaginal fistulas with an anocutaneous flap in patients with Crohn's disease. Int J Colorectal Dis. 1993;8(1):51–4.
12. Ellis CN, Clark S. Effect of tobacco smoking on advancement flap repair of complex anal fistulas. Dis Colon Rectum. 2007;50(4): 459–63.
13. Ellis CN, Clark S. Fibrin glue as an adjunct to flap repair of anal fistulas: a randomized, controlled study. Dis Colon Rectum. 2006; 49(11):1736–40.
14. Chew SS, Adams WJ. Anal sphincter advancement flap for low transsphincteric anal fistula. Dis Colon Rectum. 2007;50(7):1090–3.
15. Amin SN, Tierney GM, Lund JN, Armitage NC. V-Y advancement flap for treatment of fistula-in-ano. Dis Colon Rectum. 2003; 46(4):540–3.
16. Penninckx F, Moneghini D, D'Hoore A, Wyndaele J, Coremans G, Rutgeerts P. Success and failure after repair of rectovaginal fistula in Crohn's disease: analysis of prognostic factors. Colorectal Dis. 2001;3(6):406–11.
17. Koehler A, Risse-Schaaf A, Athanasiadis S. Treatment for horseshoe fistulas-in-ano with primary closure of the internal fistula opening: a clinical and manometric study. Dis Colon Rectum. 2004;47(11):1874–82.
18. Del Pino A, Nelson RL, Pearl RK, Abcarian H. Island flap anoplasty for treatment of transsphincteric fistula-in-ano. Dis Colon Rectum. 1996;39(2):224–6.

Ligation of Intersphincteric Fistula Tract (LIFT)

Ariane M. Abcarian

Introduction

The main tenets in treating fistula in ano are the amount of sphincter involved and the acceptable risks of incontinence. These considerations have led to the development of various sphincter sparing options throughout the years. This chapter will focus on the ligation of intersphincteric fistula tract (LIFT) procedure.

The LIFT procedure was initially described by Rojanasakul in 2007 [1]. The operation is appropriate for transsphincteric fistulas with length sufficient enough to perform the procedure. In Rojanasakul's initial paper the LIFT technique is impressive in its simplicity [2]. A probe is passed through the fistula tract to identify and connect the external and internal openings. A curvilinear incision is made approximately 1 cm from and parallel to the anal canal (Fig. 16.1a). The fibers of the internal and external sphincter are separated and the intersphincteric groove is entered. The fistula tract is identified (Fig. 16.1b). The tract is isolated, severed, and suture ligated at both ends and severed after removal of the fistula probe (Fig. 16.1c, d). The medial ligature obliterates the internal opening. If the tract length warrants, a portion of the tract may be excised, increasing the distance between the two suture-ligated ends (Fig. 16.1e). The internal and external sphincter are reapproximated; the skin is closed loosely. The external opening is enlarged and left open to drain and heal secondarily (Fig. 16.1f). Illustrations of the original LIFT procedure, including our variation, are shown in Fig. 16.1a–f [3]. Intraoperative photos are shown in Fig. 16.2a–d.

Subtle variations of the original technique are described. We prefer to remove a portion of the tract if the length allows it [3]. The closure of the tract after suture ligation may be

tested, either with direct probing or with injection of hydrogen peroxide or saline [2, 4, 5]. Postoperative admission for observation is not necessary. Several series report discharging patients with a week of oral antibiotics [2, 4, 5]. There is no consensus on the use of seton preoperatively. As a standard, at our institution, setons are used to drain all infection prior to undertaking definitive surgical repair of the fistula and many of the other series do so as well. There is anecdotal evidence that when the seton is left in place 8–12 weeks prior to LIFT, the tract fibroses nicely, making it easily identifiable and, in many cases, easier to dissect free from the surrounding tissues ensuring a successful ligation [3, 6]. Routine diagnostic imaging preoperatively or postoperatively with either MRI or endorectal ultrasound is not necessary. Diagnosis of fistula and treatment failures can be decided clinically.

This operation may be performed in prone jackknife or lithotomy position, under either regional or general anesthesia. Some surgeons use lithotomy or prone jackknife position depending on the location of the fistula [7]. Bowel preparation consists of two phospho soda enemas the day before surgery. Patients are administered only a single dose of appropriate peri-operative antibiotics intravenously, usually cefoxitin, or ciprofloxacin/metronidazole if the patient is penicillin-allergic. At the end of the procedure, a dibucaine-coated piece of gelfoam is rolled and gently inserted into the anal canal for analgesia. The patients are not admitted for observation and are sent home directly from the recovery unit on oral analgesics and stool softeners [3].

Results/Discussion

Rojanasakul's initial LIFT series in 2007 was a prospective observational study of 18 patients with fistula in ano [1]. He reported 94.4 % (17/18) healing, and one non-healing at 4 weeks of follow-up. There was no reported incontinence [1]. These impressive results set the mark for LIFT to become a promising option in treating fistula in ano, particularly

A.M. Abcarian, M.D. (✉)
Department of Surgery, University of Minnesota,
1055 Westgate Drive, Ste 190, St. Paul, MN 55114, USA
e-mail: cjensen@crsal.org

H. Abcarian (ed.), *Anal Fistula: Principles and Management*, DOI 10.1007/978-1-4614-9014-2_16,
© Springer Science+Business Media New York 2014

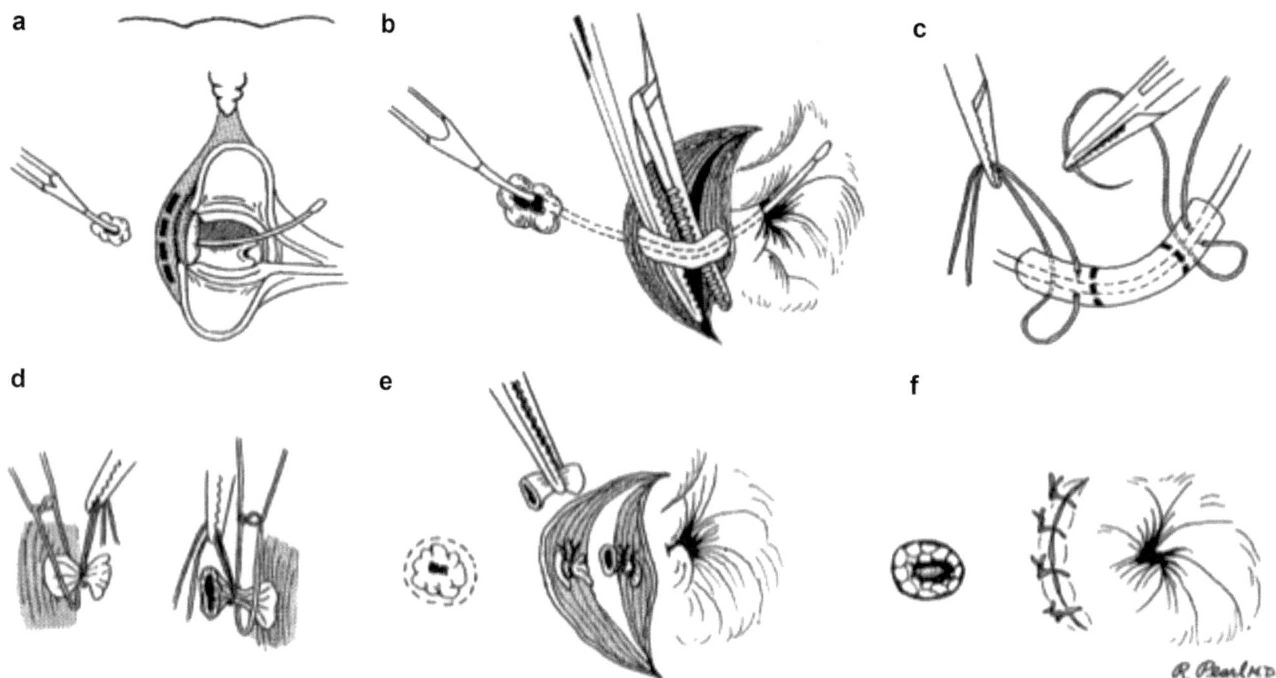

Fig. 16.1 Ligation of intersphincteric fistula tract. Reprinted with permission [3]. (**a**) Introduction of fistula probe through the tract. (**b**) Dissection of intersphincteric groove and identification of fibrotic fistula tract. (**c**) Suture ligation of fistula tract proximally and distally. (**d**) Additional ligature reinforcing tract closure. (**e**) Division of fistula tract; if tract is quite long, a segment of the tract is excised. (**f**) LIFT wound is closed loosely, and external opening of the tract is enlarged to facilitate drainage. *LIFT* ligation of intersphincteric fistula tract. Drawings courtesy of Russell K. Pearl, M.D. With permission from: Abcarian AM, Estrada JJ, Park J, et al. Ligation of intersphincteric fistula tract: early results of a pilot study. Dis Colon Rectum. 2012 Jul;55(7):778–782 © Wolters Kluwer

since the other available sphincter sparing options have variable success rates of 31–80 % at best [8–11]. Utilizing a new procedure that could offer >90 % success rate was exciting and many centers began to learn and perform the procedure, observing their results along the way.

The next published series came from Shanwani et al. [4], Bleier et al. [12], and Ooi et al. [13] which were collected prospectively as observational studies, and a retrospective review from Aboulian et al. [5]. These early reports suggested a healing rate of 57–82 % at 9–24 weeks follow-up, suggesting, as Rojanasakul had proposed, that larger series with longer term follow-up were needed to fully assess the success and limitations of the LIFT as a new surgical tool [4, 5, 12, 13]. In our series we reported overall healing of 74 % at 18 weeks with some preliminary data suggesting success rate of 90 % could be possible when LIFT was used as the first fistula procedure after seton placement [3]. Sileri et al. published a prospective study on 18 patients with complex fistulas. Following their LIFT procedure, they reported 83 % healing at median follow-up of 4 months [14].

Aboulian et al. recently published a longer follow-up of their initial cohort. Overall primary healing was reported at 61 %. They found that 80 % of failures were early, i.e., in the first 6 months following LIFT, and 20 % occurred after the first 6 months. One failure was reported at 12 months post-LIFT. No subjective incontinence was reported [15].

Wallin et al. published 93 patients and with an overall success rate of 40 % after initial LIFT at median of 19 months follow-up [16]. When including patients who underwent repeat (salvage) LIFT and/or intersphincteric fistulotomy, the success rates were 47 % and 57 %, respectively. Incontinence was observed and tracked using Wexner incontinence scores and patients with successful fistula healing were found to have a CCFFI score of 1.0 [16]. This study illustrates the desirable points of any novel sphincter sparing technique, i.e., reasonable success rates with good functional outcome and minimal risk of incontinence. Table 16.1 summarizes the published LIFT series to date.

Special Populations

The LIFT can be safely performed on any transsphincteric fistula of suitable length. The presence of inflammatory bowel disease or HIV should not preclude using the LIFT as an option. In the series by Abcarian et al., one patient had Crohn's disease and LIFT resulted in successful healing of that patient's ano-introital fistula. Additionally, in the same series, one patient with HIV also healed [3]. Population analysis will need to be performed on a larger group undergoing LIFT procedures. Other populations at risk for poor healing (cigarette smokers, obese patients) are also suitable

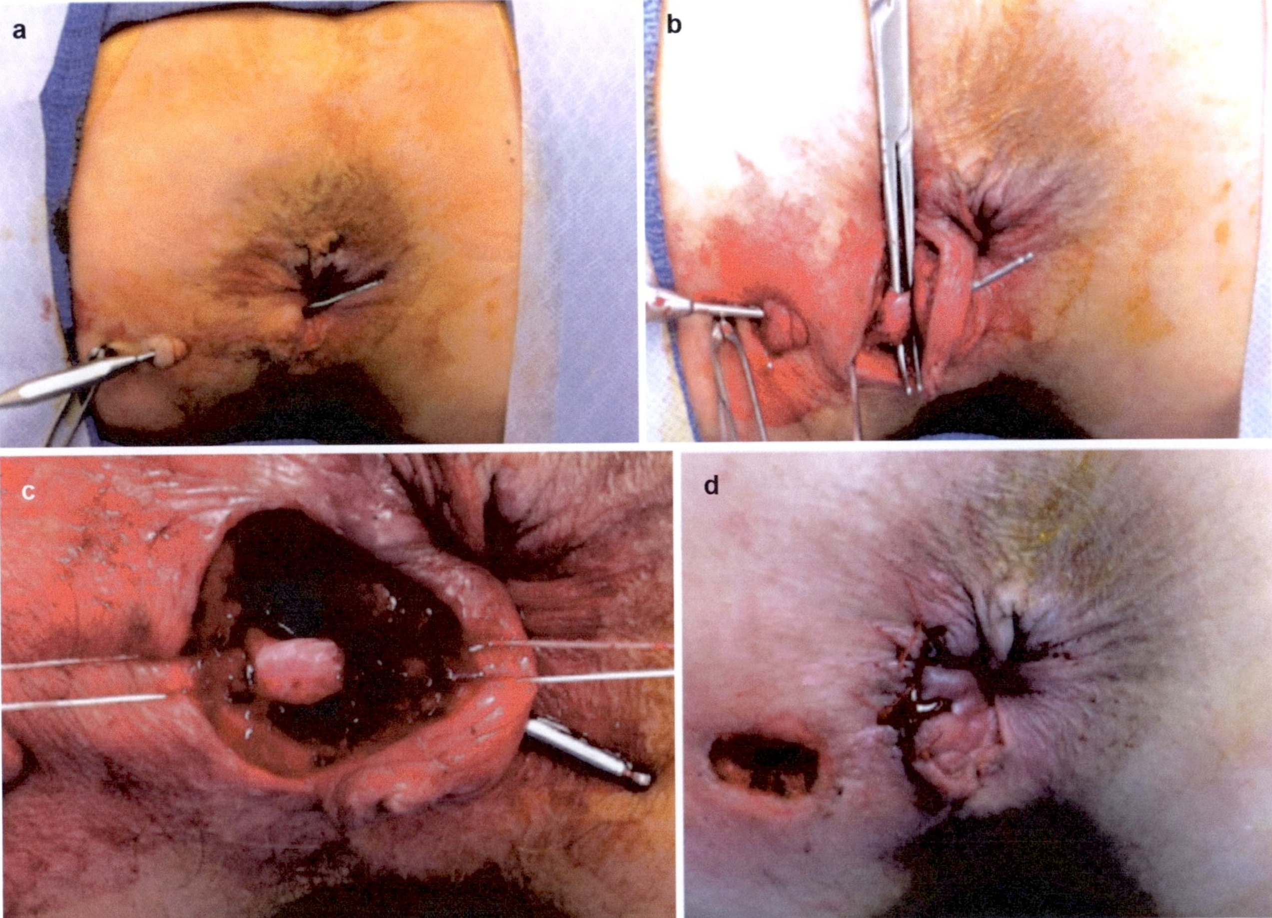

Fig. 16.2 Intraoperative photos of the original LIFT procedure, including our variation. (**a**) Passage of fistula probe through the transsphincteric tract. (**b**) Dissection to fibrotic fistula tract from surrounding muscle fibers. (**c**) Suture ligation of fistula tract proximally and distally. Probe should be removed prior to suture ligation. (**d**) LIFT wound closed loosely; external opening enlarged to facilitate drainage

to undergo LIFT. Anecdotally the procedure carries as much risk for non-healing and complications as other sphincter sparing procedures for fistula [8–11].

Failures

When utilizing a novel procedure, one must consider how to manage failures. Studies have been undertaken to examine the LIFT failures. Typically, LIFT failures fall into two broad categories: early (procedural failure) and late (recurrence). One may categorize early failures as a technical problem and late failures as a disease process. Patients who fail LIFT can still undergo other treatments for fistulas such as simple lay-open fistulotomy, salvage LIFT, or various flap procedures.

Tan et al. [6] reported that, when unsuccessful, a failed LIFT can "downstage" a transsphincteric fistula to an intersphincteric fistula, thereby allowing simple lay-open fistulotomy without risk of incontinence. The failed LIFT medializes the external opening to the intersphincteric incision and these subsequent failures were treated with fistulotomy,

repeat LIFT, or anocutaneous (dermal) advancement flap. The results have been promising. They examined their LIFT patients after a median of 23 weeks. The study differentiated between recurrences and failures. In patients in whom endo-anal ultrasound revealed failure resulting in a simple fistula, the patients were successfully treated with application of silver nitrate or fistulotomy. In the patients who recurred after initial LIFT success, the majority underwent fistulotomy and the remainder underwent either repeat LIFT or anocutaneous advancement flap. The series reports an overall freedom of failure or recurrence of 78 % at 1 year, validating what many surgeons had earlier observed when their LIFT patients did not heal. Medialization of the external opening and shortening the amount of sphincter involved in the tract allow opportunity for reoperation with various sphincter sparing techniques contributing to overall success of 78 % at 1 year [6].

van Onkelen et al. published a series of 22 patients, 82 % of whom underwent LIFT and healed at median follow-up of 19.5 months. The study also observed the four patients in whom the LIFT failed, had their transsphincteric fistula

Table 16.1 Summary of published LIFT series

Authors	Number of patients	Healing rate (success), %	Follow-up time	Measured continence scores Y/N	Type of study
Rojanasakul et al. [1]	18	94	4 weeks	N	Prospective
Shanwani et al. [4]	45	82	9 months	N	Prospective
Bleier et al. [12]	39	57	20 weeks	N	Prospective
Aboulian et al. [5]	25	68	24 weeks	N	Retrospective
Sileri et al. [14]	18	83	4 months	N	Prospective
Ooi et al. [13]	25	68	22 weeks	Y	Prospective
Abcarian et al. [3]	39	74	18 weeks	N	Prospective
van Onkelen et al. [20]	22 (low transsphincteric)	82	19.5 months	Y	Prospective
Wallin et al. [16]	93	40	19 months	Y	Retrospective
Liu et al. [15]	38	61	26 months	N	Retrospective

converted to an intersphincteric fistula, and underwent subsequent fistulotomy. Including these patients in the overall healing percentage, they observed a 100 % healing rate. Furthermore, the incontinence score after 6 months was unchanged [17]. This study illustrates the success of the LIFT itself, successful management of failures, and unchanged incontinence scores. The advantage of the LIFT procedure should be measured in all three of these data points.

Incontinence

Most of the early series were collected retrospectively and, therefore, pre- and postoperative incontinence scores were not collected. Later studies, to varying degrees, have collected incontinence scores using validated methods. Studies that look at incontinence with scores are highlighted in Table 16.1. None of the early studies reported any subjective postoperative incontinence, and rates of incontinence published in later studies are minimal and on par with other sphincter sparing techniques.

Other Techniques

Subsequent studies have validated the success rates of the initial technique (see Table 16.1). Other series have been published examining LIFT plus bioprosthetic grafts—the "BioLIFT" [18], LIFT plus the use of a bioprosthetic plug [19], and LIFT plus transanal advancement flap [20]. These series have varying healing rates; however, they are small series and none of them have been validated or duplicated. They are referred to simply for the sake of completeness.

Conclusion

The LIFT procedure became popular due to its early published successes. Large randomized trials have yet to study this operation in comparison with other established methods of sphincter sparing technique. The production of large, randomized trials is hindered by the suitability of the procedure to which the LIFT should be randomized to. No "gold-standard" sphincter sparing technique exists [21]. Furthermore, the 100 % healing rate achieved with fistulotomy comes at the risk of incontinence, which patients find unacceptable, thereby making fistulotomy as a randomization arm impossible.

The beauty of the LIFT is not only in its initial healing rates, but that the procedure itself, even when unsuccessful, may predispose a patient to subsequent healing without risk of incontinence. The LIFT has variable healing rates reported as high as 94 % with an actual healing rate equal to, or better than, other sphincter sparing procedures. Reoperation for LIFT has healing rates as high as 100 % with little reported incontinence [6]. Performing a LIFT does not exclude the possibility of subsequent operations and may even aid in final healing due to medialization of fistula tract from transsphincteric to intersphincteric. Like other sphincter sparing techniques, the operation itself is very much dependent on the biologic characteristics of the fistula itself, much of which awaits further scientific discovery. Multicenter, randomized trials on large cohorts with long follow-up are needed to produce evidence to tailor LIFT, as potentially the best operation, to the patient.

References

1. Rojanasakul A, Parranaarun J, Sahakirungruaung C, et al. Total anal sphincter saving technique for fistula-in-ano; the ligation of intersphincteric fistula tract. J Med Assoc Thai. 2007;90(3):581–6.

2. Rojanasakul A. LIFT procedure: a simplified technique for fistula-in-ano. Tech Coloproctol. 2009;13(3):237–40. doi:10.1007/s10151-009-0522-2. Epub 2009 Jul 28.

3. Abcarian AM, Estrada JJ, Park J, et al. Ligation of intersphincteric fistula tract: early results of a pilot study. Dis Colon Rectum. 2012;55(7):778–82. doi:10.1097/DCR.0b013e318255ae8a.

4. Shanwani A, Nor AM, Amri N. Ligation of the intersphincteric fistula tract (LIFT): a sphincter-saving technique for fistula-in-ano. Dis Colon Rectum. 2010;53(1):39–42. doi:10.1007/DCR.0b013e3181c160c4.

5. Aboulian A, Kaji AH, Kumar RR. Early result of ligation of the intersphincteric fistula tract for fistula-in-ano. Dis Colon Rectum. 2011;54(3):289–92. doi:10.1097/DCR.0b013e318203495d.

6. Tan KK, Tan IJ, Lim FS, et al. The anatomy of failures following the ligation of intersphincteric tract technique for anal fistula: a review of 93 patients over 4 years. Dis Colon Rectum. 2011;54(11):1368–72. doi:10.1007/DCR.0b013e31822bb55e.

7. Mushaya C, Bartlett L, Schulze B, Ho YH. Ligation of interpshinceric fistula tract compared with advancement flap for complex anorectal fistulas requiring initial seton drainage. Am J Surg. 2012;204(3):283–9. doi:10.1016/j.amjsurg.2011.10.025. Epub 2012 May 19.

8. Loungnarath R, Dietz DW, Mutch MG, et al. Fibrin glue treatment of complex anal fistulas has low success rate. Dis Colon Rectum. 2004;47(4):432–6. Epub 2004 Feb 25.

9. McGee MF, Champagne BJ, Stulberg JJ, et al. Tract length predicts successful closure with anal fistula plug in cryptoglandular fistulas. Dis Colon Rectum. 2010;53(8):1116–20. doi:10.1007/DCR.0b013e3181d972a9.

10. Soltani A, Kaiser AM. Endorectal advancement flap for cryptoglandular or Crohn's fistula-in-ano. Dis Colon Rectum. 2010;53(4):486–95. doi:10.1007/DCR.0b013e3181ce8b01.

11. Nelson R. Anorectal abscess fistula: what do we know? Surg Clin North Am. 2002;82(6):1139–51, v–vi.

12. Bleier JI, Moloo H, Godberg SM. Ligation of the intersphincteric fistula tract: an effective new technique for complex fistulas. Dis Colon Rectum. 2010;53(1):43–6. doi:10.1007/DCR.0b013e3181bb869f.

13. Ooi K, Skinner I, Croxford M, et al. Managing fistula-in-ano with ligation of the intersphincteric fistula tract procedure: the Western Hospital experience. Colorectal Dis. 2012;14(5):599–603. doi:10.1111/j.1463-1318.2011.02723.x.

14. Sileri P, Franceschilli L, Angelucci GP, et al. Ligation of the intersphincteric fistula tract (LIFT) to treat anal fistula: early results from a prospective observational study. Tech Coloproctol. 2011;15(4):413–6. doi: 10.1007/s10151-011-0779-0. Epub 2011 Nov 11.

15. Liu WY, Aboulian A, Kaji AH, Kumar RR. Long-term results of ligation of intersphincteric fistula tract (LIFT) for fistula-in-ano. Dis Colon Rectum. 2013;56(3):343–7. doi:10.1097/DCR.0b013e318278164c.

16. Wallin UG, Mellgren AF, Madoff RD, Goldberg SM. Does ligation of the intersphincteric fistula tract raise the bar in fistula surgery? Dis Colon Rectum. 2012;55(11):1173–8. doi:10.1097/DCR.0b013e318266edf3.

17. van Onkelen RS, Gosselink MP, Schouten WR. Ligation of the intersphincteric fistula tract in low transsphincteric fistulas: a new technique to avoid fistulotomy. Colorectal Dis. 2012. doi:10.1111/codi.12030. [Epub ahead of print].

18. Ellis CN. Outcomes with the use of bioprosthetic grafts to reinforce the ligation of the intersphincteric fistula tract (BioLIFT procedure) for the management of complex anal fistulas. Dis Colon Rectum. 2010;53(10):1361–4. doi:10.1007/DCR.0b013e3181ec4470.

19. Han JG, Yi BQ, Wang ZJ et al. Ligation of the intersphinceric fistula tract plus bioprosthetic anal fistula plug (LIFT-Plug): a new technique for fistula-in-ano. Colorectal Dis. 2012. doi: 10.1111/codi.12062. [Epub ahead of print].

20. van Onkelen RS, Gosselink MP, Schouten WR. Is it possible to improve the outcome of transanal advancement flap repair for high transsphincteric fistulas by additional ligation of the intersphincteric fistula tract? Dis Colon Rectum. 2012;55(2):153–6. doi:10.1097/DCR.0b013e31823c0f74.

21. Abcarian H. Letter to the editor on "The management of fistula-in-ano: a plea for randomized trials and standard reporting of a case series with adequate follow up. Dis Colon Rectum. 2013;56:e1. doi:10.1097/DCR.0b013e31827421b5.

Video-Assisted Anal Fistula Treatment (VAAFT)

Piercarlo Meinero and Lorenzo Mori

Introduction

The video-assisted anal fistula treatment (VAAFT) is a new technique performed for the surgical treatment of complex anal fistulas and their recurrences. Until now all technical procedures to treat anal fistulas included a "blind" preliminary gentle probing of the tract in order to explore it and to locate the internal opening. VAAFT works on the principle of "putting an eye" on the probe and exploring the tract from the inside under direct vision. This allows precise identification of secondary tracts and abscess cavities and minimizes the risk of creating false passages on the way to reaching the internal opening. After this a diatermocoagulation of the fistula walls and a hermetic closure of the internal opening are performed. The accurate anatomic definition and the precise identification of the internal opening, the drainage of associated sepsis, the destruction of the tract, and the closure of the internal opening itself are the rationale principles of anal fistula surgery and VAAFT respects all of them. This technique comprises two phases: (1) a diagnostic one and (2) an operative one.

Materials

Karl Storz GmbH Video Equipment (Tuttlingen, Germany) is used (Fig. 17.1). The operating kit includes a fistuloscope (Fig. 17.2), an obturator, a unipolar electrode (Fig. 17.3), an endobrush (Fig. 17.4), and forceps. The fistuloscope has an 8° angled eyepiece, its diameter is 3.3×4.7 mm and it is equipped with an optical channel and also a working and irrigation channel. The operative length is 18 cm without a

P. Meinero, M.D. • L. Mori, M.D. (✉)
Sestri Levante Hospital, ASL 4 Chiavarese, Via Arnaldo Terzi 43, Sestri Levante, Genoa, 16039, Italy
e-mail: morilorenzo67@gmail.com

removable handle. With the handle the effective length is reduced to 14 cm. The fistuloscope has two taps one of which is connected to a 5,000 mL bag of glycine–mannitol 1 % solution. Which tap is used depends on the position of the fistula. Also in the kit are a semicircular or linear stapler and 0.5 mL of synthetic cyanoacrylate (Glubran 2, GEM, Viareggio, Italy) with a tiny catheter (Fig. 17.5). The optimal patient positioning is the lithotomic position. Spinal anesthesia is required. The fistuloscope is connected to the Karl Storz equipment and to the washing solution bag.

The Diagnostic Phase

The purpose of this phase is to find the main and secondary tracts and abscess cavities and to correctly locate the internal fistula opening. At the beginning of the procedure insert a syringe in the external orifice and inject low-pressure saline solution in order to obtain a fistula tract dilatation. Any scar tissue around the external opening can be removed by electrosurgical knife for ease of entry of the fistuloscope tip and the excised tissue may be sent for histopathological examination. During the insertion, the washing solution is already running, providing a clear view of the fistula pathway, which appears on the screen (Figs. 17.6 and 17.7). At this point, it is very important to be patient and wait for an adequate dilation of the tract. Since the fistuloscope is rigid, it helps to guide it using a trans-anally inserted finger. If the tract is very tortuous, the positioning of a Kocher's forceps on the external opening, allows it to be straightened by a counter traction. Blocking tissue in the tract can be removed using the 2 mm forceps to facilitate the progression of the fistuloscope. The orientation of the fistuloscope is correct when the obturator appears in the lower part of the screen. The surgeon follows the fistula pathway using slow left-right and up-down movements. Any force used at this stage may lead to the fistuloscope entering the fatty tissue of the buttock and rupturing the fistula, causing severe edema, and the procedure may have to be abandoned. These maneuvers are aided

H. Abcarian (ed.), *Anal Fistula: Principles and Management*, DOI 10.1007/978-1-4614-9014-2_17,
© Springer Science+Business Media New York 2014

by the complete relaxation of the surrounding tissue induced by the spinal anesthesia. At this point, the finger in the anus helps to straighten the fistula tract by combined movements between the finger and the fistuloscope. Optimum vision of the inside of the fistula is assured by the continuous jet of the washing solution to the point where you reach the end of the fistula pathway which is the internal fistula opening (Fig. 17.8). Dimming the lights in the operating theatre enables an easy localization of the fistuloscope light in the rectum. The assistant can insert an anal retractor in order to localize the internal fistula opening by looking for the light of the telescope in the rectum or anal canal. When the

fistuloscope exits through the internal opening, the rectal mucosa clearly appears on the screen. The fistuloscope usually goes out through the internal opening but sometimes it is not so easy, as the internal opening might be very narrow: in that case, its location is found by viewing the fistuloscope light behind the rectal mucosa. At this point, it's useful to put

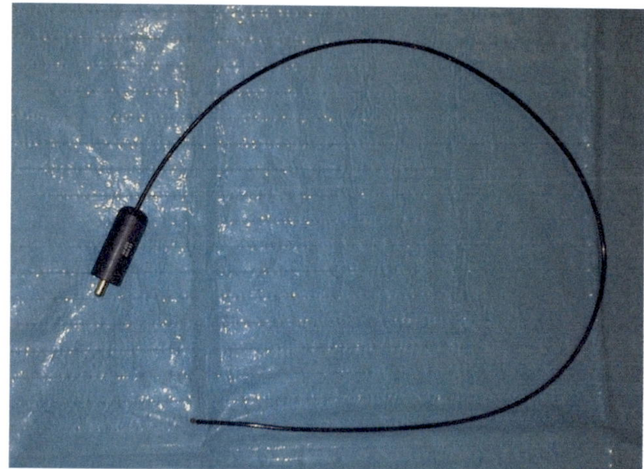

Fig. 17.3 The unipolar electrode

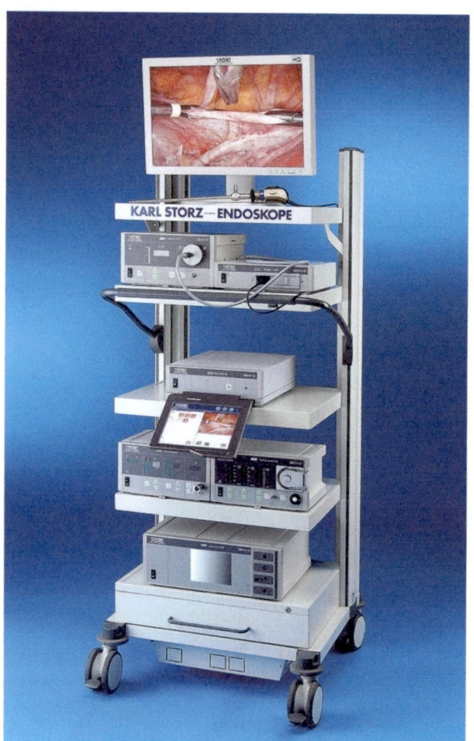

Fig. 17.1 The Karl Storz video equipment

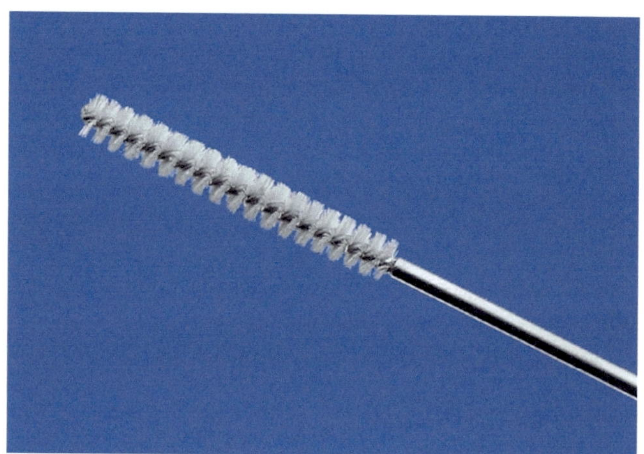

Fig. 17.4 The endobrush

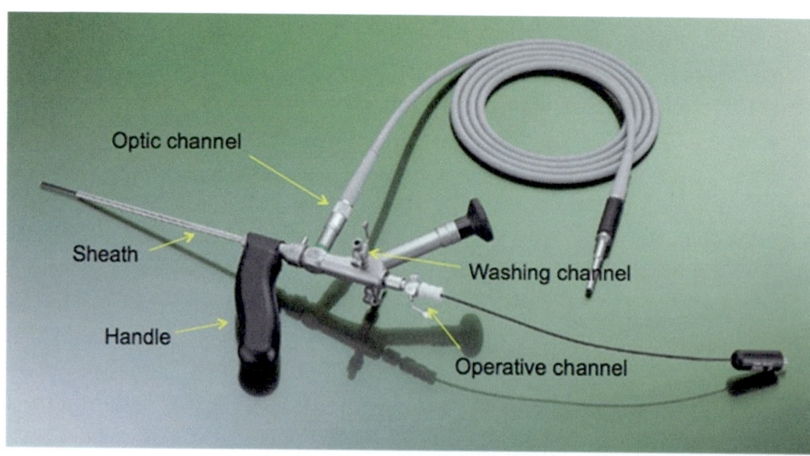

Fig. 17.2 The Meinero fistuloscope

two or three stitches in two opposite points of the internal opening margin in order to isolate and, above all, not to lose it (Figs. 17.9 and 17.10). The stitches must not be knotted because the internal opening must remain open to allow the flowing out of the waste material during the operative phase.

The Operative Phase

The purpose of this phase is the destruction of the fistula from the inside, followed by the fistula canal being cleaned/the waste material removed and the internal opening closed hermetically. We start destroying the fistula under vision using a unipolar electrode, which is connected to the electro-surgical power unit (Fig. 17.11) and is passed through the operative channel of the fistuloscope. Starting at the internal fistula opening, all fragments of the whitish material adhering to the fistula wall and all granulation tissue are coagulated. This phase of the operation is completed centimeter by

centimeter, from the internal opening to the external opening not forgetting any abscess cavities. The necrotic material is removed under vision using the fistula brush (Fig. 17.12). Until that time, the isolated internal fistula opening remains open to allow the flowing out of waste and washing material into the rectum. At this point, the fistuloscope is completely removed. The assistant stretches the threads holding the internal fistula opening, towards the internal rectal space or the anal canal using a straight forceps in order to lift the internal fistula opening at least 2 cm into the shape of a

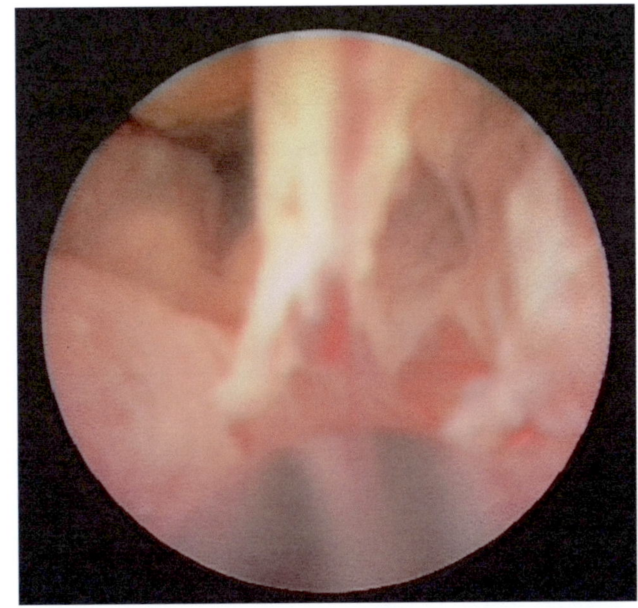

Fig. 17.7 The fork between the main tract and a secondary one

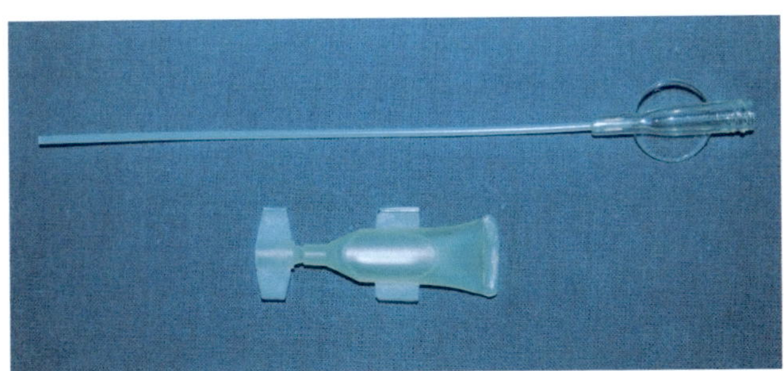

Fig. 17.5 The synthetic cyanoacrylate (GLUBRAN 2, GEM)

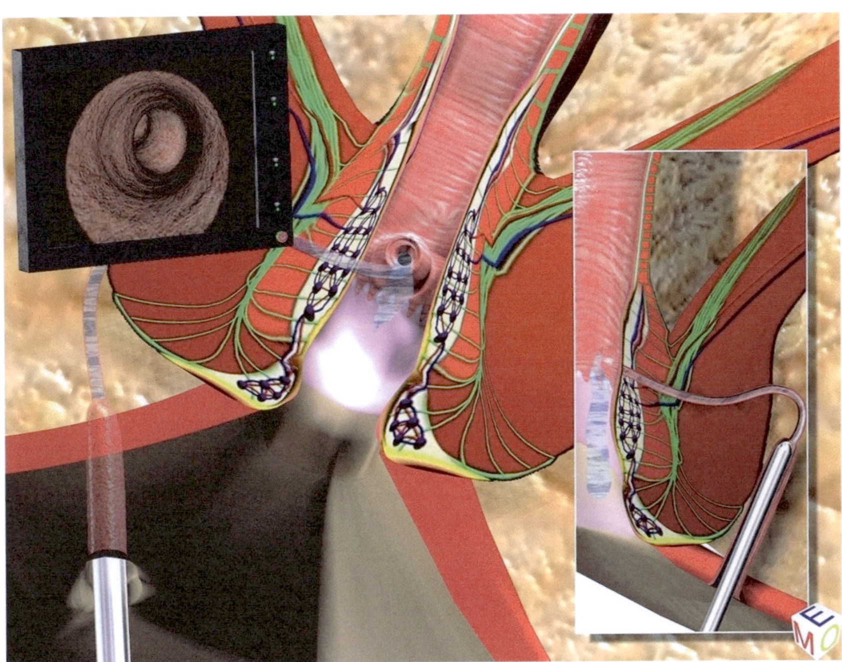

Fig. 17.6 The insertion of the fistuloscope with the glycine–mannitol 1 % solution already running; in the box the fistula pathway appears on the screen

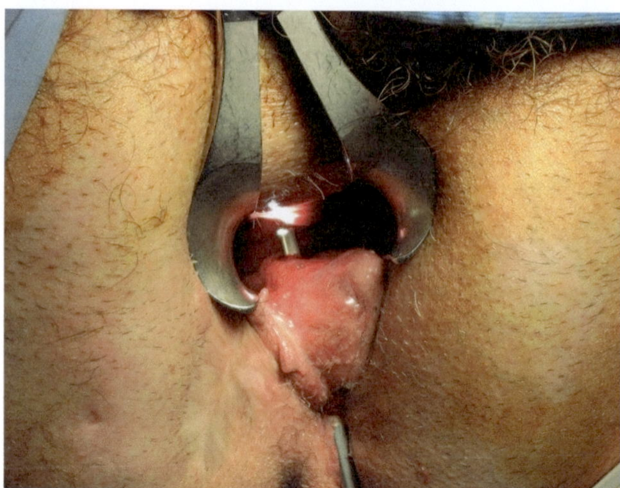

Fig. 17.8 The fistuloscope has reached the internal orifice and the tip is in the rectum

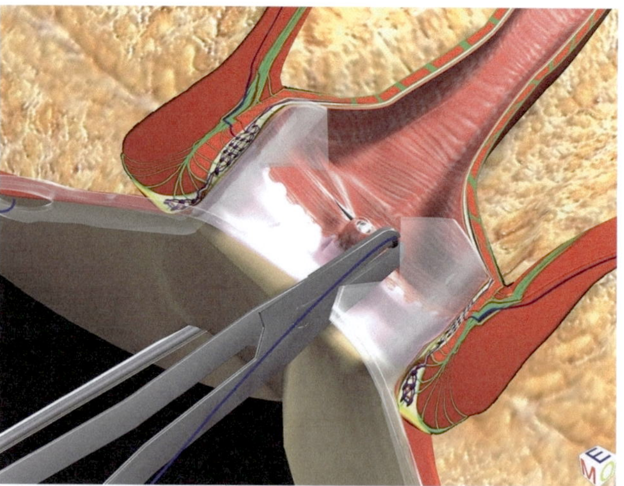

Fig. 17.9 The isolation of the internal orifice with two stitches in opposite points

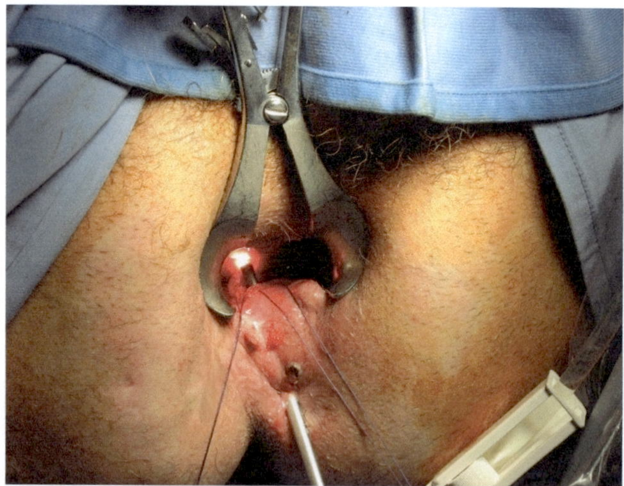

Fig. 17.10 The isolation of the internal orifice with two stitches in opposite points

volcano. We then insert a semicircular or a linear stapler at the volcano's base and complete the mechanical cutting and suturing. The choice of the stapler also depends on the internal opening position. Using a semicircular stapler, the suture will be horizontal (Fig. 17.13). Using a linear stapler, the suture will be vertical (Figs. 17.14 and 17.15). When the tissue in the area of the internal opening is not sclerotic and allows the formation of a good "volcano," the stapler can be used; however, if the tissue around the internal opening is too rigid and sclerotic, the use of the stapler might be difficult. In this case a cutaneous or an endorectal advancement flap would be preferred (Fig. 17.16). As a last step, we insert 0.5 mL of synthetic cyanoacrylate (GLUBRAN 2, GEM) immediately behind the suture/staple line via the fistula pathway to further reinforce the suture (Fig. 17.17). In this way the use of the synthetic cyanoacrylate behind the suture line or behind the flap assures the perfect closure of the opening. It is essential to keep in mind that not the whole fistula tract is filled up with the synthetic cyanoacrylate; only a small amount is inserted directly below the suture line. That's why the fistula pathway has to stay open to allow the passage of secretions. This procedure assures a perfect excision and a hermetic closure of the internal fistula opening, excluding the risk of stool passage. Since the suture is situated tangential to the sphincter, the postoperative pain is low even if the suture falls both in the anal canal and the rectum.

Results

From May 2006 to February 2012, 203 patients with a complex anal fistula were managed with this technique. Any fistula that could not be adequately treated by simple fistulotomy was considered "complex." Our series consisted of 124 males and 79 females, with a median age of 40 years (range 21–77 years). Exclusion criteria included Crohn's disease and cases of simple fistulas. Preoperative assessment included blood tests, virtual or traditional colonoscopy, and a chest X-ray where appropriate. Approval was obtained from the Ethics Committee of our Institution and all patients provided informed consent. Fifty-two patients did not require any additional diagnostic investigations, and preoperative assessment of the fistula anatomy was based on clinical grounds alone. Sixty patients underwent magnetic resonance imaging (MRI) or endoanal ultrasonography at our institution, while 91 underwent fistula imaging (MRI, ultrasonography or CT) prior to referral and did not require further testing. One hundred fourty-nine patients had already undergone prior surgery for complex anal fistula. Eleven patients had a diverting colostomy. Follow-up was conducted at 2, 6, and 12 months after VAAFT and subsequently, once per year. Forty-two patients were contacted by phone interview after the first year of follow-up. One hundred fifty-five out of the 203 patients were followed up for a minimum of 6 months

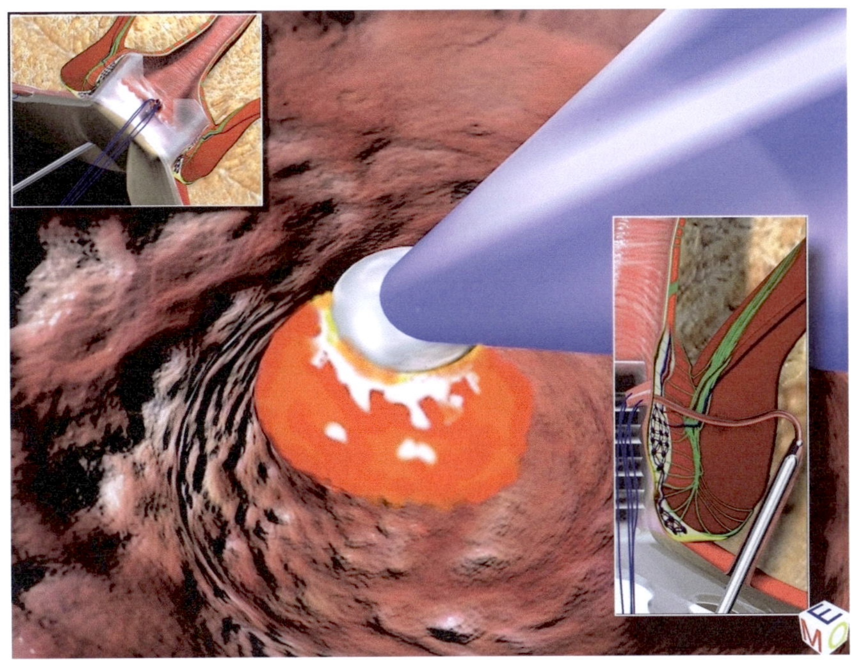

Fig. 17.11 The rectal wall is visually cauterized by a unipolar electrode

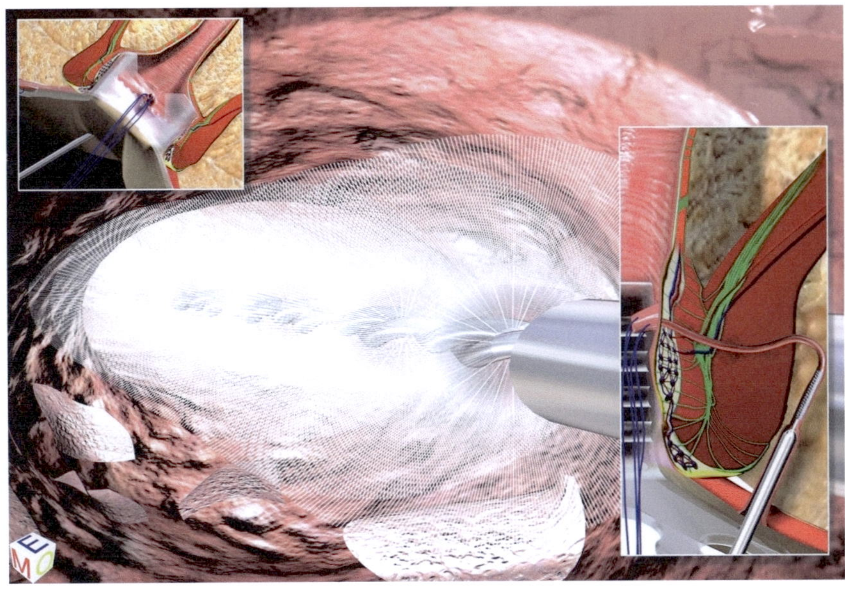

Fig. 17.12 The tract is cleaned under vision by an endobrush

with a median duration of follow-up of 15 months (range 6–69 months). In 121 cases (59.6 %), secondary tracts and abscesses were found. In 36 cases (17.7 %), the internal fistula opening was located in the anal canal, in 152 cases (74.8 %) at the level of the dentate line and in 15 cases (7.4 %) in the rectum. In 171 patients (84.2 %), the internal opening of the fistula was located in less than 5 min. In the other 32 (15.8 %), it was found by viewing the fistuloscope light in the rectum. The operative time was progressively reduced (from 2 h to 30 min) following improvement in the learning curve. No major complications occurred and no infection or bleeding was observed; however, there were two

cases of postoperative urinary retention. In one case, scrotal edema was observed, caused by the infiltration of the irrigation solution after rupture of the fistula wall. Two cases of allergy to the synthetic cyanoacrylate were reported. One patient was discharged after 6 days because of headache related to the spinal anesthesia; all the other patients were discharged within 24 h. Most patients reported that postoperative pain was acceptable both in the early and in the later postoperative period. Pain control was based on the visual analogue scale (VAS) score with a mean value of 4.0 (on a scale of 1–10) during the first 48 h. None of the patients reported pain after the first postoperative week. Thirty-six

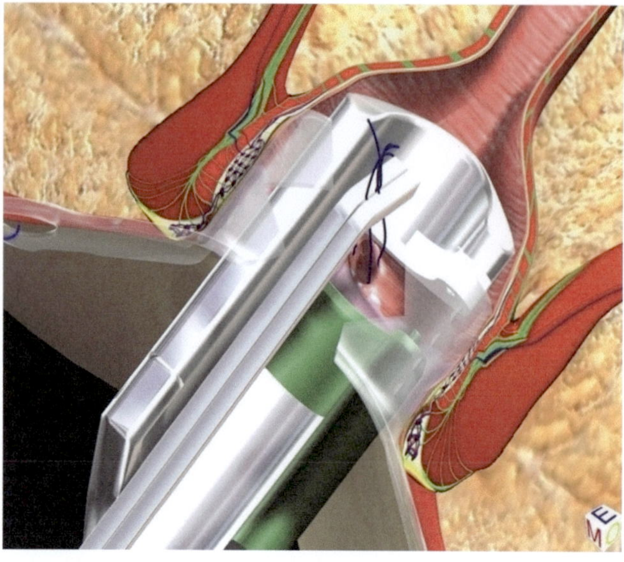

Fig. 17.13 Closure of the internal opening by a semicircular stapler

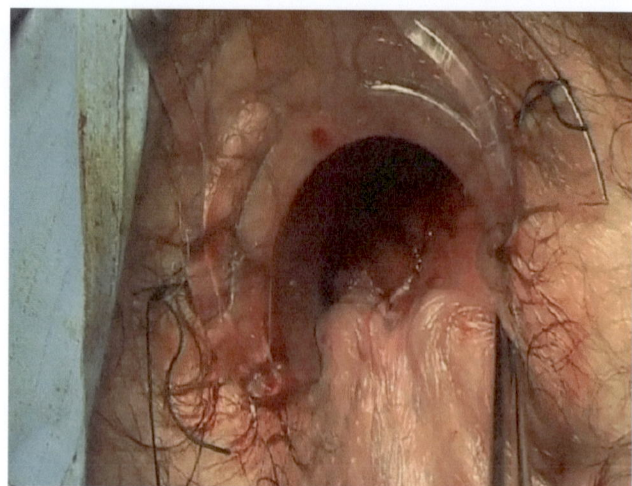

Fig. 17.15 Vertical suture after linear stapler closure

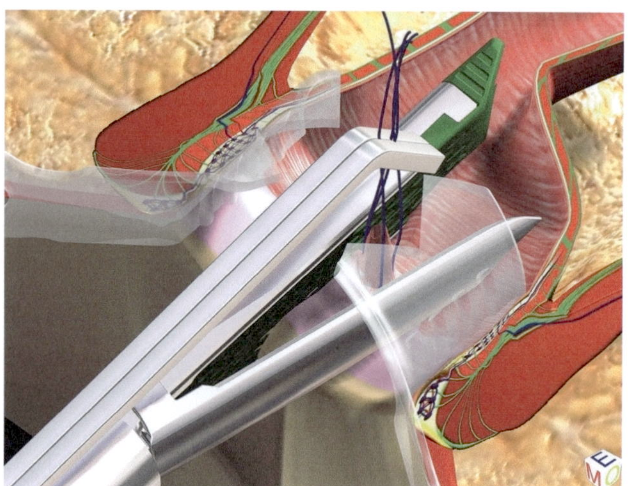

Fig. 17.14 Closure of the internal opening by a linear stapler

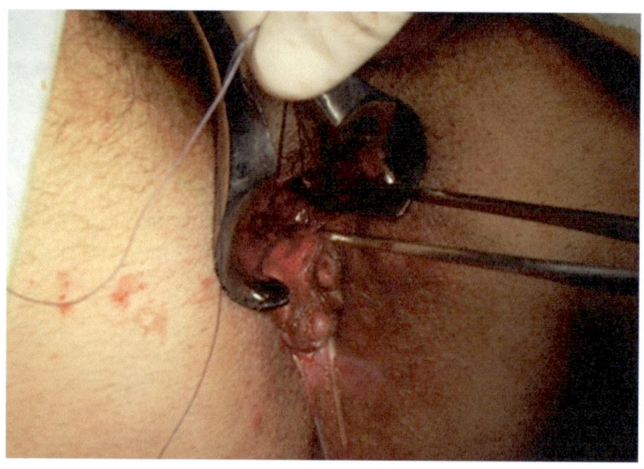

Fig. 17.16 Closure by endorectal advancement flap

patients (17.8 %) did not require analgesics whereas 141 patients (69.4 %) needed Ketorolac trimetamine for 3–4 days and only 26 (12.8 %) needed Ketorolac trimetamine for a week. In the group of 155 patients with a follow-up >6 months primary healing was achieved in 118 patients (73.5 %) within 2–4 months after surgery; in 37 patients (23.9 %), no wound healing was observed. Thirty-one of the 37 underwent reoperation with VAAFT (six patients were lost at follow-up) and 17 (45.9 %) of them healed whereas 14 have had a recurrence. Overall (first VAAFT and successive VAAFT retreatment) healing was obtained in 135/155 patients (87.1 %). Seventy-four patients were followed up for at least 12 months, of which 69 (93.2 %) had primary healing of their fistula. We did not formally evaluate anal continence in our patients with a validated score before and

after surgery. Our aim was only to determine whether the operation might have worsened patients' continence, and this was evaluated by simply asking the patients about continence problems. All patients denied worsening of fecal continence postoperatively. Among those who had an active job, the longest time off work was 3 days.

Comments

In the last few years the traditional seton treatment of complex anal fistulas has been associated with a risk of anal sphincters impairment and a recent review reports an incontinence rate as high as 12 % [1]. Many alternative attempts have been made to treat high anal fistulas [2] and in all cases

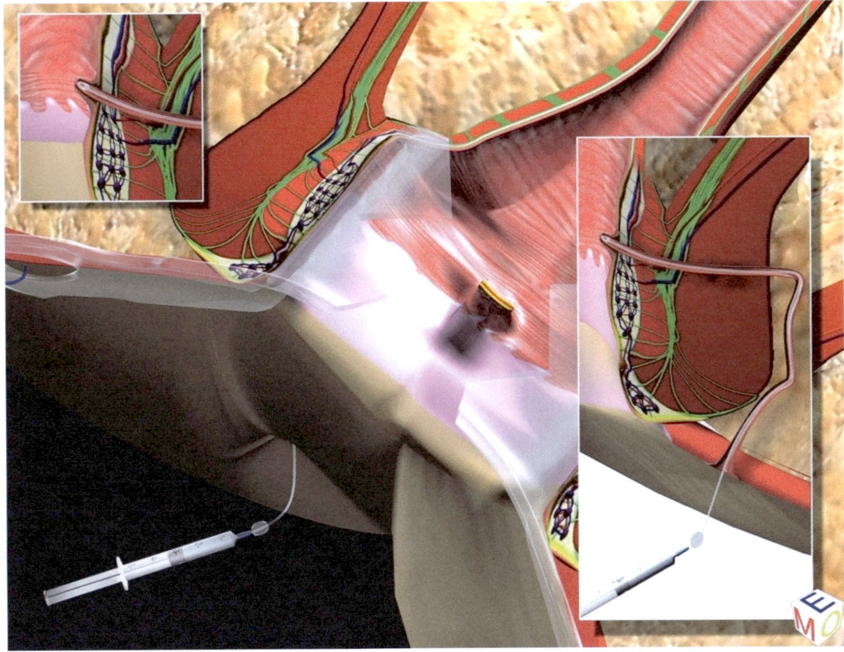

Fig. 17.17 Injection of synthetic cyanoacrylate directly below the suture line through a tiny catheter

the blind probing of the tract was the first step in order to define the fistula course and to locate the internal opening. Therefore the probe introduction and the progression maneuver remained a difficult technique that a coloproctologist had to sharpen thanks to his progressively wider experience. Every surgeon knows that correct location of the internal opening offers the best opportunities to successfully cure anal fistulas; on the other hand, the accidental creation of false passages is a sure sign that the fistula will not heal. VAAFT's main innovation is the possibility to explore the fistula tract from the inside: the blind "burglar like" probing is replaced by a complete endoluminal "under vision" evaluation that includes, in addition to the main tract, secondary tracts, and abscess cavities. The fistuloscopy minimizes the risk of rupture of the fistula and plays a fundamental role in understanding the course of a complex fistula. The effectiveness of this approach is emphasized when patients have been operated on many times and many unpredictable pathways and multiple orifices have to be located. Sometimes in these types of fistulas there is no longer a single internal orifice and the chronic suppuration is supported by large, undrained, abscess cavities, and secondary tracts: the operation of the fistuloscope allows the surgeon to find them and to directly cauterize their walls under vision. In the VAAFT-operative phase, all tracts can be treated by the monopolar electrode and the brush in order to destroy pyogenic tissue and to stimulate the processes of fibrosis and regeneration. This treatment is optimal to prepare the closure of the internal orifice. As regards this step, VAAFT describes different options, a semicircular or a linear stapling or an advancement flap rein-

forced by a half milliliter of synthetic cyanoacrylate immediately behind the suture. We must consider that the closure could also be achieved by other techniques—i.e., ligation of the intersphincteric tract (LIFT), plugs of different shape and materials, fibrin glue—and there is an unexplored field of potential association with our video-assisted approach. The true revolutionary concept of VAAFT procedure is it being carried out visually and it can be considered compatible with instead of alternative to other different recent sphincter sparing techniques. Recently many authors report experience of treating high anal fistulas by many different associated techniques [3, 4]. We believe that our preliminary published results [5] will be improved and the endoluminal video-assisted approach will be a winning choice. These considerations are confirmed by the preliminary experience of Schwandner who adopted VAAFT to treat 11 patients with perianal Crohn disease suffering from complex fistulas and reported an 82 % success rate after a mean follow-up of 9 months [6]. These results on complex fistula treatment in Crohn disease are confirmed in our preliminary experience in few cases: the cauterization and cleaning of fistula tracts allows even its closure or, however, obtains a temporary healing and drainage avoiding the insertion of a seton. The advantages of the VAAFT technique are evident: surgical wounds on the buttocks or in the perianal region are very small (Fig. 17.18), there is complete certainty in the localization of the internal fistula opening (a key point in all fistula surgical treatments), and the fistula can be completely destroyed from the inside. There is no requirement to previously know the kind of fistula and no preoperative

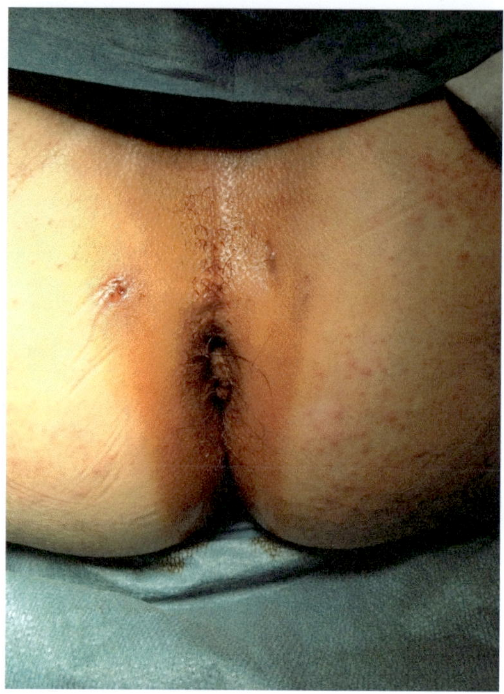

Fig. 17.18 The scar resulting at the end of the procedure

examination is necessary because VAAFT has a diagnostic phase, thanks to the fistuloscopy. Operating from the inside no damage is caused to the anal sphincters so the risk of postoperative fecal incontinence is excluded. Moreover, the patient have no need for dressing and he can start working again after a few days since the VAAFT technique can be performed in day surgery. The patients' quality of life with VAAFT is so much better than after traditional techniques. That's why, even in case of recurrence the patient requests VAAFT again.

References

1. Ritchie RD, Sackier JM, Hodde JP. Incontinence rates after cutting seton treatment for anal fistula. Colorectal Dis. 2009;11(6): 564–71.
2. Blumetti J, Abcarian A, Quinteros F, Chaudhry V, Prasad L, Abcarian H. Evolution of treatment of fistula in ano. World J Surg. 2012;36(5):1162–7.
3. van Onkelen RS, Gosselink MP, Schouten WR. Is it possible to improve the outcome of transanal advancement flap repair for high transsphincteric fistulas by additional ligation of the intersphincteric fistula tract? Dis Colon Rectum. 2012;55(2):163–6.
4. Han JG, Yi BQ, Wang ZJ, Zheng Y, Cui JJ, Yu XQ, Zhao BC, Yang XQ. Ligation of the intersphincteric fistula tract plus bioprosthetic anal fistula plug (LIFT-Plug): a new technique for fistula-in-ano. Colorectal Dis. 2013;15(5):582–6. doi:10.1111/codi.12062.
5. Meinero P, Mori L. Video-assisted anal fistula treatment (VAAFT): a novel sphincter-saving procedure for treating complex anal fistulas. Tech Coloproctol. 2011;15(4):417–22.
6. Schwandner O. Video-assisted anal fistula treatment (VAAFT) combined with advancement flap repair in Crohn's disease. Tech Coloproctol. 2012;17(2):221–5.

Stem Cell Application in Fistula Disease

Damian Garcia-Olmo and Hector Guadalajara-Labajo

The Rationale for Cell Therapy to Treat Anal Fistula

Cell therapy has emerged as a new tool to improve wound healing in a number of settings. In mammals, wound healing begins when a number of different cell types that arrive at the wound area in a step known as the "cellular phase." There are pathological situations in which this cell supply is deficient and wound healing may be delayed or not achieved, this is the case of anal fistula.

Stem cell transplantation provides a way of increasing the number of cells locally in this critical phase with the aim of restoring normal wound healing. In the case of anal fistula, wound healing is a critical item. Even treatment of a simple fistula is complicated as the surgeon will need to access the sphincter and, in doing so, may compromise its integrity leading to fecal incontinence. Limited surgical treatment often results in high recurrence whereas extensive surgical treatment may cause fecal incontinence [1]. Surgical flaps and other surgical techniques have the handicap of healing in a septic environment. Recurrence is almost always due to occult sepsis that has initially escaped surgical detection and has, thus, gone untreated. Recurrent fistulas pose a notoriously difficult surgical challenge and multiple failed operations are the rule rather than the exception in these patients. Such a state of affairs complicates matters as the perianal scarring and distortion that inevitably accompanies multiple surgical attempts at cure makes the preoperative assessment more and more complicated, which further complicates identification of unsuspected areas of sepsis. The inevitable result is that these individuals are progressively more difficult to treat with both patient and surgeon becoming ever more

D. Garcia-Olmo, M.D., Ph.D. (✉) • H. Guadalajara-Labajo, M.D.
Colorectal Surgery Unit, La Paz University Hospital,
Universidad Autonoma de Madrid,
Paseo de la Castellana 261, 28046 Madrid, Spain
e-mail: damian.garcia@uam.es

exasperated [2]. Moreover, continuous suppuration in the anal region in unhealed or recurrent fistulas leaves the patient at risk of acute infection with abscess formation, which will require urgent surgical drainage. Importantly, chronic fistulas could lead to tumor development (mainly anal epithelial carcinoma) due to the irritation caused by constant suppuration.

In the case of anal fistula associated to Crohn's disease, recent improvements in medical treatment (e.g., infliximab and adalimumab) add to expert surgical management, have decreased the need for complicated surgery [3–5], but many patients are not cured completely and fecal incontinence remains a problem [6–8].

In this scenario, cell therapy is envisaged as an effective alternative to surgery. The promising preclinical and clinical data that we will review below suggest that cell therapy could represent a major advance in the clinical management of this difficult problem.

Choosing Type of Stem Cells

Stem cells (SCs) are generally defined by being undifferentiated, with a capacity for long-term self-renewal and the potential to undergo multilineage differentiation from a single cell. Some authors include in vivo production of functional tissues as another defining characteristic [9]. They can undergo facultative symmetric or asymmetric division in which they simultaneously perpetuate themselves and give rise to a second daughter cell programmed to differentiate. Different SC types have been considered for preclinical and clinical applications in digestive tract diseases, unfortunately, in the clinical practise an optimal SC type has not been found [10].

To the date, only mesenchymal stem cells (MSCs) have been used to treat anal fistula. Nevertheless the place of extraction of this kind of cells can be different. MSCs were initially described as a bone marrow-derived mononuclear cell population that, when cultured ex vivo, adhered to plastic

H. Abcarian (ed.), *Anal Fistula: Principles and Management*, DOI 10.1007/978-1-4614-9014-2_18,
© Springer Science+Business Media New York 2014

with a fibroblast-like morphology. MSCs exist in the bone marrow and other tissues such as fat. The International Society for Cellular Therapy (ISCT) established three minimal criteria that MSCs must fulfill in vitro: adherence to plastic, specific surface antigen expression pattern (CD73+ CD90+ CD105+ CD34– CD45– CD11b– CD14–CD19– CD79a– HLA-DR–) and differentiation potential (osteogenic, chondrogenic, and adipogenic lineages) (Revised by García-Gómez et al. [11]).

MSCs have been reported to be immunoprivileged cells. Although the mechanisms underlying the immunosuppressive effects of MSCs have not been clearly defined, it seems that MSCs modulate the function of different cells involved in the immune response. The therapeutic potential of MSCs is currently being explored in a number of clinical trials. At present time only three Phase III clinical trials have been concluded for graft-versus-host disease (GVHD), Crohn's disease, and perianal fistula [11].

Since ex vivo-expanded MSCs have become a good option in a clinical setting, it is necessary to pay attention to the safety of cellular therapies. To achieve this aim, optimized culture conditions and isolation protocols are being developed. Additionally, precise genetic stability studies have been developed to ensure the quality and biosafety of MSCs in clinical practice. Overall, we are seeing how the evolution of stem cell research in the last decade is converting the MSCs into a new medical product that can be useful to treat anal fistula.

Fat appears as a great source of stem cells; liposuction can achieve large quantities of stem cells, and then can be harvested with minimal adverse effects.

Mechanism of Action of Stem Cell to Improve Healing

Somehow, we can say that the basis for fistula recurrence is a defect in the wound healing process. There is much scientific and clinical interest in the potential of MSCs to stimulate wound repair. Mesenchymal stem cell-based therapies represent a new treatment for preventing morbidity and disability associated with chronic wounds, an unresolved clinical problem that has shown little improvement over the past decades [12]. Healing of a cutaneous wound requires a well-orchestrated integration of complex, biological, and molecular events and such processes may be impaired in many chronic diseases [13]. Functional characteristics of MSCs, like their ability to migrate to the site of injury [14] or inflammation and to stimulate proliferation and differentiation of resident progenitor cells through growth factor secretion and matrix remodeling, and their immunomodulatory and anti-inflammatory effects, may benefit wound healing.

Recent studies have demonstrated that treatment of cutaneous wounds with bone marrow MSCs accelerates wound healing kinetics and increases epithelialization and angiogenesis [15–17], suggesting that MSCs enhance wound repair by at least two different mechanisms: differentiation and paracrine interactions with specific cell types in the cutaneous wound [18]. Considered together, the MSC treatments for delayed wound healing are associated with dermal rebuilding in addition to remodeling, an increase in wound vascularity, and reduced fibrosis or scarring [19].

MSCs from fat injected in the site of inflammation recognize proinflammatory cytokines, like IFN-gamma, and consequently activate IDO enzyme. We showed that tryptophan breakdown products such as kynurenine and 3-hidroxyanthranilic acid (3-HAA) can inhibit lymphocyte proliferation. These data suggest that IDO exerts its effect through the local accumulation of tryptophan metabolites, creating a microenvironment able to suppress the proliferation of activated lymphocytes including T cells and NK cells [20]. Once the proliferation of reactive lymphocytes is controlled, the pro-inflammatory mediators are reduced (TNF-a, IL6, IL12, IL1-b, etc.), the anti-inflammatory mediators are increased (IL-10) and the inflamed environment is restored. In summary, the proposed mechanism of action of this kind of cells for the treatment of anal fistula is primarily based on anti-proliferative and anti-inflammatory effects. According to this mechanism, eASCs deliver immunomodulatory signals that suppress inflammatory molecules and reactive lymphocyte proliferation, diminishing the inflammatory environment allowing the fistula tract to heal (Fig. 18.1) [20].

The application of MSC therapy in human wounds show excellent results from studies in the last years [15, 21, 22] and hence, in the treatment of complex perianal fistulas as we describe below.

Routes of Stem Cells Administration to Treat Anal Fistula

In clinical practise, most of experiences have been directed to treat anal fistula related with Crohn's disease. In this context two routes of administration have been tried: intravenous (systemic) and intralesional.

Intravenous injection has been used by the Group sponsored by Osiris Therapeutics that, to the date, do not provide publications of the results (*A Phase III, Multicenter, Placebo-controlled, Randomized, Double-blind Study to Evaluate the Safety and Efficacy of PROCHYMAL[tm] Intravenous Infusion for the Induction of Remission in Subjects Experiencing Treatment-refractory Moderate-to-severe Crohn's Disease.* Responsible Party: Osiris Therapeutics. ClinicalTrials.gov Identifier: NCT00482092; http://www.clinicaltrials.gov/). They are using intravenous infusion of suspension of allogenic

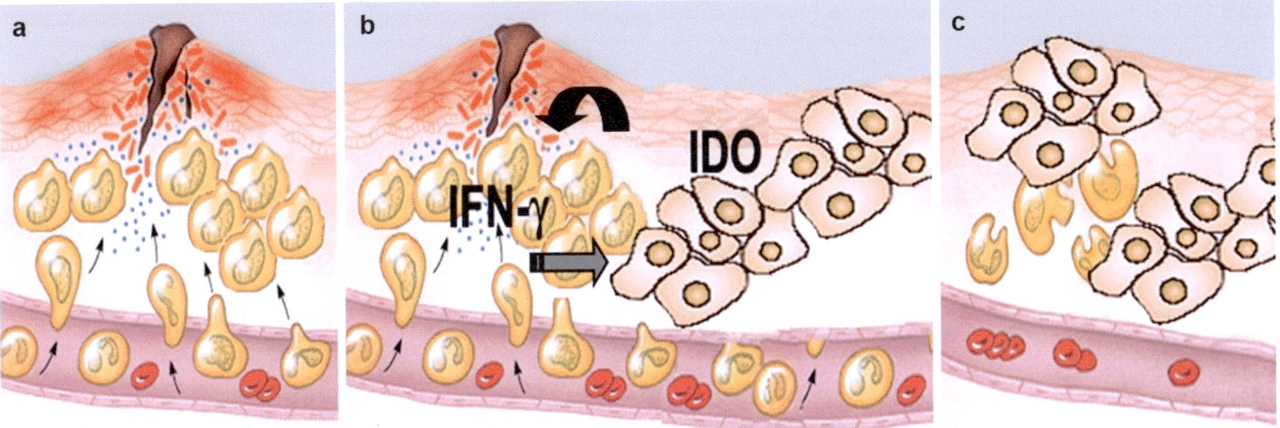

Fig. 18.1 Scheme of the mechanism of action of allogeneic eASCs in the tract of the anal fistula: anti-inflammatory and antiproliferative effect in an inflamed local environment (Courtesy of María Pascual). (**a**) MSCs from fat injected in the site of inflammation recognize proinflammatory cytokines. (**b**) IDO enzyme exerts its effect suppressing the proliferation of activated lymphocytes including T cells and NK cells. Once the proliferation of reactive lymphocytes is controlled, the proinflammatory mediators are reduced (TNF-a, IL6, IL12, IL1-b, etc.). (**c**) The anti-inflammatory mediators are increased (IL-10) and the inflamed environment is restored

adult human MSCs, total of 1,200 million (high dose) or 600 million (low dose) cells infused in four visits over 2 weeks. These adult human stem cells are manufactured from healthy, volunteer donors, extensively tested, and are stored to be available as needed. According with the Osiris information, human and animal studies have shown that the cells do not require any donor–recipient matching. The cells may have both immunosuppressive and healing benefits in Crohn's disease. The cells naturally migrate specifically to sites of inflammation, so their effects are believed to be local and self-limiting rather than systemic. Currently, they are enrolling subjects to evaluate the ability of PROCHYMAL to induce remission in subjects with moderate-to-severe disease (Crohn's disease activity index—CDAI—of between 250 and 450, inclusive) who have failed or been intolerant of at least one drug in each of the steroid, immunosuppressant, and biologic classes (http://www.clinicaltrials.gov/). Although publications are not available is important to remark that this protocol is now running as a Phase III clinical trial (http://www.clinicaltrials.gov/).

The rest of the experiences using stem cells to treat fistulas have been designed using cells in intralesional way. One of them is using autologous MSCs from bone marrow [23] and the others from fat (autologous and allogenic) as we describe ahead (see Tables 18.1, 18.2, 18.3, and 18.4).

Cells from bone marrow are isolated after an aspiration and MSCs were expanded ex vivo to be used for to treat fistula [23]. Cells from fat are named adipose-derived stem cells (ASCs) and are a suspension of living adult stem cells of mesenchymal origin extracted from adipose tissue of subdermal origin obtained in a liposuction procedure (Fig. 18.2). Subdermal adipose tissue has a heterogeneous cell component comprising mast cells, endothelial cells, pericytes, fibroblasts, and the stem cells of interest with multilineage capacity

(ASCs). The ASCs are isolated by digesting the adipose tissue with collagenase, followed by differential centrifugation and adherence to tissue culture plates with subsequent in vitro expansion [24]. The phenotype and the cell growth kinetic data demonstrate that the ex vivo expansion of ASCs does not alter their biological properties significantly as regards their proliferation capacity, morphological characteristics, and surface marker expression pattern and potency. The cell population present in the final product has therefore remained essentially unchanged throughout the whole expansion procedure [24].

Protocols of intra-fistula cell injections include the following steps: tract curettage, closure of internal opening, and cell injection. To be exact, after the initial experiences in 2002 [25, 26], the protocol described in 2009 [27] is currently followed by our Team and has 5–6 steps (Fig. 18.3):

1. Tract identification, with special emphasis on location of the internal opening.
2. Tract curettage with special emphasis on intersphincteric tracts.
3. Closure of the internal opening, if possible, with a Vicryl 2/0 (Ethicon) stitches.
4. Cell suspension and immediate use to prevent cells from settling.
5. Injection of cell suspension through a long fine needle (e.g., Abocatt 20; Terumo) into the tract walls, with half of the total cells being placed in the intersphincteric tracts and those adjacent to the internal opening and the other half being placed in the tract walls in the direction of the external opening. Injections were very superficial, no deeper than 2 mm.
6. In some cases we performed a sealing of the fistulous tract with fibrin adhesive.

Table 18.1 Published clinical experiences of stem cells treatments of anal fistula (Part 1)

Investigators	Year of publication	Trial code	Location	Condition	Study design	Cells source	Expanded	Cells number
García-Olmo et al. [25]	2003	NA	Spain	Recto-vaginal fistula in Crohn's disease	Case report	Autologous fat	Yes	$1 \times 10e7$
García-Olmo et al. [26]	2005	Not registered	Spain	Enterocutaneous, recto-vaginal, perianal fistula in Crohn's disease	Phase I	Autologous fat	Yes	$1–3 \times 10e7$ resuspended in fibrin glue
García-Olmo et al. [27]	2009	NCT0011 5466	Spain	Perianal fistula with or without Crohn's disease	Phase II	Autologous fat	Yes	Not specified
García-Olmo et al. [31]	2010	NA	Spain	Recto-vaginal fistula in Crohn's disease	Case report	Allogeneic fat	Yes	Not specified
Ciccocioppo et al. [23]	2011	NA	Italy	Enterocutaneous and complex perianal fistula in Crohn's disease	Case report	Autologous bone marrow	Yes	$5 \times 10e7$
Cho et al. [32]	2012	NCT0099 2485	Korea	Perianal fistula in Crohn's disease	Phase I	Autologous fat	Yes	Not specified
Herreros et al. [28]	2012	NCT0047 5410	Spain	Complex perianal fistula without Crohn's disease	Phase III	Autologous fat	Yes	$2 \times 10e7$ then $4 \times 10e7$ when no effect
Herreros et al. [28]	2012	NCT0102 0825	Spain	Complex perianal fistula without Crohn's disease	Observational	Autologous fat	Yes	$2 \times 10e7$ then $4 \times 10e7$ when no effect
Guadalajara et al. [33]	2012	Not registered	Spain	Perianal fistula with or without Crohn's disease	Observational	Autologous fat	Yes	Not specified
de la Portilla et al. [34]	2012	NCT0137 2969	Spain	Perianal fistula in Crohn's disease	Phase I/II	Allogeneic fat	Yes	$2 \times 10e7$ then $4 \times 10e7$ when no effect

It is important to remark that the technical items were showed as a key point, because after a Phase III clinical trial [27], we could observe objective evidence that the surgical expertise using cell therapy in anal fistula is a major item, i.e., our results in the Phase II study [27], the healing rate was of 70 %, whereas we achieved a healing rate of 83.3 % in the Phase III, although the baseline characteristics of the patients were similar in both [28].

Other techniques are described in uncompleted clinical trials, like successive injections in site without surgery.

The number of cells applied to the patients in the published studies is still low. The first step is to prove a safe profile of this treatment. This number is rising gradually, expecting that the success of the therapy is a matter of volume of cells.

Evidence Related to the Use of Stem Cells to Treat Anal Fistula

In order to analyze evidences about the safety and efficacy of stem cells in the treatment of anal fistulas, we have performed two different systematic reviews. The first one includes all published clinical data in Medline (keyword: fistula, stem cells) and the other one reviews all data available in ClinicalTrials.gov (A service of the U.S. National Institutes of Health (http://www.clinicaltrials.gov/)).

Systematic Review of Published Clinical Data (Tables 18.1 and 18.2)

We identify ten papers published that include data about clinical treatment of the anal fistula using stem cells. The first one was published in 2003 [25] and the last one recently, in 2012 [34]. Eight of them are from Spanish groups and the other two, one from Korea [32] and the other one from Italy [23]. Mostly are directed to treat anal fistula related with Crohn's disease. Only one study [23] treated fistulas using bone marrow as a cell source. The rest of the studies are using autologous or allogenic cells from fat. In all studies, cells were expanded with a wide range of doses (Table 18.1). Except the Italy study [23], procedures include the internal opening closure but in all cases the cell injections were intralesional. About 300 patients have been enrolled in this studies and the more important result is directed to assure that the safety profile of the stem cells are excellent: no serious adverse events related with cells were described. Regarding efficacy results show very different profiles, but we can say that about 40–60 % of patients achieve healing (Table 18.2).

Table 18.2 Published clinical experiences of stem cells treatments of anal fistula (part 2)

Investigator	Intervention model	Masking	Procedure	Enrolled	Number of treated patients	Healed	Follow up (months)	Recurrence	SAE[a]
García-Olmo et al. [25]	Single arm	Open label	Closure of IO. Without fibrin glue. Injection in site	1	1	1	3	0	0
García-Olmo et al. [26]	Single arm	Open label	Cells resuspended in fibrin glue. Injection in site	9	9	6	12	Not specified	0
García-Olmo et al. [27]	Two arms: fibrin glue, fibrin glue+ASCs	Open label	Closure of IO. Injection in site	50 (35 with Crohn's disease, 15 without Crohn's disease)	Fibrin glue: 25 Fibrin glue+ASCs: 24	Fibrin glue: 3 Fibrin glue+ASCs: 17	12	Fibrin glue: 0 Fibrin glue+ASCs: 2	4 (only one related to Fibrin glue, others not related)
García-Olmo et al. [31]	Single arm	Open label	Closure of IO. Without fibrin glue. Injection in site	1	1	1	36	1	0
Ciccocioppo et al. [23]	Single arm	Open label	Four injections in site	12	10	7	12	0	0
Cho et al. [32]	Single arm: dose escalation study	Open label	Closure of IO. Fibrin glue. Injection in site	10	9	3 of 9	15	0	0
Herreros et al. [28]	Three arms: fibrin glue, ASCs, fibrin glue+ASCs	Double blind (subject, Outcomes Assessor)	Closure of IO. Injection in site	214	ASCs: 64 Fibrin glue+ASCs: 60 Fibrin glue: 59	ASCs: 27 Fibrin glue+ASCs: 24 Fibrin glue: 23	6	ASCs: 0 Fibrin glue+ASCs: 4 Fibrin glue: 0	4 Unrelated to study treatment
Herreros et al. [28]	Three arms: fibrine, ASCs, fibrin glue+ASCs	Double blind (subject, Outcomes Assessor)	Closure of IO. Injection in site	135	Not specified	ASCs: 57 % Fibrin glue+ASCs: 52.4 %Fibrin glue: 37.3 %	12	Not specified	1 Unrelated to study treatment
Guadalajara et al. [33]	Two arms: fibrin glue, fibrin glue+ASCs	Open label	Closure of IO. Injection in site	34	Fibrin glue: 13 Fibrin glue+ASCs: 21	Fibrin glue: 3 Fibrin glue+ASCs: 10	38	Fibrin glue: 1 Fibrin glue+ASCs: 5	0
de la Portilla et al. [34]	Single arm	Open label	Closure of IO. Without fibrin glue. Injection in site	34	24	9	4	Not specified	2 Unrelated to study treatment

ASCs adult stem cells, *SAE* serious adverse events
[a]Requiring hospital admission longer than 24 h

Table 18.3 Ongoing clinical trials using stem cells for treatment of anal fistula (part 1)

Trial code	Condition	Sponsor	Investigator	Study start date	Location
NCT01157650	Enterocutaneous, recto-vaginal, perianal fistula in Crohn's disease	Clínica Universidad de Navarra, Universidad de Navarra	Prosper F	2010	Spain
NCT00999115	Recto-vaginal fistula in Crohn's disease	Instituto de Investigación Hospital Universitario la Paz	García-Olmo D	2009	Spain
NCT01314092	Complex perianal fistula without Crohn's disease	Anterogen Co., Ltd.	You CS	2011	Korea
NCT01586715	Extremely complex perianal fistula	Instituto de Investigación Hospital Universitario la Paz	García-Olmo D	2012	Spain
NCT01440699	Perianal fistula in Crohn's disease	Anterogen Co., Ltd.	Kim TI	2011	Korea
NCT01623453	Complex perianal fistula without Crohn's disease	Anterogen Co., Ltd.	Park KJ	2011	Korea
NCT01144962	Perianal fistula in Crohn's disease	Leiden University Medical Center	Hommes DW	2010	the Netherlands
NCT01011244	Perianal fistula in Crohn's disease	Anterogen Co., Ltd.	You CS	2010	Korea
NCT01548092	Recto-vaginal fistula in Crohn's disease	Instituto de investigación Hospital Universitario la Paz	Herreros MD	2011	Spain
NCT01584713	Enterocutaneous fistula with or without Crohn's disease	Instituto de Investigación Hospital Universitario la Paz	García-Arranz M	2011	Spain
NCT01314079	Perianal fistula in Crohn's disease	Anterogen Co., Ltd.	You CS	2011	Korea
NCT01541579	Perianal fistula in Crohn's disease	Tigenix	Not specified	2012	Europe, Israel
NCT00482092	Crohn's disease (reduction in number of draining fistulas)	Osiris Therapeutics	Custer L	2007	USA, Australia, Canada, New Zealand

Source: Clinicaltrials.gov (http://www.clinicaltrials.gov/)

Table 18.4 Ongoing clinical trials using stem cells for treatment of anal fistula (part 2)

Trial code	Cells source	Expanded	Cells number	Status	Phase	Intervention model	Masking	Estimated enrollment
NCT01157650	Autologous fat	Yes	Not specified	Recruiting	1, 2	Single arm	Open label	15
NCT00999115	Allogeneic fat	Yes	2×10e7, when no effect 4×10e7	Completed	1, 2	Single arm	Open label	10
NCT01314092	Autologous fat	Yes	1×10e7 or 2×10e7. Additional double dose when no effect	Recruiting	2	Two arms: low dose, high dose	Single blind (subject)	40
NCT01586715	Autologous fat	Yes	Not specified	Recruiting	2	Single arm	Open label	10
NCT01440699	Allogeneic fat	Yes	1×10e7 or 3×10e7	Recruiting	1	Single arm	Open label	6
NCT01623453	Autologous fat	Yes	1×10e7 or 2×10e7. Additional double dose when no effect	Active, not recruiting	2 (Follow-up)	Two arms: low dose, high dose	Single blind (subject)	40
NCT01144962	Allogeneic bone marrow	Yes	1×10e7, 3×10e7, 90×10e7	Recruiting	1, 2	Four arms: control group, ASCs	Double blind	21
NCT01011244	Autologous fat	Yes	Depending on the surface area of fistula	Completed	2	Single arm	Open label	40
NCT01548092	Autologous fat	No	Not specified	Recruiting	1, 2	Single arm	Open label	10
NCT01584713	Autologous fat	No	Not specified	Recruiting	1, 2	Single arm	Open label	10
NCT01314079	Autologous fat	Yes	Depending on the surface area of fistula	Ongoing, not recruiting	2 (Follow-up)	Single arm	Open label	40
NCT01541579	Allogeneic fat	Yes	12×10e7	Recruiting	3	Two arms: (ASCs, Placebo)	Double blind	208
NCT00482092	Allogeneic bone marrow	Yes	1,200 million or 600 million cells infused in four visits	Recruiting	3	Three arms: placebo, high dose and low dose	Double blind	270

ASCs adult stem cells

Source: Clinicaltrials.gov (http://www.clinicaltrials.gov/)

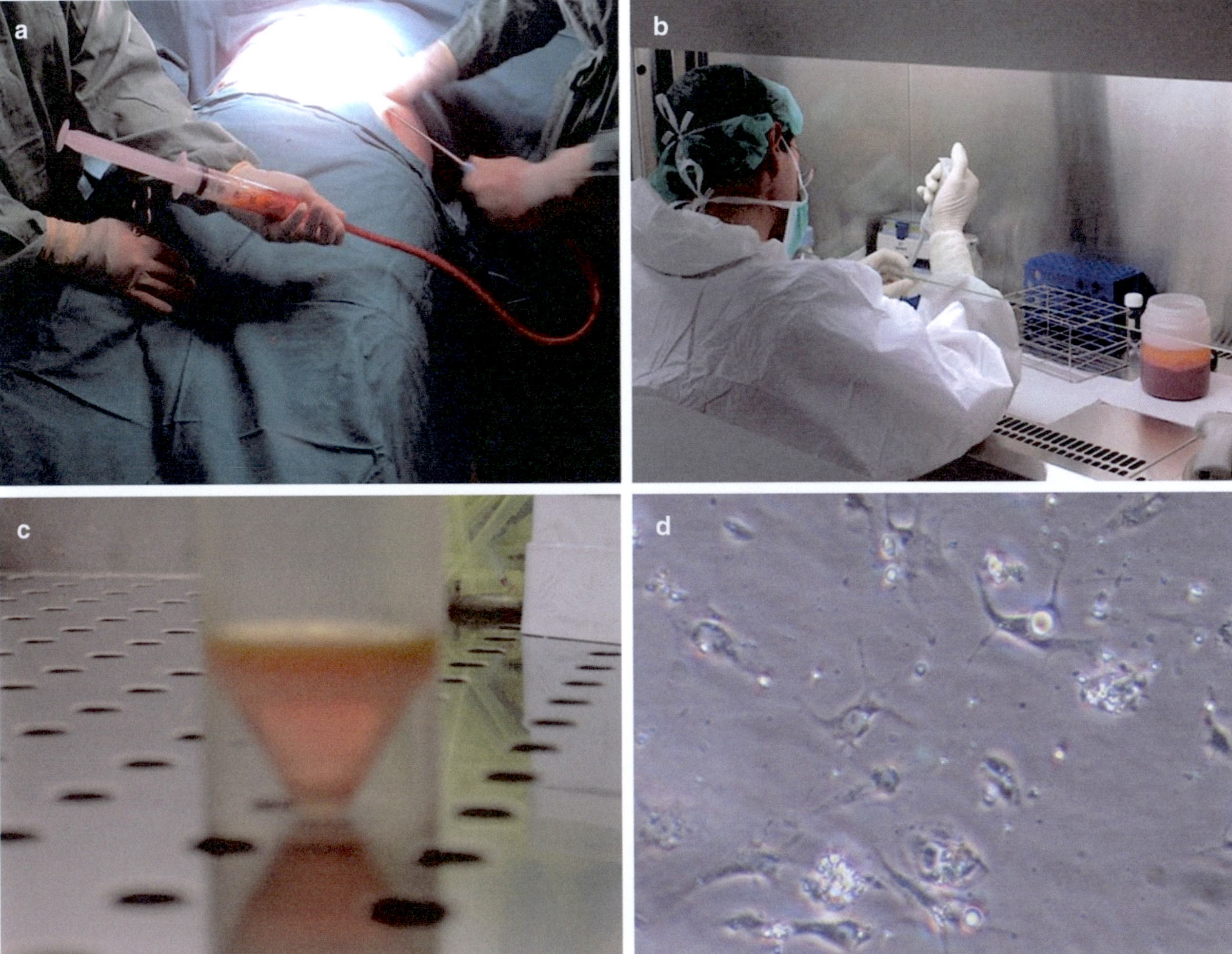

Fig. 18.2 Process of extraction of cells from fat (ASCs). (**a**) Liposuction with local anesthesia and little incision. (**b**) The ASCs are isolated by digesting the adipose tissue with collagenase, followed by differential centrifugation and adherence to tissue culture plates with subsequent in vitro expansion. (**c**) Stromal vascular fraction: subdermal adipose tissue has a heterogeneous cell component comprising mast cells, endothelial cells, pericytes, fibroblasts, and the stem cells of inter-est with multilineage capacity. (**d**) Microscope picture of ASCs before expansion. The phenotype and the cell growth kinetic data demonstrate that the ex vivo expansion of ASCs does not alter their biological properties significantly as regards their proliferation capacity, morphological characteristics, and surface marker expression pattern and potency. The cell population present in the final product has therefore remained essentially unchanged throughout the whole expansion procedure

Ongoing Clinical Trials (Tables 18.3 and 18.4)

To the date, 13 trials directed to treat anal fistula using stem cells were identified in Clinicaltrials.gov (http://www.clinicaltrials.gov/). Twelve of them are focused exclusively in Crohn's disease. Korea and Spain have registered five and the Netherlands one, all of them in Phase I or II. The other two clinical trials are multinational studies in Phase III. One of them is developing in Europe and Israel under Tygenix SL sponsorship. The other Phase III clinical trial is running in the USA, Australia, Canada, and New Zealand under Osiris Therapeutics sponsorship (Table 18.3).

Autologous or allogenic fat is the cells source in 11 studies and the two others use bone marrow as a cell source in an allogenic mode (Table 18.4). Two of these clinical trials have been completed (NCT00999115 and NCT01011244) but to the date data have not been published. The total estimated patient enrollments are 270 patients and the majority of results are expected by 2015.

From Present Experiences: A Look to the Future

Indeed, new approaches are therefore needed in the treatment of anal fistula due to outcomes are far from ideal given the problems of fecal incontinence in the case of aggressive surgery or recurrence in the case of less aggressive surgery.

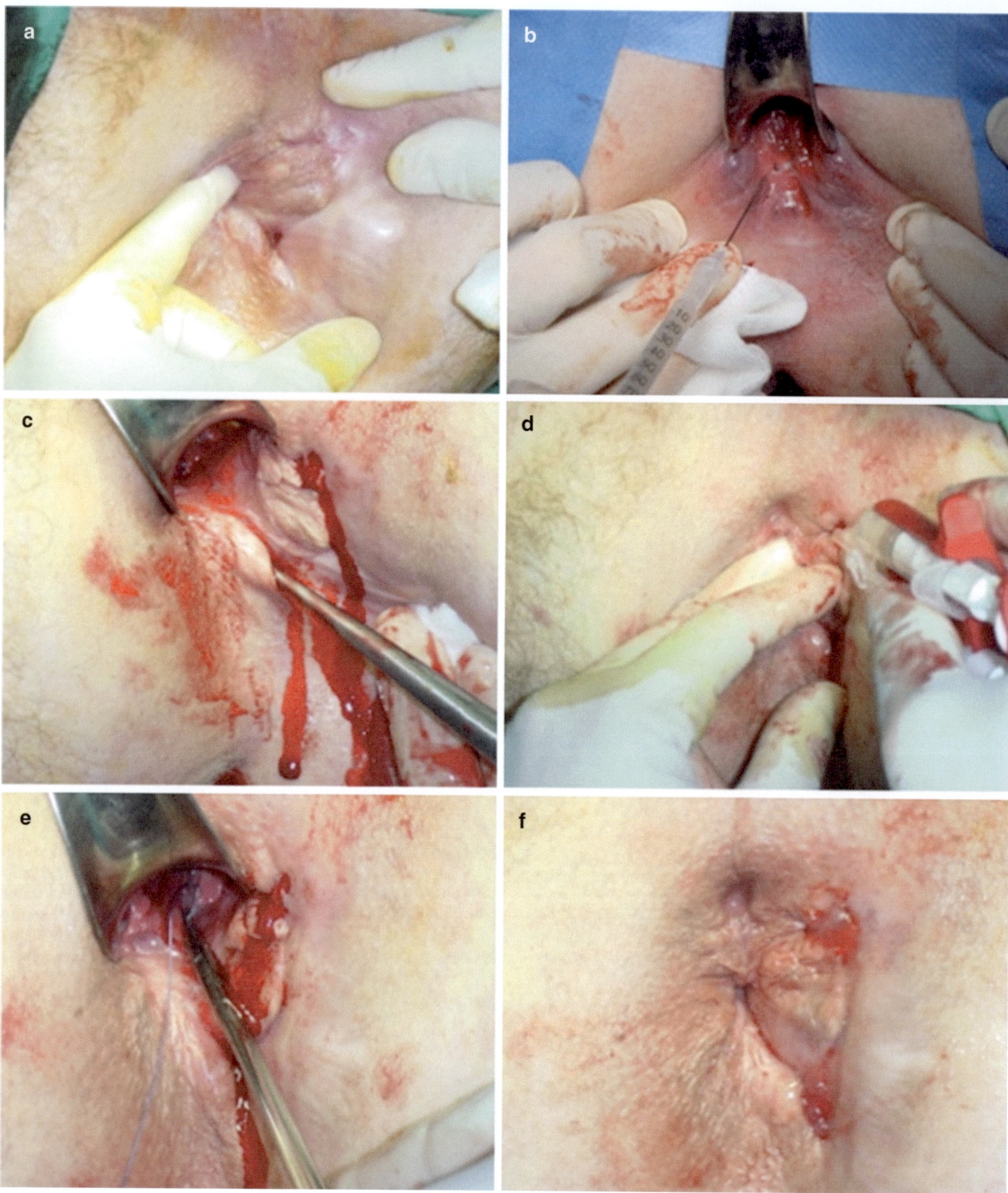

Fig. 18.3 Surgical protocol for intra-fistula cells injection. (**a**) Tract identification; (**b**) cells injection in internal opening; (**c**) curettage; (**d**) tract sealant; (**e**) internal opening closure; (**f**) final view

Stem cells appear to be a novel tool for the repair of damaged tissues. Their use exploits two coordinated biological effects, namely, immunoregulation and the local suppression of inflammation on the one hand and the proliferation and differentiation of cells on the other.

Randomized controlled studies using stem cells to treat anal fistula has been conducted, and all of them show an excellent safety profile. Nevertheless, the real efficacy is hard to assess. The outcome of the only Phase III clinical trial published [28] was negative in that the primary outcome measure was not met, but there are certain indications, in line with the preceding studies, suggesting that the procedure can be effective in the right conditions. Furthermore, long-term results showed that the healing rate at 1 year was double for the use of ASCs with or without fibrin in comparison with fibrin glue alone. That's one of the reasons why further studies should be performed to better define the most beneficial scenario for stem cell therapy in patients with anal fistula.

Is this approach to treat complex anal fistula worth pursuing? Any decision will be influenced by the fact that surgery is the only accepted effective treatment for complex anal fistula. Despite healing rates above 60 %, surgery is associated with incontinence rates between 10 and 35 % and recurrence rates between 11 and 45 % [29, 30]. With cell therapy, there is no injury to the anal sphincter because tract resection is not required and repeated doses can be used to increase the chance of healing. In addition, adult stem cell therapy is not subject to the major ethical concerns. On the other hand, the cost of therapy with stem cells is difficult to ascertain at present. For our Phase II study [27], the cost of producing pharmaceutical grade cells (i.e., Good Manufacturing Practice (GMP) compliant) was in the range of dollars 8,000–12,000. However, this estimate corresponds to an experimental production cost, and economies of scale would be expected for industrial production.

Other treatments for perianal fistulas that may be in clinical development have yet to be tested in randomized trials, and so we do not anticipate other products coming onto the market in the near future. Once available, for the reasons outlined earlier in the chapter, we believe the stem cells will fulfill a clear unmet medical need and will help improve the healing and hence the quality of life of patients with anal fistula.

Summary

- Cell therapy has emerged as a new tool to improve wound healing in a number of settings. There are pathological situations in which this cell supply is deficient and wound healing may be delayed or not achieved, this is the case of anal fistula. Stem cells exploit two coordinated biological effects, namely, immunoregulation and the local suppression of inflammation. The promising preclinical and clinical data that we will review in this chapter suggest that stem cells could represent a major advance in the clinical management of this difficult problem.
- With cell therapy, there is no injury to the anal sphincter because tract resection is not required and repeated doses can be used to increase the chance of healing. Importantly, in a clinical setting, fat appears as a great source of stem cells.
- The immunoregulation effect and the local suppression of inflammation, make of patients with perianal Crohn's disease perfect candidates for this treatment.

- For the reasons outlined in this chapter, we believe the stem cells will fulfill a clear unmet medical need and will help improve the healing and hence the quality of life of patients with anal fistula.

Acknowledgment The authors thank Maria Pascual Martinez for her support during drafting of this chapter.

Disclosure UAM and Cellerix SL/Tygenix SL share patents rights in cell products. García-Olmo is a member of the scientific advisory board of Tygenix. Damian García-Olmo is inventor in two patents related to cell products entitled "Identification and isolation of multipotent cells from non-osteochondral Mesenchymal tissue" (10157355957US) and "Use of adipose tissue-derived stromal stem cells in treating fistula" (US11/167061). The authors have received no payment in preparation of this manuscript.

References

1. Garcia-Aguilar J, Davey CS, Le CT, et al. Patient satisfaction after surgical treatment for fistula-in-ano. Dis Colon Rectum. 2000; 43(9):1206–12.
2. Halligan S, Buchanan G. MR imaging of fistula-in-ano. Eur J Radiol. 2003;47(2):98–107.
3. Sands BE, Anderson FH, Bernstein CN, et al. Infliximab maintenance therapy for fistulizing Crohn's disease. N Engl J Med. 2004; 350(9):876–85.
4. Present DH, Rutgeerts P, Targan S, et al. Infliximab for the treatment of fistulas in patients with Crohn's disease. N Engl J Med. 1999;340(18):1398–405.
5. Sandborn WJ, Rutgeerts P, Enns R, et al. Adalimumab induction therapy for Crohn disease previously treated with infliximab: a randomized trial. Ann Intern Med. 2007;146(12):829–38.
6. Whiteford MH, Kilkenny 3rd J, Hyman N, et al. Practice parameters for the treatment of perianal abscess and fistula-in-ano (revised). Dis Colon Rectum. 2005;48(7):1337–42.
7. Van Bodegraven AA, Sloots CE, Felt-Bersma RJ, Meuwissen SG. Endosonographic evidence of persistence of Crohn's disease-associated fistulas after infliximab treatment, irrespective of clinical response. Dis Colon Rectum. 2002;45(1):39–45; discussion 45–6.
8. Van Assche G, Vanbeckevoort D, Bielen D, et al. Magnetic resonance imaging of the effects of infliximab on perianal fistulizing Crohn's disease. Am J Gastroenterol. 2003;98(2):332–9.
9. Verfaillie CM. Adult stem cells: assessing the case for pluripotency. Trends Cell Biol. 2020;12:502–8.
10. Trebol Lopez J, Georgiev Hristov T, García-Arranz M, García-Olmo D. Stem cell therapy for digestive tract diseases: current state and future perspectives. Stem Cells Dev. 2011;20(7):1113–29.
11. García-Gómez I, Elvira G, Zapata AG, Lamana ML, Ramírez M, Castro JG, Arranz MG, Vicente A, Bueren J, García-Olmo D. Mesenchymal stem cells: biological properties and clinical applications. Expert Opin Biol Ther. 2010;10(10):1453–68.
12. Boulton AJM, Vileikyte L, Ragnarson-Tennvall G, Apelqvist J. The global burden of diabetic foot disease. Lancet. 2005;366:1719–24.
13. Singer AJ, Clark RAF. Cutaneous wound healing. N Engl J Med. 1999;341:738–46.
14. Chapel A, Bertho JM, Bensidhoum M, Fouillard L, Young RG, Frick J, Demarquay C, Cuvelier F, Mathieu E, Trompier F, Dudoignon N, Germain C, Mazurier C, Aigueperse J, Borneman J, Gorin NC, Gourmelon P, Thierry D. Mesenchymal stem cells home to injured tissues when co-infused with hematopoietic cells to treat a radiation-induced multi-organ failure syndrome. J Gene Med. 2003;5:1028–38.

15. Falanga V, Iwamoto S, Chartier M, Yufit T, Butmarc J, Kouttab N, Shrayer D, Carson P. Autologous bone marrow derived cultured mesenchymal stem cells delivered in a fibrin spray accelerate healing in murine and human cutaneous wounds. Tissue Eng. 2007; 13:1299–312.

16. McFarlin K, Gao X, Liu YB, Dulchavsky DS, Kwon D, Arbab AS, Bansal M, Li Y, Chopp M, Dulchavsky SA, Gautam SC. Bone marrow-derived mesenchymal stromal cells accelerate wound healing in the rat. Wound Repair Regen. 2006;14:471–8.

17. Wu Y, Chen L, Scott PG, Tredget EE. Mesenchymal stem cells enhance wound healing through differentiation and angiogenesis. Stem Cells. 2007;25:2648–59.

18. Chen L, Tredget EE, Wu PYG, Wu Y. Paracrine factors of mesenchymal stem cells recruit macrophages and endothelial lineage cells and enhance wound healing. PLoS One. 2008;3(4):e1886.

19. Hanson SE, Bentz ML, Hematti P. Mesenchymal stem cell therapy for nonhealing cutaneous wounds. Plast Reconstr Surg. 2010;125: 510–6.

20. DelaRosa O, Lombardo E, Beraza A, Mancheño-Corvo P, Ramirez C, Menta R, Rico L, Camarillo E, García L, Abad JL, Trigueros C, Delgado M, Büscher D. Requirement of IFN-gamma-mediated indoleamine 2,3-dioxygenase expression in the modulation of lymphocyte proliferation by human adipose-derived stem cells. Tissue Eng Part A. 2009;15(10):2795–806.

21. Lataillade JJ, Doucet C, Bey E, Carsin H, Huet C, Clairand I, Bottollier-Depois JF, Chapel A, Ernou I, Gourven M, Boutin L, Hayden A, Carcamo C, Buglova E, Joussemet M, de Revel T, Gourmelon P. New approach to radiation burn treatment by dosimetry-guided surgery combined with autologous mesenchymal stem cell therapy. Regen Med. 2007;2:785–94.

22. Yoshikawa T, Mitsuno H, Nonaka I, Sen Y, Kawanishi K, Inada Y, Takakura Y, Okuchi K, Nonomura A. Wound therapy by marrow mesenchymal cell transplantation. Plast Reconstr Surg. 2008;121: 860–77.

23. Ciccocioppo R, Bernardo ME, Sgarella A, Maccario R, Avanzini MA, Ubezio C, Minelli A, Alvisi C, Vanoli A, Calliada F, Dionigi P, Perotti C, Locatelli F, Corazza GR. Autologous bone marrow-derived mesenchymal stromal cells in the treatment of fistulising Crohn's disease. Gut. 2011;60(6):788–98.

24. Garcia-Olmo D, Garcia-Arranz M, Herreros D. Expanded adipose-derived stem cells for the treatment of complex perianal fistula including Crohn's disease. Expert Opin Biol Ther. 2008;8(9): 1417–23.

25. García-Olmo D, García-Arranz M, García LG, Cuellar ES, Blanco IF, Prianes LA, Montes JA, Pinto FL, Marcos DH, García-Sancho L. Autologous stem cell transplantation for treatment of rectovaginal fistula in perianal Crohn's disease: a new cell-based therapy. Int J Colorectal Dis. 2003;18(5):451–4.

26. García-Olmo D, García-Arranz M, Herreros D, Pascual I, Peiro C, Rodríguez-Montes JA. A phase I clinical trial of the treatment of Crohn's fistula by adipose mesenchymal stem cell transplantation. Dis Colon Rectum. 2005;48(7):1416–23.

27. Garcia-Olmo D, Herreros D, Pascual I, Pascual JA, Del-Valle E, Zorrilla J, De-La-Quintana P, Garcia-Arranz M, Pascual M. Expanded adipose-derived stem cells for the treatment of complex perianal fistula: a phase II clinical trial. Dis Colon Rectum. 2009;52(1):79–86.

28. Herreros MD, Garcia-Arranz M, Guadalajara H, De-La-Quintana P, Garcia-Olmo D. Autologous expanded adipose-derived stem cells for the treatment of complex cryptoglandular perianal fistulas: a phase III randomized clinical trial (FATT 1: fistula Advanced Therapy Trial 1) and long-term evaluation. Dis Colon Rectum. 2012;55(7):762–72.

29. Ortiz H, Marzo J. Endorectal flap advancement repair and fistulectomy for high trans-sphincteric and suprasphincteric fistulas. Br J Surg. 2000;87:1680–3.

30. Abbas MA, Lemus-Rangel R, Hamadani A. Long-term outcome of endorectal advancement flap for complex anorectal fistulae. Am Surg. 2008;74:921–4.

31. García-Olmo D, Herreros D, De-La-Quintana P, Guadalajara H, Trébol J, Georgiev-Hristov T, García-Arranz M. Adipose-derived stem cells in Crohn's rectovaginal fistula. Case Report Med. 2010;2010:961758.

32. Cho YB, Lee WY, Park KJ, Kim M, Yoo HW, Yu CS. Autologous adipose tissue-derived stem cells for the treatment of Crohn's fistula: a phase I clinical study. Cell Transplant. 2013;22(2):279–85. doi:10.3727/096368912X656045.

33. Guadalajara H, Herreros D, De-La-Quintana P, Trebol J, Garcia-Arranz M, Garcia-Olmo D. Long-term follow-up of patients undergoing adipose-derived adult stem cell administration to treat complex perianal fistulas. Int J Colorectal Dis. 2012;27:595–600.

34. de la Portilla F, Alba F, García-Olmo D, Herrerías JM, González FX, Galindo A. Expanded allogeneic adipose-derived stem cells (eASCs) for the treatment of complex perianal fistula in Crohn's disease: results from a multicenter phase I/IIa clinical trial. Int J Colorectal Dis. 2013;28(3):313–23. doi:10.1007/s00384-012-1581-9.

James Fleshman and Rachel Tay

Background

Perianal and anovaginal fistulas represent a very challenging problem in 20–30 % of patients with Crohn's disease. Of these patients, 80 % will also have or develop intestinal disease. Perianal fistulas are more likely to develop in patients with Crohn's disease involving the colon or rectum as opposed to those with isolated ileocolic disease. Men, those who develop Crohn's at a younger age, and non-Caucasians are also at an increased risk of developing perianal disease. The development of perianal fistulas is oftentimes a poor prognostic indicator and portends a worse course of disease in patients who are afflicted. The priority for physicians treating patients with Crohn's fistulas of the anus should be preservation of the anal sphincter and avoidance of a permanent ostomy.

Types of Fistulas

The classification of fistulas of common (cryptoglandular) anal fistulas was described by Parks and Gordon in 1976. There are four types of fistulas within this classification (Fig. 19.1). Intersphincteric fistulas are the most common, and comprise approximately 45 % of all fistulas. These fistulas only traverse the internal anal sphincter and connect to the perianal skin. Transsphincteric fistulas comprise 30 % of fistulas and involve both the external and internal anal sphincters. A small portion of the external anal sphincter is usually involved. Suprasphincteric fistulas comprise 20 % of anal fistulas and cross the internal anal sphincter, then pass upwards and around the majority of the external anal sphincter

back to the skin. Extrasphincteric fistulas encompass the entire sphincter complex and open internally into the bowel above the anus. They are the least common type and represent only 2–5 % of all fistulas. The most common cause is iatrogenic injury to the levator plate when draining a large suprasphincteric abscess. They are very often related to an intra-abdominal intestinal source in patients with Crohn's disease, which will respond only to bowel resection.

Fistula classification and location can be very important with regard to selecting the appropriate treatment options in both cryptoglandular and Crohn's disease patients. Fistulas rarely follow these rules of classification in patients with Crohn's disease. Even so, males with a low, intersphincteric, posterior Crohn's fistula may be treated successfully with primary fistulotomy with good success and minimal risk of incontinence. In contrast, women with anterior fistulas have a high risk of incontinence even when treated with superficial fistulotomy and will often require an alternative form of surgical therapy such as a sliding flap repair. Regardless of the position of the fistula around the circumference of the anal canal, high fistulas are less likely to heal, more likely to result in incontinence after treatment, and may require diversion.

Cryptoglandular Fistulas Versus Crohn's Disease

It may be difficult at times to distinguish between cryptoglandular and Crohn's fistulas even though the pathogenesis and natural history are very different. This distinction is important to make, as the treatment of these diseases is very different. Fistulas which develop in an atypical location or do not heal regardless of multiple attempts with medical and surgical treatment point to a diagnosis of Crohn's fistula. Cryptoglandular fistulas are thought to arise from the blockage and infection of one of the anal glands at the dentate line. The gland normally empties into the anal crypt. Abscess formation results in the development of an anal fistula in up

J. Fleshman, M.D., F.A.C.S., F.A.S.C.R.S. (✉) • R. Tay, M.D.
Department of Surgery, Baylor University Medical Center,
3500 Gashan Ave, Dallas, TX 75204, USA
e-mail: fleshman@wudosis.wustl.edu

H. Abcarian (ed.), *Anal Fistula: Principles and Management*, DOI 10.1007/978-1-4614-9014-2_19,
© Springer Science+Business Media New York 2014

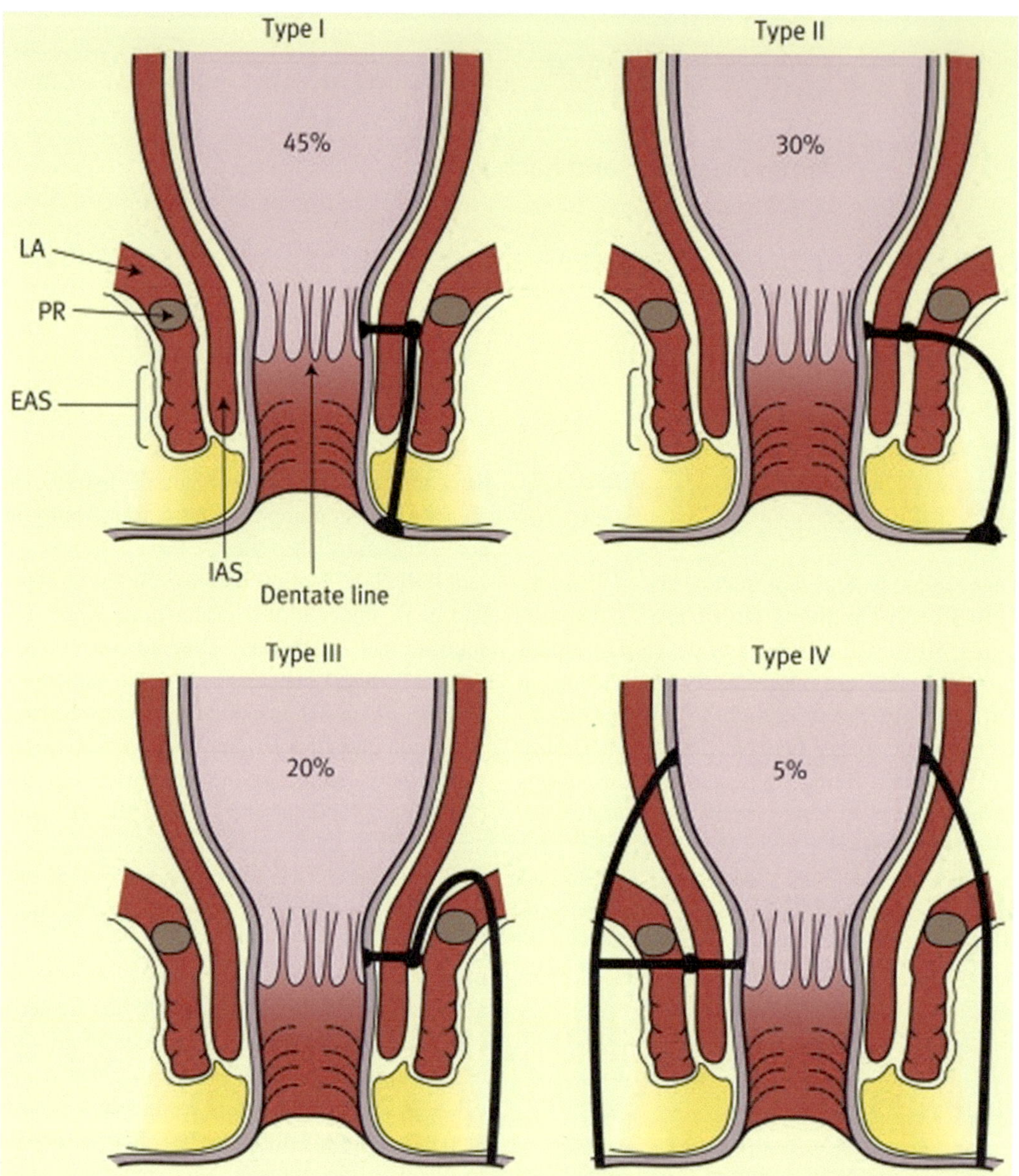

Fig. 19.1 Parks' classification of fistula-in-ano. Type I, intersphincteric; Type II, transsphincteric; Type III, suprasphincteric; Type IV, extrasphincteric. The terms trans-, supra-, and extra- refer to the external sphincter mass. *EAS* external anal sphincter, *IAS* internal anal sphincter, *LA* levator ani, *PR* puborectalis. (With permission from: Tiernan JP, Brown Sr. Benign anal conditions: haemorrhoids, fissures, perianal abscess, fistula-in-ano, and pilonidal sinus. Surgery (Oxford) 2011;29(8):382–386)

to 1/3 of patients. The pathogenesis of Crohn's fistulas remains poorly understood but is thought to be different than that of the cryptoglandular form. One theory is that a deep anorectal ulcer forms, which subsequently becomes invaded by fecal material and bacteria. The tract is then created by the pressure from the anorectum. Crohn's fistulas are generally more complex with branching and multiple tracts, which do not follow the typical pattern of cryptoglandular fistulas or Goodsall's Rule. Unlike patients with cryptoglandular fistulas, Crohn's fistulas usually do not respond to operative therapy alone. A different algorithm of treatment must be followed with a stronger emphasis on optimal medical management to control rectal disease and reduce the autoimmune inflammatory component of the fistulization.

The possibility that fistulas are due to Crohn's disease should trigger a search for active disease in the colon or small bowel. Even if intestinal disease is not present, it is possible to distinguish Crohn's from cryptoglandular fistulas by identifying granulomas in the curettings from the fistula tract or areas of undermined skin. Perianal skin tags may also yield pathognomonic non-caseating granulomas. Zawadzki and colleagues in Sweden reported a unique imaging characteristic on 3D endoanal ultrasound (EUS) for Crohn's fistulas. This was defined as a hypoechogenic fistula track surrounded by a hyperechogenic area extending into the perianal tissue with a thin, regular hypoechogenic edge. They noted that 20 of 29 (69 %) patients with Crohn's had a positive Crohn ultrasound fistula sign (CUFS) while 125 out of 128 (98 %) patients with cryptoglandular fistulas did not [1]. This may be a useful, noninvasive method which helps to distinguish Crohn's fistulas from other forms of perianal disease.

Differential Diagnosis

It is not uncommon ($\approx$20 %) for patients to present with perianal Crohn's disease as their first symptom. As already mentioned, it can be difficult to distinguish between this and other etiologies of perianal disease. Hidradenitis is a common diagnosis which may be confused with Crohn's fistulas and may also occur in association with severe perianal Crohn's disease. Clues to a diagnosis of hidradenitis include additional tracts or abscesses within the groin or armpit, multiple tracts in the perianal skin without connection to the anal canal, and severe disease at onset rather than a gradual worsening in severity over time. Other diagnoses within the differential include cryptoglandular fistula, pilonidal cysts, sexually transmitted diseases, anal fissure, Kaposi's sarcoma, and anal squamous cell cancer. Knowledge of each of these and heightened suspicion are necessary as one evaluates a patient with unusual findings or presentations.

Clinical Manifestations and Diagnosis

Undiagnosed patients may present with constant anal pain, pain with defecation, a painless draining perianal skin opening, a painful persistent abscess in the perineum, or unexplained fever. Proper evaluation of the patient includes taking a thorough history with regard to any prior episodes in the past as well as other symptoms of Crohn's disease including abdominal pain, diarrhea (with or without blood), tenesmus, fevers, or weight loss. A perianal and rectal exam should be performed in the prone jackknife position, looking for fistula tracts, fluctuance, erythema, strictures, or skin tags. An exam under anesthesia (EUA) is necessary if the patient does not tolerate the in-office exam and an anal probe would be used to identify and define the tract and location of the internal opening. If there is difficulty delineating the tract, dilute hydrogen peroxide or betadine may be injected through the external opening in order to aid in locating the internal opening. EUA has long been recognized as the gold standard for identifying tracts and delineating the extent of disease in fistula disease. A lighted Buie Hirschman anoscope is essential

to provide good vision in the office while the half circle Hill Ferguson retractor usually gives adequate exposure and vision with reflected light in the operating room. Lighted Hill Ferguson retractors are also available.

A complete evaluation of the rectum should also be performed using either flexible sigmoidoscopy or rigid proctoscopy. Documentation of rectal mucosa involvement is essential to planning treatment. Eventually, colonoscopy should be performed to evaluate the rest of the colon.

Imaging

EUS, MRI, CT, fistulography, and endoscopy have been used in diagnosing and evaluating Crohn's fistulas. Fistulography is an older imaging modality which involves the injection of contrast into the visible external opening, with subsequent radiography. This technique has fallen out of favor for use in perianal disease as it has been shown to have a low accuracy rate. A retrospective study showed that it was accurate in only four of 25 patients in delineating fistulas compared to operative findings. Fistulography may be helpful in the circumstance of extrasphincteric disease or when used with other modalities. CT has been used for fistula imaging; however, it is limited by lower resolution, artifact, image blurring, streaking due to fistula contents, and an inconsistency identifying the levator ani. CT has not been useful to classify fistulas or guide appropriate treatment [2, 3].

MRI is a proven technique for detecting and delineating fistula tracts. The internal and external anal sphincters are well characterized, and therefore the relationship of the fistula tract to these structures can be determined. Endoanal coils may be used to enhance the resolution of the MRI, though this technique may be limited by patient discomfort. For patients suspected to have complex disease extending into the pelvis, such as in suprasphincteric fistulas, 1 mL of glucagon may be administered intramuscularly to help decrease bowel motion [4]. Fibrotic fistulous tracts will appear hypo-intense on T1- and T2-weighted images and enhance with administration of gadolinium (Fig. 19.2). Fluid and granulation tissue will both appear hyper-intense but only granulation tissue will enhance with gadolinium (Figs. 19.3 and 19.4). Buchanan found that disease recurrence after surgery in patients with fistula-in-ano was decreased by 75 % in those who underwent preoperative MRI [5].

EUS of the anal canal was introduced in the 1980s [6, 7], and multiple studies have shown this technique to be accurate in defining fistula anatomy with greater ease and lower cost than MRI. Injection of peroxide into the fistula tract has been found to help accurately (95 %) delineate fistula tracts [8]. The tract will become hyper-echoic on ultrasound with this technique. Accuracy may be improved further by using

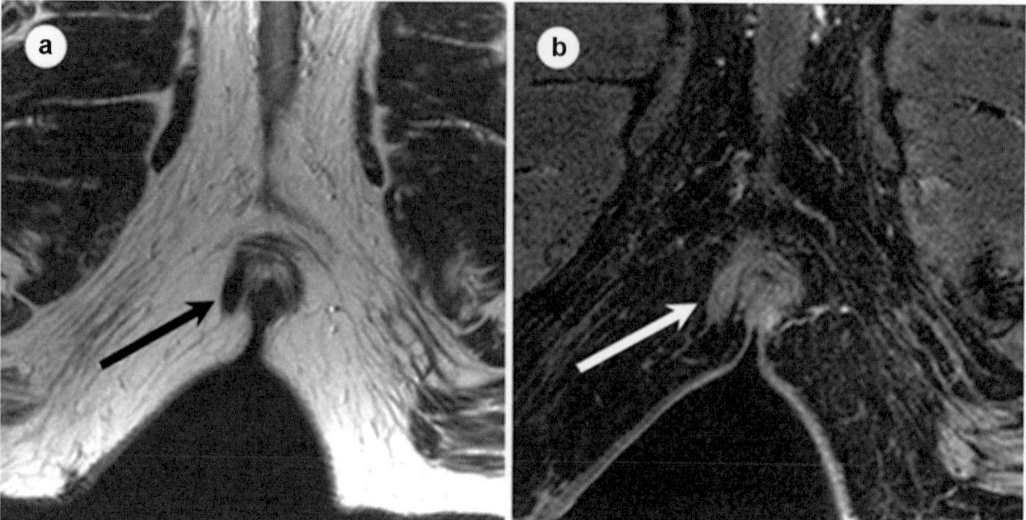

Fig. 19.2 Appearance of fibrotic fistula track at MR. Sixty-three-year-old male with right lateral fibrotic intersphincteric fistula track. Axial T2 FSE (**a**) and axial T1W SPGR postgadolinium images with fat saturation (**b**) obtained at 1.5 T below the level of the anal sphincters. Fibrotic tracks at MR appear as bands of homogenous low signal intensity at T2W1 (*black arrow* in **a**). After the administration of gadolium, enhancement is homogenous throughout the fibrotic track (*white arrow* on **b**). *FSE* fat spin echo, *SPGR* spoiled gradient recalled echo. (Adapted from Sun MR, Smith MP, Kane RA. Current techniques in imaging of fistula in ano: 3D endoanal ultrasound and magnetic resonance imaging. Semin Ultrasound CT MRI 2008;29:454–471, with permission)

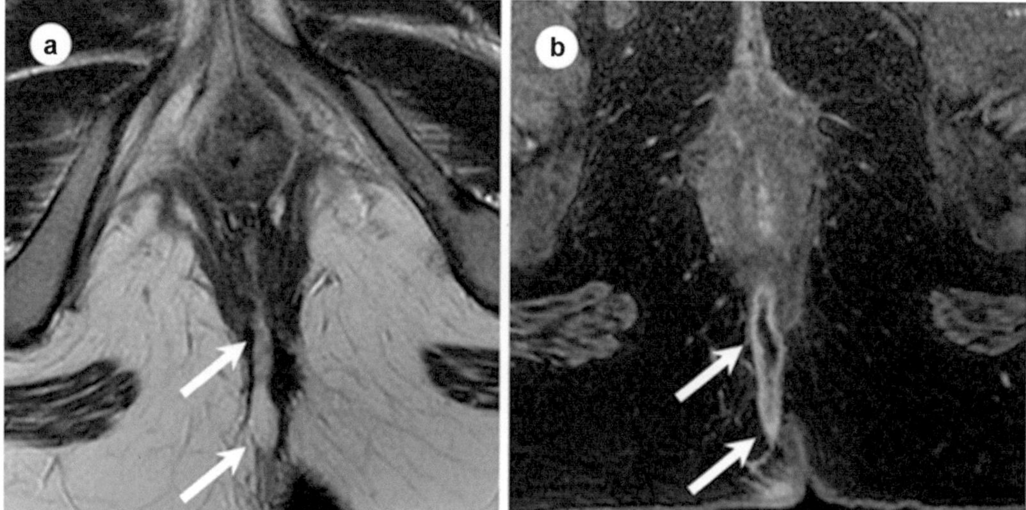

Fig. 19.3 Appearance of fluid-containing track at MR. Twenty-five-year-old female with posterior transsphincteric fistula. Axial T2 FSE (**a**) and postgadolinium T1W SPRG (**b**) images obtained at 1.5 T. Fluid-containing tracks show peripheral low signal intensity and linear central high signal intensity on T2WI (*arrows* in **a**). After the administration of intravenous gadolinium the track enhances peripherally but the fluid within the track lumen does not enhance (*arrow* in **b**). *FSE* fat spin echo, *SPGR* spoiled gradient recalled echo. (Adapted from Sun MR, Smith MP, Kane RA. Current techniques in imaging of fistula in ano: 3D endoanal ultrasound and magnetic resonance imaging. Semin Ultrasound CT MRI 2008;29:454–471, with permission)

the 3D EUS (Fig. 19.5). EUS is less accurate in detecting disease extending into the pelvis or ischiorectal fossa [9]. Crohn's patients especially are less likely to tolerate the endoanal probe due to pain or the presence of stricture and this may limit the usefulness of EUS. The accuracy rate of EUS remains, in part, operator-dependent [10]. Multiple studies comparing EUS with MRI provide no clear consensus regarding superiority. Schwartz prospectively demonstrated equivalent accuracy between MRI, EUS, and EUA (87 %, 91 %, and 91 %, respectively) for determining fistula anatomy in Crohn's disease patients. Combining MRI and EUS was noted to have a near 100 % accuracy rate for the detection and delineation of fistula tracts [11]. Sahni et al. found MRI to be superior to EUS with regard to specificity and sensitivity

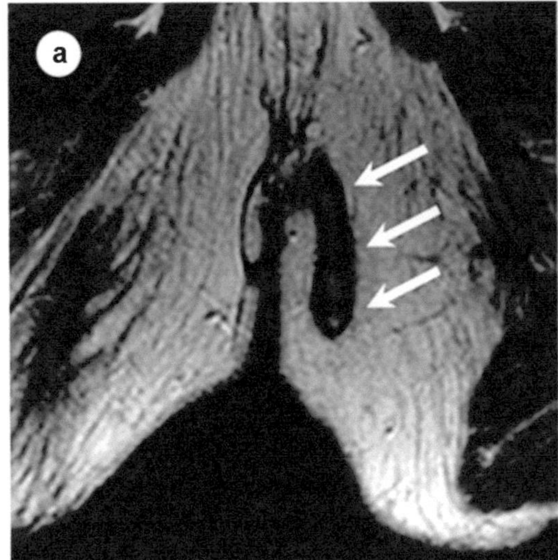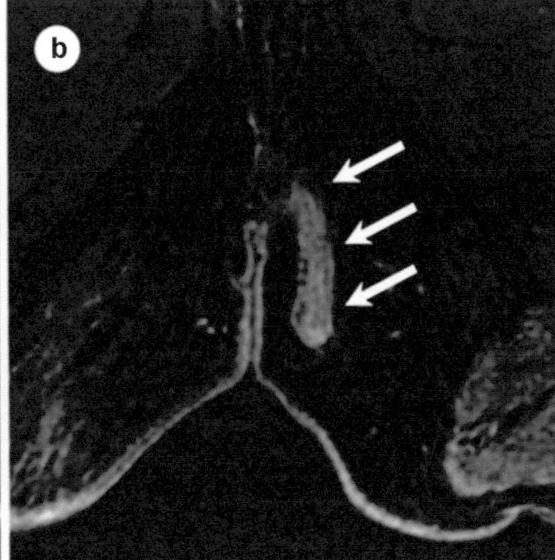

Fig. 19.4 Fistula track containing granulation tissue at MR. Seventy-seven-year-old male with transsphincteric fistula track containing granulation tissue. Axial T2 FSE (**a**) and axial T1W SPGR postgadolinium (**b**) images, obtained at 1.5 T. Granulation tissue within a fistula track appears similar to fluid within a track on T2WI, visible as a linear area of hyperintensity at T2WI (*arrows* in **a**). However, after the administration of intravenous gadolinium, granulation tissue enhances (*arrows* in **b**), while fluid within a track does not. *FSE* fast spin echo, *SPGR* spoiled gradient recalled echo. (Adapted from Sun MR, Smith MP, Kane RA. Current techniques in imaging of fistula in ano: 3D endoanal ultrasound and magnetic resonance imaging. Semin Ultrasound CT MRI 2008;29:454–471, with permission)

(97 % and 96 % vs. 92 % and 85 %, respectively) [12]. Selective use of MRI and EUS in conjunction with EUA is probably the best approach.

Medical Therapy

Once a diagnosis of Crohn's fistula is made, it is important to have a treatment strategy planned. Crohn's fistulas are often very complex, and the initial treatment modality should always be with medical therapy combined with drainage if necessary. Medical therapy may include appropriate antibiotics, immunosuppressive agents, or biologic agents. There is no role for corticosteroids in the treatment of perianal Crohn's disease.

Ciprofloxacin and Metronidazole

Ciprofloxacin and metronidazole have a role in the treatment of Crohn's perianal fistulas. West prospectively compared ciprofloxacin in conjunction with infliximab vs. infliximab alone, and found that the response rate (50 % reduction in the number of draining fistulas) was 8 of 11 (73 %) in the combination therapy group vs. 5 of 13 (39 %) with infliximab alone [13]. However, this difference was not significant due to the small number of patients in the groups. Bernstein found that, in a series of 21 patients treated with metronidazole 20 mg/kg/day for 6–8 weeks, all patients noticed less

discomfort, and 56 % had complete healing. However, the fistulas recurred in 75 % of patients on stopping the drug [14] and severe side effects included nausea and peripheral neuropathy. A small randomized, double blinded, placebo-controlled pilot trial at the Mayo clinic showed that remission and response occurred more frequently (but not significantly) in patients treated with ciprofloxacin [15]. The use of ciprofloxacin and metronidazole remains widespread for the treatment of this disease, despite the lack of conclusive evidence of their benefit.

Immunosuppressants

6-Mercaptopurine (6-MP) and Azathioprine (AZT) have been used in the treatment of intestinal Crohn's disease for many years. However, there have been no randomized controlled trials testing their efficacy in the treatment of perianal fistulas as a primary endpoint. Several reports have shown improvement or complete healing in up to 70 % of patients [16–19]. Ochsenkühn et al. combined azathioprine, 6-MP, and infliximab in patients with Crohn's fistulas refractory to conventional management [20]. The 14 patients with perianal fistulas received 3–4 infusions of infliximab followed by long-term therapy with 6-MP and azathioprine. Complete closure of the fistula occurred in 13 patients for more than 6 months. They concluded that 6-MP and azathioprine may prolong the fistula closure achieved with infliximab.

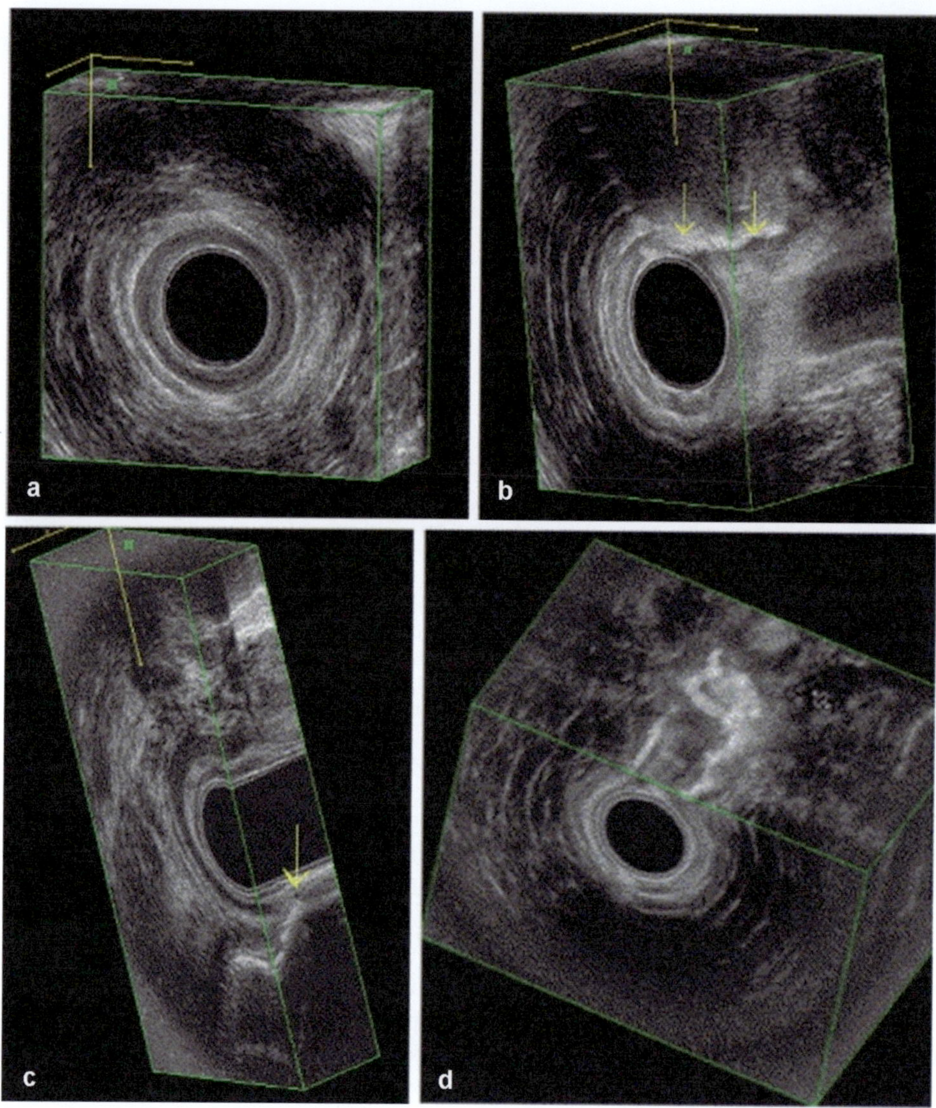

Fig. 19.5 Anal endosonography. Normal anatomy of the anal sphincter and puborectal muscle in 3D imaging: (**a**) frontal view of puborectal muscle (PR); (**b**) frontal view of the anal sphincters; (**c**) lateral view; and (**d**) coronal view. *SM* submucosa, *IAS* internal anal sphincter, *EAS* external anal sphincter. (Adapted from Felt-Bersma RJF. Endoanal ultrasound in perianal fistulas and abscesses. Digestive and Liver Disease 2006;38(8):537–543)

TNFα Inhibitors: Biologics

Monoclonal antibody therapy against T cells has become the mainstay in medical treatment of perianal Crohn's fistulas. Infliximab is a monoclonal antibody with mouse origin against TNFα which was initially approved for the treatment of intestinal Crohn's disease in 1998 [21]. Infliximab is administered intravenously typically at 6–8 week intervals. The first randomized, double blind, placebo-controlled trial of infliximab for the treatment of Crohn's fistulas was done in 1999 by Present and associates [22]. This study included 94 patients with both intra-abdominal and perianal fistulas. At a dose of 5 mg/kg, there was a complete response with fistula closure in 55 % of the patients treated with infliximab vs. 13 % of patients receiving placebo. The most frequent adverse events occurring were headache, abscess, upper respiratory infection, and fatigue.

Adalimumab is a human-derived monoclonal antibody against TNFα. The CHOICE trial evaluated the safety and efficacy of adalimumab in patients who had failed to respond or lost response to infliximab therapy in 673 patients with Crohn's fistula [23]. Approximately 40 % of these patients demonstrated healing of their fistulas by their last follow-up visit (ranging from 4 to 36 weeks). They concluded that adalimumab was an effective treatment for patients who failed therapy with infliximab.

This illustrates the largest problem with trials evaluating medical therapy. The usual follow-up in the study is less than 6 months. Typical follow-up for surgical treatment is greater than a year. This is even too short since fistula recurrence happens up to 5–10 years later. Short follow-up has limited our knowledge regarding medical treatment of fistulas. The true value of medical treatment may be reduction of active Crohn's disease in the rectum and anal canal to allow definitive closure of the internal opening of the anal fistula.

Certolizumab pegol is a monoclonal antibody against TNFα combined with polyethylene glycol to prolong its half-life, allowing the drug to be administered monthly. PRECiSE 2, a multicenter, randomized controlled trial, evaluated the response to certolizumab pegol in 668 patients with moderate to severe Crohn's. This trial showed certolizumab to be effective in inducing a clinical response in 58 of 100 patients with anal fistulas. After 6 weeks, additional analysis was done separately on those patients with draining fistula. These patients were randomized to either maintenance therapy with certolizumab or placebo. A significantly greater number of patients maintained a 100 % fistula closure in the maintenance vs. placebo group (36 % vs. 17 %). The authors concluded that continuous treatment with certolizumab improves outcomes when compared with placebo [24].

Biologic agents are significantly more expensive and have some serious side effects including abscess formation and upper respiratory infections. Nevertheless, there is strong evidence that this group of drugs is more efficacious than antibiotics or immunosuppressants. The 2011 London Position Statement of the World Congress of Gastroenterology provided guidelines for the use of biologic agents in Crohn's disease. Biologic agents are recommended for the treatment of complex fistulas. Infliximab should be regarded as the first line biologic agent for fistulizing Crohn's at this time. All abscesses must be drained prior to initiation of a biologic agent as this can result in worsening perianal sepsis [25]. Adalimumab and certolizumab pegol may be reserved for treatment failures with infliximab.

Surgical Management

If optimum medical therapy fails, the patients may require more definitive surgical management of their disease. The first step in surgical management is to manage and treat perianal sepsis. Abscesses should be appropriately and thoroughly drained. A non-cutting seton using an inert material such as a silastic vessel loop may be placed for continued drainage and to mark the fistula for future surgical procedures. Appropriate antibiotics and medical therapy to control any active Crohn's disease should be initiated. With appropriate drainage and control of perianal sepsis, fistulas may heal without any further surgical treatment, though the recurrence rates are high. Setons are generally effective in helping to control perianal sepsis but may be associated with recurrence after removal in up to 31 % of patients [26].

There are multiple other techniques for treating fistulas if simple drainage and medical management fails. Choosing the optimal surgical management requires consideration of the type of fistula involved. A proposed treatment algorithm is shown in Fig. 19.6. A low intersphincteric fistula may be treated with fistulotomy or fistulectomy. Excision of the tract leads to larger surgical wounds, and therefore fistulotomy of the superficial fibers of distal internal sphincter is preferred in most circumstances.

High transsphincteric fistula tracts are best treated with the ligation of the intersphincteric fistula tract (LIFT) technique or rectal wall advancement flaps, as the incidence of minor incontinence is less. Suprasphincteric fistulas start out as an intersphincteric abscess with a cephalad extension which then drains through the rectal outer wall and levator ani into the ischiorectal fossa and then to the buttock skin. Unroofing or drainage of the tract lateral to the external sphincter should be performed, and the remaining intersphincteric tract can be incised from the dentate line to the upper extent of the fistula. Setons are not recommended for suprasphincteric fistulas. Final closure with a sliding flap or proximal diversion may be required.

Extrasphincteric fistulas in Crohn's disease are most often the result of a connection with intra-abdominal intestine. In this case, fistulotomy will not definitively treat the disease. Resection of the diseased portion of intestine is the only effective manner to bring about healing and eliminate recurrences of these fistulas.

Fistulotomy and Fistulectomy

The first step in performing a short fistulotomy for the low intersphincteric fistula is to identify the external opening. A probe is then placed through the opening and into the tract in order to try to identify the internal opening within the anal canal and document the amount of muscle encircled by the fistula. Once the probe is in place, the tissue overlying the probe may be divided using a scalpel blade or the cutting current of a cautery device. No external sphincter should be divided. If a diagnosis of Crohn's disease is suspected but not confirmed, curettings from the tract may be sent at this time.

If fistulectomy is chosen, the external opening is located and a stay suture is placed. The tissue around the fistula may be injected with local anesthetic and epinephrine to minimize bleeding. The skin surrounding the external opening is then divided. Scissors are used to core out the tissue surrounding the fibrous tract while the stay suture is retracted downwards. If the tract penetrates the external anal sphincter low, the muscle may be divided; however, if the tract is high

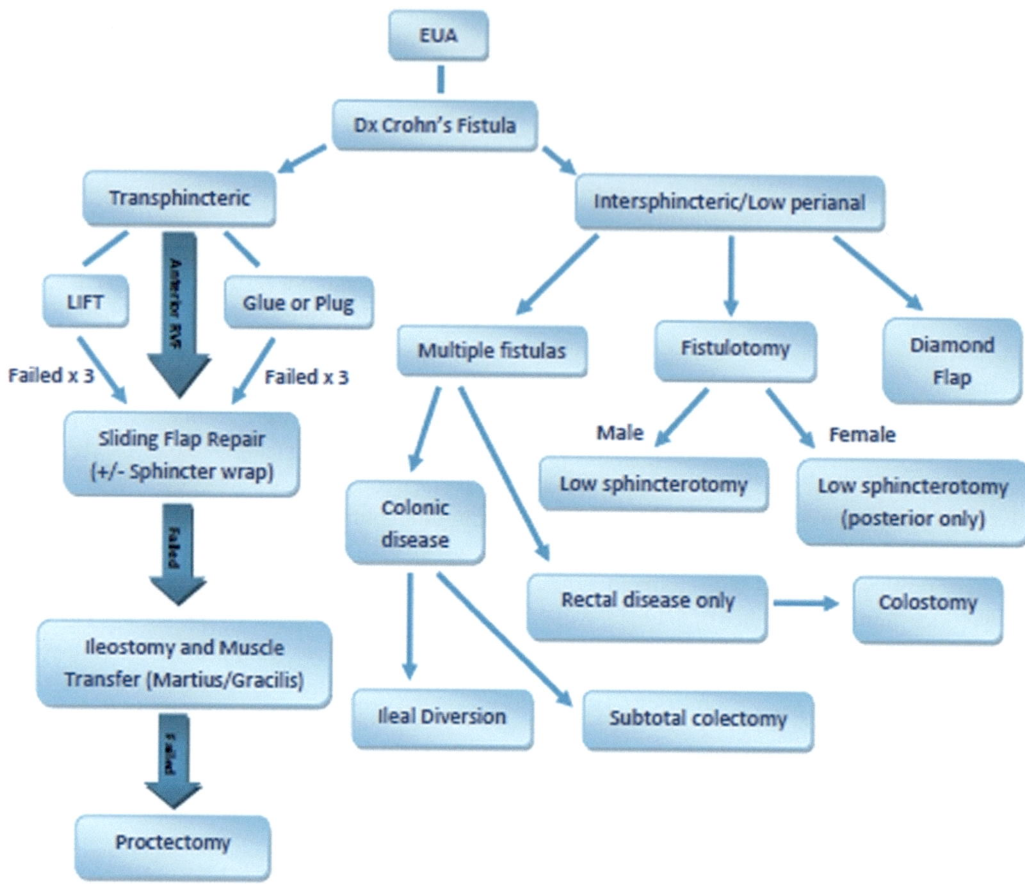

Fig. 19.6 Treatment algorithm for Crohn's perianal fistula

or the patient already has other risk factors for incontinence, dissection should proceed in a meticulous fashion, coring out the track from the muscle and leaving most of the external anal sphincter intact. The defect may then be allowed to heal by secondary intention or may be closed with a suture or an advancement flap. The internal opening should be closed with figure of eight closure.

Fistulotomy or fistulectomy is not appropriate in females with anterior fistulas as the risk of incontinence is very high. Patients with a history of obstetric injury should not undergo either of these procedures. High transsphincteric or supra-sphincteric fistulas involve a large portion of the external sphincter. Cutting through the sphincters at this level is associated with high rates of total incontinence. Preexisting scar in the rectovaginal septum which is involved by Crohn's fistula may be injured and result in rectovaginal fistula (RVF) after fistulotomy or fistulectomy.

Postoperative care after fistulotomy or fistulectomy includes appropriate analgesia, tub baths with the water stream hitting the perineum at least three times a day, stool softeners as needed, and frequent follow-up visits. Packing the wound is not necessary. Marsupialization of the edges of the wound rarely lasts and there is very little difference from closure by delayed secondary intention. Some degree of leakage or lack of control may occur, and 90 % of cases will spontaneously resolve. Other postoperative complications include urinary retention, bleeding, pain, pruritis, and poor wound healing due to active Crohn's. Anal stenosis from chronic inflammation may also occur as a late postoperative complication.

Flaps

Coverage of the internal opening with an advancement flap of the rectal wall may be considered for the treatment of anterior low rectal Crohn's fistulas in patients where fistulotomy is not an option. Prior to this procedure any perianal abscess, sepsis, or active intestinal or perianal Crohn's disease must be controlled. Although these flaps are often referred to as endorectal mucosal advancement flaps, various layers of tissue may be used including mucosal, partial thickness rectal, full thickness rectal, or perianal skin. Transanal advancement flaps close the internal opening and leave the external sphincter intact, thus they are associated with a lower risk of incontinence and recurrence. A broad-based U flap

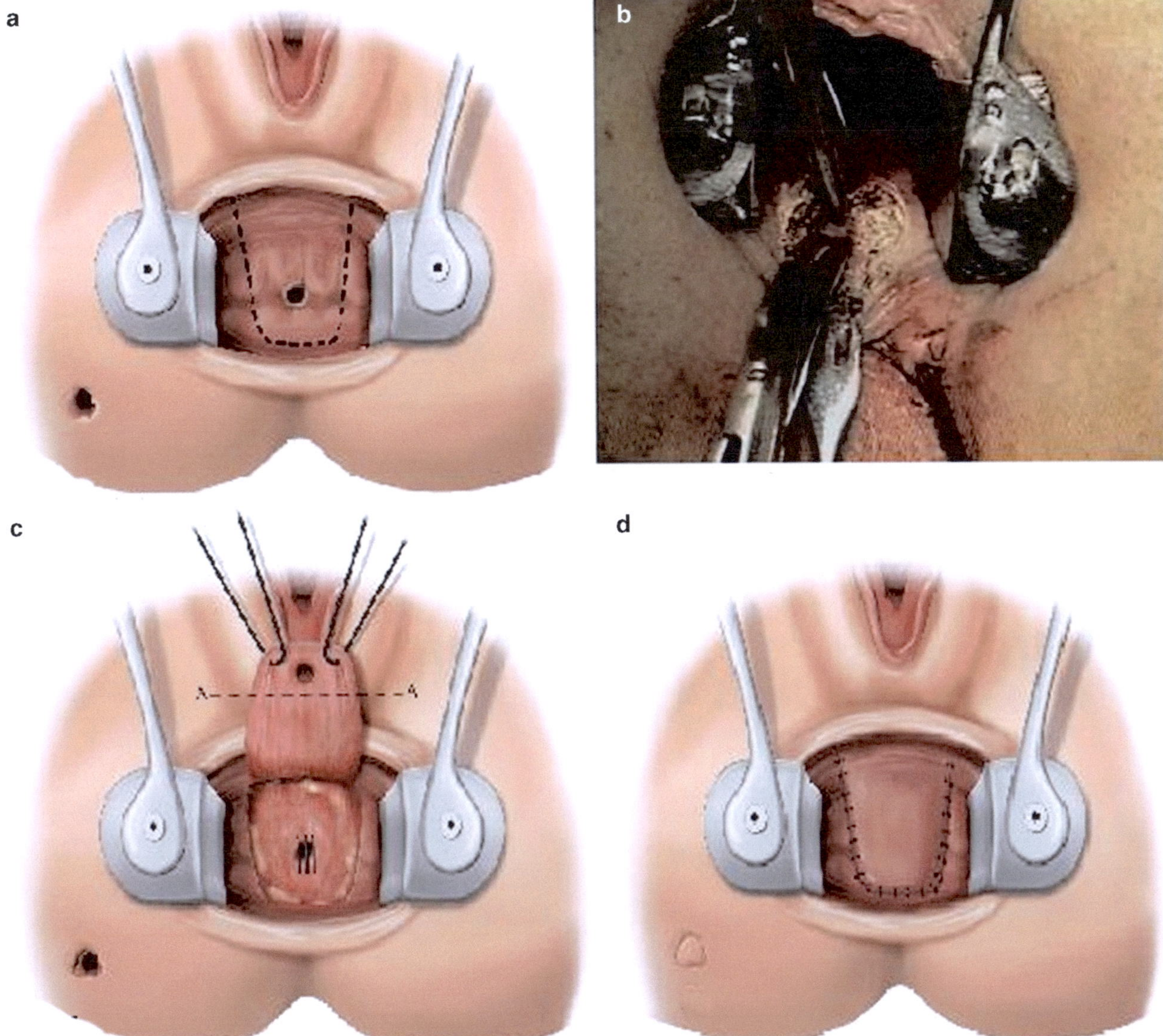

Fig. 19.7 (**a**) Line of incision for a broad-based U endorectal advancement flap (schematic), (**b**) developing the flap, in this case in the intersphincteric plane, raising a full thickness endorectal advancement flap, (**c**) fully mobilized flap retracted using two holding sutures. Internal opening excised along line A-A. Internal opening defect in the sphincter is closed with interrupted sutures (schematic), (**d**) sutured endorectal advancement flap (schematic). (Adapted from Wexner SD, Fleshman JW. Colon and rectal surgery: Anorectal operations 2012;44–46, with permission)

is raised with the apex starting approximately 5–10 mm below the internal opening and 10–15 mm in width on either side of the opening (Fig. 19.7a). The flap is raised, usually including mucosa and submucosa in the distal portion of the flap, and either partial or full thickness circular rectal wall muscle fibers (Fig. 19.7b). The length of the flap need only be enough to provide a tension-free closure after excising the fistula opening in the flap. The tract opening in the muscle and surrounding tissue is cored out and closed with interrupted absorbable monofilament sutures (Fig. 19.7c). The flap is secured over the top of the internal opening with interrupted absorbable braided sutures (Fig. 19.6d).

The external opening is left open and curetted or drained with a mushroom tip catheter. In patients with low fistulas in the setting of long-standing perianal sepsis or anal stenosis, endorectal advancement flaps are not typically successful. In these cases, an anocutaneous advancement flap may be performed. Full thickness 2×2 cm diamond of perianal skin and subcutaneous fat is elevated adjacent to the fistula internal opening, ensuring there is a broad base with good vascular supply at its lateral aspect. The internal opening and surrounding tissue is once again excised with a vertically directed elipse and the tract closed. The skin flap is advanced into the anal canal and sutured over the internal opening with

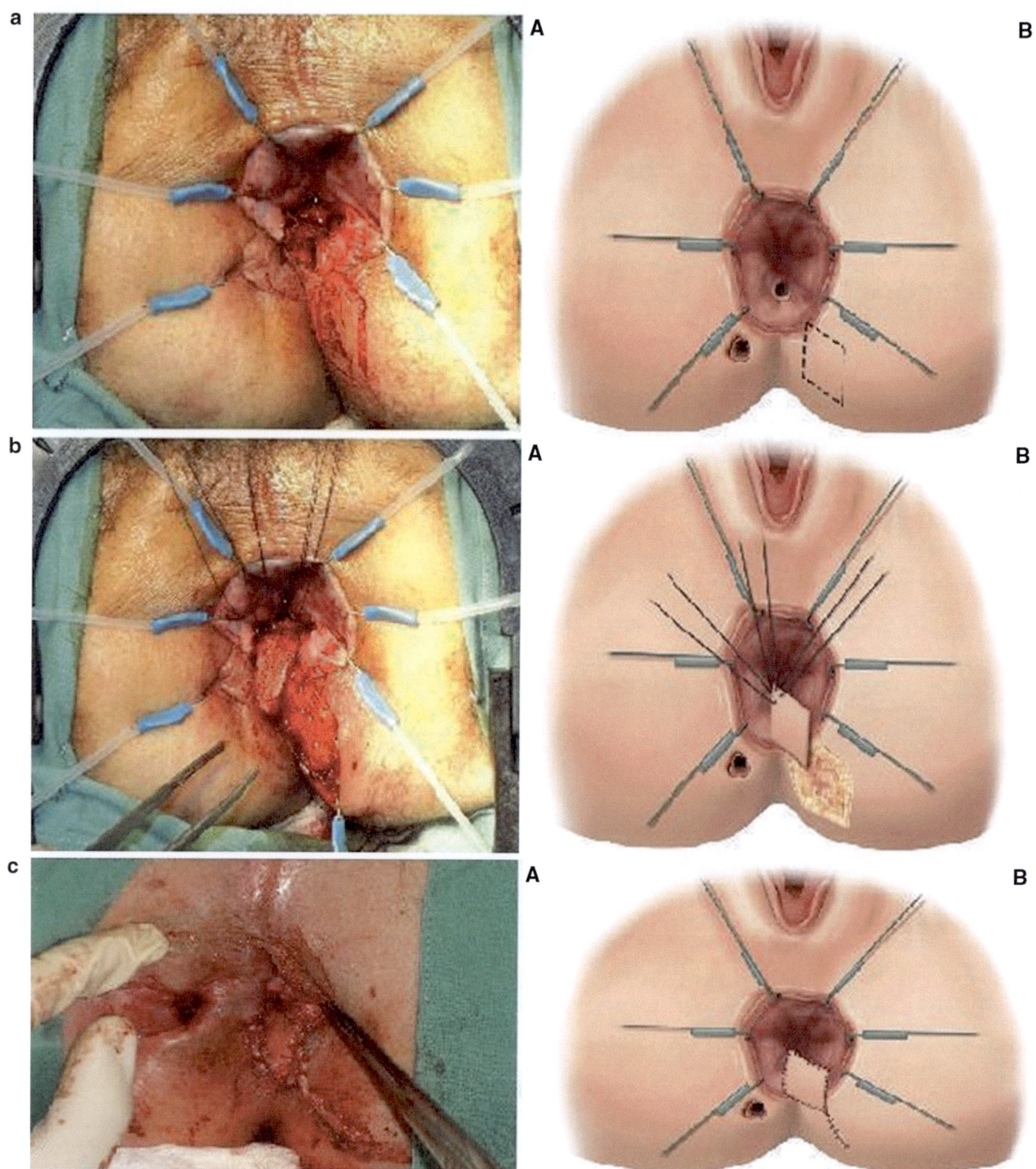

Fig. 19.8 (**a**) Incision for diamond-shaped anocutaneous advancement flap: (*A*) actual view and (*B*) schematic; (**b**) flap being advanced to cover the internal opening: (*A*) actual view and (*B*) schematic; (**c**) sutured anocutaneous advancement flap: (*A*) actual view and (*B*) schematic. (Adapted from Wexner SD, Fleshman JW. Colon and Rectal Surgery: Anorectal Operations: 2012:47–48, with permission)

absorbable braided suture. The skin defect is then closed primarily resulting in a linear suture line with the appearance of a "kite tail" extending from the anal canal (Fig. 19.8).

Postoperative care is minimal. Sitz baths are used to clean the area after a bowel movement. It is important to keep the wound clean and dry, otherwise. Postoperative complications include flap breakdown, incontinence, perianal sepsis, bleeding, ectropion, and iatrogenic fistulas. The reported efficacy rate of this technique varies. Soltani showed a reported efficacy rate of 81 % with cryptoglandular fistulas but only 64 %

with Crohn's fistulas. The rate of incontinence with this procedure in Crohn's fistula patients was nearly 10 % [27]. If the initial flap procedure fails, a second flap procedure may be successful after a period of waiting and the addition of a diverting stoma. The final success rate should be close to 90 % [28].

Glues and Plugs

Two additional options for the treatment of anal fistulas include a fistula plug and fibrin glue. Fibrin glue was first studied in the early 1990s for the treatment of fistulas and approved by the FDA in 1998. The main active ingredient in fibrin glue is fibrinogen, which when combined with thrombin, forms a fibrin clot. This subsequently undergoes fibrinolysis and promotes tissue healing. A recent randomized trial achieved an initial closure rate of 38 % (13/34) in Crohn's patients treated with fibrin glue vs. 16 % for the placebo group. Two of these patients developed recurrence at 16 weeks. Of the 21 patients who did not respond to the initial treatment, five were treated again with the glue. None went into remission [29]. This illustrates the need for long-term follow-up to assess the true efficacy of any method of treating a fistula in Crohn's disease.

Robb and Sklow reported the first use of rolled submucosal "plugs" for the treatment of fistulas. Subsequently, numerous commercial "plugs" have been developed. Initial results using these products were promising, with reported success rates up to 80–90 %. However, eventually it became apparent that recurrence rates were high, especially in patients with Crohn's disease. A recent systematic review by O'Riordan et al. concluded that the rate of closure with the fistula plug was 64 % in patients with cryptoglandular disease. The evidence regarding closure rates in patients with Crohn's disease was insufficient to provide any conclusions [30].

Plugs and glues may be placed after proper drainage of any perianal abscess and fibrosis of the fistula tract has occurred. If any evidence of active infection is present, the procedure should be postponed until this has been controlled. When using fibrin sealant, primary and secondary tracts should be identified, and the fibrin sealant injected into the secondary tracts until seen in the primary tract. Fistula plugs should be fully submerged in sterile saline for rehydration for up to 2 min. A suture may be placed through the seton within the fistula tract. The seton is then pulled out and the suture remains. The suture is then secured to the narrow external opening portion of the plug, and the plug is drawn through the fistula tract inside the rectum and secured at the wide portion of the plug which is trimmed flush to the rectal wall internal opening of the fistula using an absorbable suture. After this is in place, a small mucosal advancement flap may be created to cover the plug at the internal opening.

Postoperative complications are rare and include recurrent abscess or plug extrusion. A controversy exists over whether the fistula tract should be curetted before "setting" the plug. Care should be taken to remove all debris from the tract by repeated flushing with saline or dilute betadine or hydrogen peroxide.

Despite the low rates of remission described in recent literature with the use of anal plugs and glues, they still remain valid treatment options to consider for the treatment of Crohn's fistulas due to their minimally invasive nature and ease of use. A failure with an attempted "plug" closure does not preclude use of another method. This makes the plug an attractive early option for fistula treatment. This is especially true with Crohn's disease given its increased risk for morbidity and recurrence with surgical treatment of anal fistulas.

A recently described technique combining fibrin glue and adipose-derived stem cells (ASCs) has been reported by Garcia-Olmo and colleagues for the treatment of perianal fistulas. A small series of 14 patients with Crohn's fistulas showed healing in 71 % (5/7) of patients treated with fibrin glue and ASCs compared to 14 % (1/7) in the fibrin glue group [31]. Another series of patients treated with ASCs showed a recurrence rate of 42 % after more than 3 years in those patients who were initially treated successfully [32].

Ligation of the Intersphincteric Fistula Tract

Possibly the most innovative recent advance in fistula surgery is the LIFT procedure. This was developed and first described by Rojanasakul et al. in 2007 and has shown promising results since its introduction. The initial report was of a prospective observational study in cryptoglandular disease with 17/18 patients successfully treated and no incontinence [33]. Sileri et al. subsequently showed healing rates of 83 % in patients with cryptoglandular fistulas without recurrence, though median follow-up was only 4 months [34]. However, Tan et al. reported a retrospective comparison of advancement flaps and the LIFT procedure for treatment of cryptoglandular fistulas and found that the advancement flap had a significantly higher success rate (94 % vs. 63 %) [35]. Han reported a series of patients in whom the LIFT technique was used in combination with the "plug" to achieve a 95 % overall success rate with median follow-up of 14 months [36].

The technique isolates and divides the fistula tract between the internal and external anal sphincters by means of an intersphincteric dissection, which begins at the anal verge, thus preserving both anal sphincters. The procedure is performed by identifying the internal and external openings initially and placing a fistula probe to guide the dissection to the fistula tract. The space between the internal and external anal sphincters between the external and internal openings is palpated and a 2–3 cm curvilinear incision is made in the

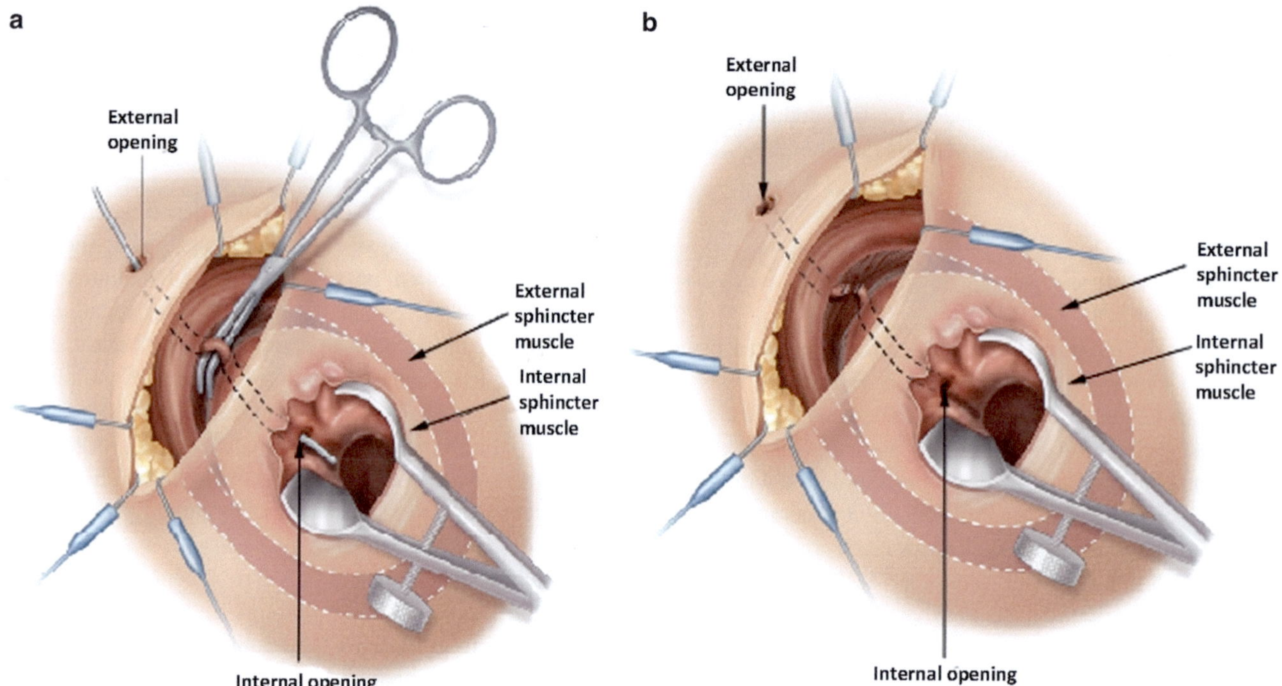

Fig. 19.9 (**a**) The fistula tract, with the probe through it for ease of identification, is dissected free in the intersphincteric space; (**b**) the probe is removed, and the fistula tract is ligated and divided. (Adapted from Wexner SD, Fleshman JW. Colon and Rectal Surgery. Anoretal Operations 2012; 82, with permission)

intersphincteric groove. Intersphincteric dissection is carried out until the fistula tract is identified. The tract is exposed circumferentially. Clamps are placed on either side of the tract as the probe is removed, and the tract is cut (Fig. 19.9). Success seems to be highest when the fistula tract feels like the "spermatic cord during a vasectomy." Alternatively, sutures are placed at each end of the exposed fistula tract to close and expose the tract. A portion of the tract centrally may be removed if desired. Each side is ligated with the absorbable suture. The external opening is generally left open. The internal opening within the rectal lumen is closed with a figure of eight suture. In some instances, such as an anterior fistula in a thin perineal body in a female or in a Crohn's fistula, a square of biomesh can be placed in the intersphincteric space to separate the cut ends of the tract. The outer edges of the muscle are approximated to capture the patch. The skin is closed in an interrupted fashion over a small section of silicone vessel loop as a drain.

The initial results of this technique are good, with minimal postoperative complications and success rates between 60 and 85 %. However, there are currently no studies specifically relating to the treatment of fistulas in Crohn's patients using the LIFT technique. Further studies with long-term follow-up, particularly relating to Crohn's patients, are needed to better evaluate the efficacy of this procedure.

Diversion

In patients with severe perianal disease, diversion coupled with a local surgical procedure may increase the success rate of these local procedures. Rehg et al. reported 85 % of fistulas healed after fecal diversion and local surgical treatment vs. 19 % with local treatment alone. Only 46 % of the diverted patients underwent stoma reversal and of these, half recurred [37]. Galandiuk et al. attempted to identify risk factors which would predict failure of local, sphincter sparing operations in patients with perianal Crohn's disease. Permanent fecal diversion was required in 49 % of this group. Risk factors for failure included anal stricture, the need for ileocolic resection, and the presence of colonic Crohn's disease [38]. For these patients, and patients with complex, high anal fistulas, it may be helpful to construct a diverting stoma. However, it is important that the patient understands that there is a significant chance that this may be a permanent stoma.

Proctectomy

Ultimately between 12 and 20 % of patients with refractory perianal Crohn's disease will eventually undergo a proctectomy [39]. However, 23–79 % of patients who undergo proctectomy will experience unhealed wounds following proctectomy; especially those with rectal strictures or high anal fistulas [39]. For this reason, it is our opinion that proctectomy should be reserved for situations in which all other treatment options have been exhausted and the patient continues to have debilitating perianal symptoms. This may result in the patient having multiple small procedures to manage symptoms and improve quality of life over the period of many years. In some instances the Crohn's disease will "burn out" or respond to medical therapy and allow the patient to avoid a permanent stoma. In those patients who do not respond or who have worsening disease, their decision to undergo a permanent ostomy will be made much easier and will truly improve their quality of life with the knowledge that all has been tried to avoid this outcome.

Follow-up

As stated previously, the natural history of Crohn's fistulas is such that recurrence is common, and may occur months to years after initial healing. Close follow-up and maintenance with prophylactic medications including metronidazole or ciprofloxacin, immunosuppressants, and biologic agents is imperative. It is also important to be aware that patients with long-standing Crohn's fistulas have an increased risk of anal cancer, both squamous cell and adenocarcinoma. The mechanism is unknown, but is thought to be related to constant inflammation and regeneration of mucosal cells. Ky et al. reported an estimated 0.7 % incidence of carcinoma arising in Crohn's anal fistulas [40]. On average, development of carcinoma in Crohn's fistula has been reported 15–20 years after disease onset [40, 41] in ages 47–51 [40]. Early detection is critical; therefore, patients with Crohn's fistulas must be followed with frequent, thorough physical examinations including EUA if needed.

Rectovaginal Fistulas

Background

RVFs are most commonly associated with a history of rectovaginal trauma (i.e., episiotomy), and have been reported in 3–9 % of women with Crohn's disease [42–44]. Symptoms include dyspareunia, passage of fecal matter or stool from the vagina, or recurrent urinary tract infections. Multiple classification symptoms exist, and may be based on their relationship to the anal sphincter, the complexity of disease, and their etiology. However, no clear consensus has been reached on the usefulness of these classifications except that high fistulas require more complex repair efforts than low fistulas.

Diagnosis

Diagnosis of RVFs includes a thorough physical examination. The rectal opening may be readily visible on anoscopy, though this is not always the case. A methylene blue exam may be done in which a tampon is inserted into the patients vagina, and the patient is given an enema with methylene blue. Staining on the tampon would suggest a RVF is present. Shobeiri et al. described another method of diagnosis using vaginal fistulography. A cone tip catheter is used to locate possible fistula openings within the vagina. Contrast is then injected slowly under fluoroscopy, and if a fistula tract is found, a guidewire is introduced through the vaginal opening into the rectum to delineate the tract. This technique reportedly aided in diagnosing 5 of 9 RVFs which had not been found otherwise [44].

MRI and EUS have also been used for diagnosing RVFs. Stoker compared EUS and MRI for diagnosing RVFs and found that these tests had comparable positive predictive values (100 % and 92 %, respectively) [45]. Maconi et al. evaluated transperineal ultrasound as an alternative diagnostic technique in detecting perianal fistulas and RVFs and found that they had a similar positive predictive value as well [46]. Transperineal ultrasound may be beneficial for patients with anal stenosis or those who are unable to tolerate EUS. No consensus has been reached regarding the superiority of these imaging studies.

Anal manometry, EUS, and pudendal nerve latencies are used in evaluating patients with fecal incontinence and RVFs. Diarrhea is common in active Crohn's disease and must be controlled, as it can cause incontinence even in patients with normal sphincter function. Mean resting pressure in normal individuals is 40–70 mmHg, and is influenced most by the internal anal sphincter [47]. An advancement flap is likely to be effective for treatment of a RVF in a patient with normal sphincter function [48]. Sphincteroplasty and flap advancement with or without diversion is recommended in a patient with abnormal sphincter function. The addition of moving viable muscle across the thin rectovaginal septum adds thickness to the tissue between vaginal and rectal openings. The repair of the sphincter defect may also improve control of stool.

Medical Therapy

RVFs can be very difficult to treat. Similar to perianal Crohn's fistulas, treatment depends on symptoms, and a combination of medical and surgical therapy is commonly warranted. The principles of medical therapy are largely similar to those for all perianal fistulas. The treatment focuses on control of the underlying disease, particularly in the rectum. Unfortunately the contamination of the urethral meatus requires a more urgent approach to the fistula. There are few studies which specifically evaluate medication ability to close Crohn's RVFs. Sands performed a post hoc analysis after the Accent II trial (a Crohn's disease clinical trial evaluating infliximab in a new long-term treatment regimen in patients with fistulizing Crohn's disease) to determine the effect of infliximab specifically on RVFs. At weeks 10 and 14, 60.7 % and 44.8 % of RVFs were closed, respectively [43]. Duration of closure was longer in patients who were treated with maintenance therapy.

Surgical Therapy

Initial surgical management includes treatment of perianal sepsis, which may include drainage and seton placement followed by appropriate medical management. If the underlying rectal disease has been appropriately treated and controlled but the RVF remains, surgical treatment options should be considered. Fistulotomy is not recommended because of the associated high rate of incontinence. Fibrin glue has not been shown to reliably close Crohn's RVFs [49, 50].

Fistula plugs may be used, though success rates are variable. The button anal fistula plug is a biologically absorbable xenograft made from the submucosa of porcine intestine which has been studied specifically in patients with RVFs. Gajsek et al. prospectively studied the button fistula plug in eight women with Crohn's RVFs, and reported four of eight of these achieved complete closure at 15 weeks. However, these results did not hold up during long-term follow-up with high rates of recurrence, and all repeat procedures failed [51].

Sphincteroplasty

Overlapping sphincteroplasty is used when there is a defect in the external anal sphincter causing incontinence in the setting of a RVF. A curvilinear incision is made at the dentate line in the anterior anal canal which includes anoderm and submucosa, extending cephalad beyond the internal opening of the fistula. The fistula tract is divided and curetted. The edges of the internal and external anal sphincters are located laterally and mobilized away from the ischiorectal fossa fat, overlapped, and sutured with nonabsorbable horizontal mattress sutures. Initial success rates reported were 86–100 % [52–54]; however, long-term maintenance of continence was worse. Gutierrez reported only 40 % of patients treated with sphincteroplasty maintained continence at 10 years [55]. Malouf et al. reported a 50 % continence rate after a minimum of 5-year follow-up in patients with obstetric trauma [56]. Nevertheless, sphincteroplasty is the procedure of choice in patients with RVFs and incontinence (Fig. 19.10).

Ligation of the Intersphincteric Fistula Tract

The LIFT procedure may also be performed for the treatment of RVFs. Ellis described the technique with the addition of a bioprosthetic material. Once the intersphincteric fistula tract is ligated, the tract openings to the vagina and rectum are sutured and closed. A bioprosthetic material is placed between the external sphincter/posterior vaginal wall and internal sphincter/rectal mucosa and sutured to the levator ani laterally, and the external sphincter distally (Fig. 19.11). He reported a 19 % recurrence rate, which was lower than the recurrence rates reported with anodermal and mucosal advancement flaps (27 % and 38 %, respectively) [57]. The most common complications are urinary retention and perianal sepsis.

Advancement Flaps

A diamond skin advancement flap may be used for very low anovaginal fistulas. As previously described, a 2×2 cm diamond of perianal skin and subcutaneous fat is elevated adjacent to the fistula internal opening. The internal opening and surrounding tissue is once again excised. The skin flap is advanced into the anal canal and sutured over the internal opening with absorbable braided suture. A cutaneous flap may also be used on the vaginal side in conjunction with the anal advancement flap [58].

An endorectal advancement flap for RVF may be performed for higher fistulas, with or without sphincteroplasty. A broad-based, U-shaped flap including mucosa, submucosa, and varying thickness of muscle is created with enough length to provide a tension-free repair. The fistula tract is debrided. The opening of the tract in the muscle is closed with figure eight sutures. The flap is sutured into place with absorbable interrupted sutures. The vaginal tract opening is left open to drain. Complications include bleeding, incontinence, perianal sepsis, and flap failure, though the risk of these should be low. Vaginal flaps are performed in much the same way. A flap of vaginal mucosa inferior to the fistula is elevated and the rectal opening of the fistula tract is closed. A levatorplasty is often done to enhance tissue coverage.

Both the transvaginal and transrectal approaches have advantages and disadvantages. One advantage to vaginal repair in patients with Crohn's disease is that non-diseased tissue is used for the repair. An advantage to the transrectal approach is that the repair is done on the high-pressured side of the fistula. Ruffolo et al. systematically reviewed transrectal vs. transvaginal repair of Crohn's RVFs and reported primary closure rates of 54.2 % and 69.4 % with transrectal and transvaginal flaps, respectively. The difference was not significant, and the recurrence rates were similar with each procedure [59].

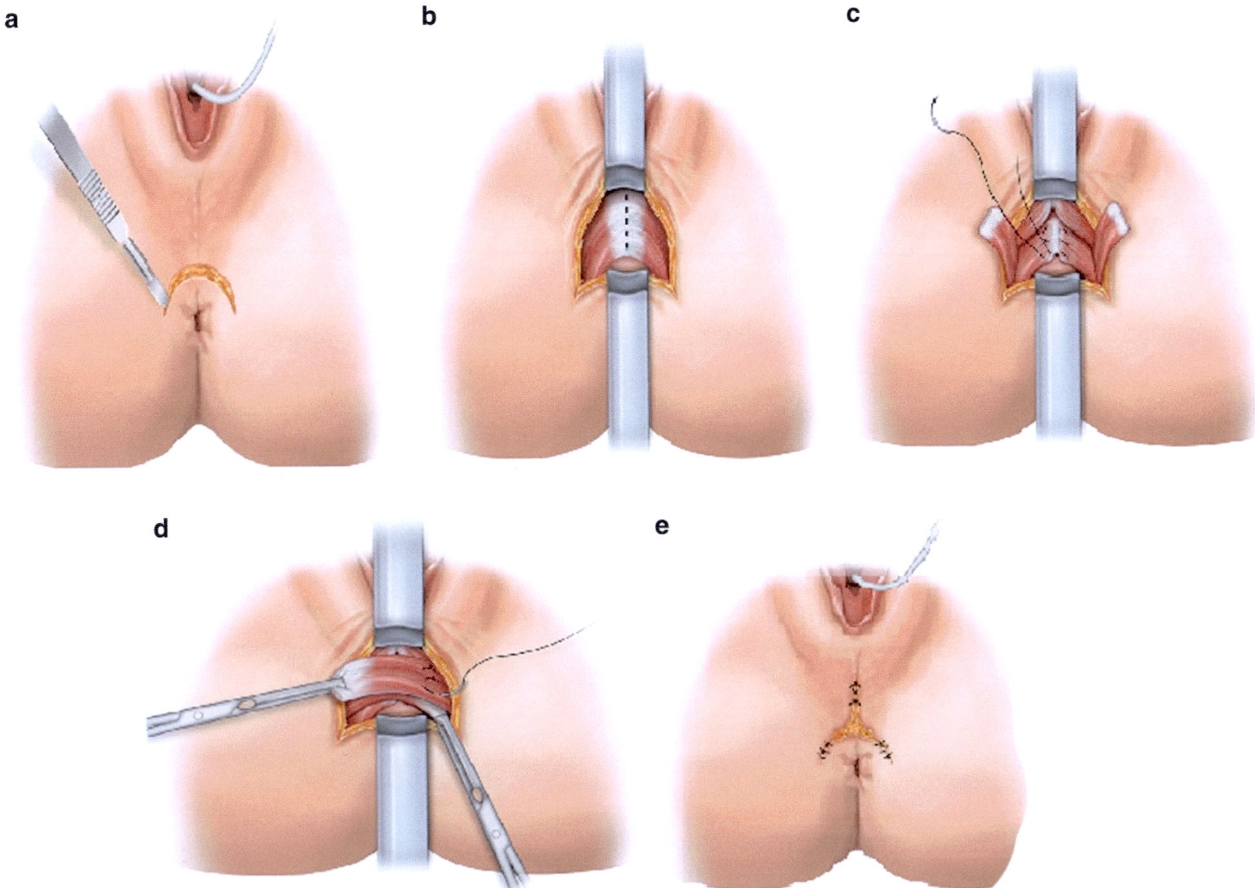

Fig. 19.10 (**a**) Curvilinear incision made along the perineal body; (**b**) the sphincter scar is divided but not excised; (**c**) the internal anal sphincter ins imbricated when a layered repair is performed; (**d**) the external anal sphincter is overlapped; (**e**) the center of the wound is left open for drainage. (Adapted from Wexner SD, Fleshman JW. Colon and Rectal Surgery. Anoretal Operations 2012; 94–97, with permission)

Birman first described rectal sleeve advancement flaps for the treatment of severe anorectal and RVFs. This technique is especially useful in patients with extensive, distal rectal circumferential ulceration or scarring, but with sparing of the more proximal rectum. Patients should undergo bowel prep prior to this procedure. A transperitoneal approach may be needed to sufficiently mobilize the rectum. A circumferential incision is made at the dentate line, extending into the submucosa. The dissection is carried proximally, becoming full thickness at the anorectal ring (at the level of the pelvic floor) and continuing cephalad to obtain mobility. The diseased anal mucosa is excised, and the rectum is pulled caudal to the dentate line and sutured to the anoderm without tension. Marchesa et al. used this technique in 13 patients with severe Crohn's perianal fistulas and RVFs (previously treated unsuccessfully with a transanal rectal advancement flap) and reported a 60 % success rate [60]. Hull reported success in 4/5 patients with Crohn's anovaginal fistulas treated with sleeve advancement flap, three of which were diverted at the time of the procedure [61].

Tissue Interposition

Tissue interposition grafts bring healthy, non-diseased, well vascularized tissue into the diseased region for repair. There are multiple different types of tissue interposition grafts. Gracilis transposition grafts are performed by mobilizing the muscle, detaching it from the tibia, and tunneling the muscle subcutaneously to the perineum. Furst et al. reported fistula closure in 11 of 12 patients with recurrent Crohn's RVFs treated with gracilis transposition, with a mean follow-up of 3.4 years. All patients were diverted, and 11 of 12 were reversed [62]. The gracilis muscle is not ideal for this purpose since the distal end of the muscle is narrow and does not cover a large area.

Martius flaps were initially used for the treatment of vesicovaginal fistulas, and have undergone various modifications over the years. The Martius flap initially referred to tissue interposition using bulbocavernosus muscle, but has more recently been used to describe either a labial fat pad graft, or a combination of muscle and fat pad. The procedure is

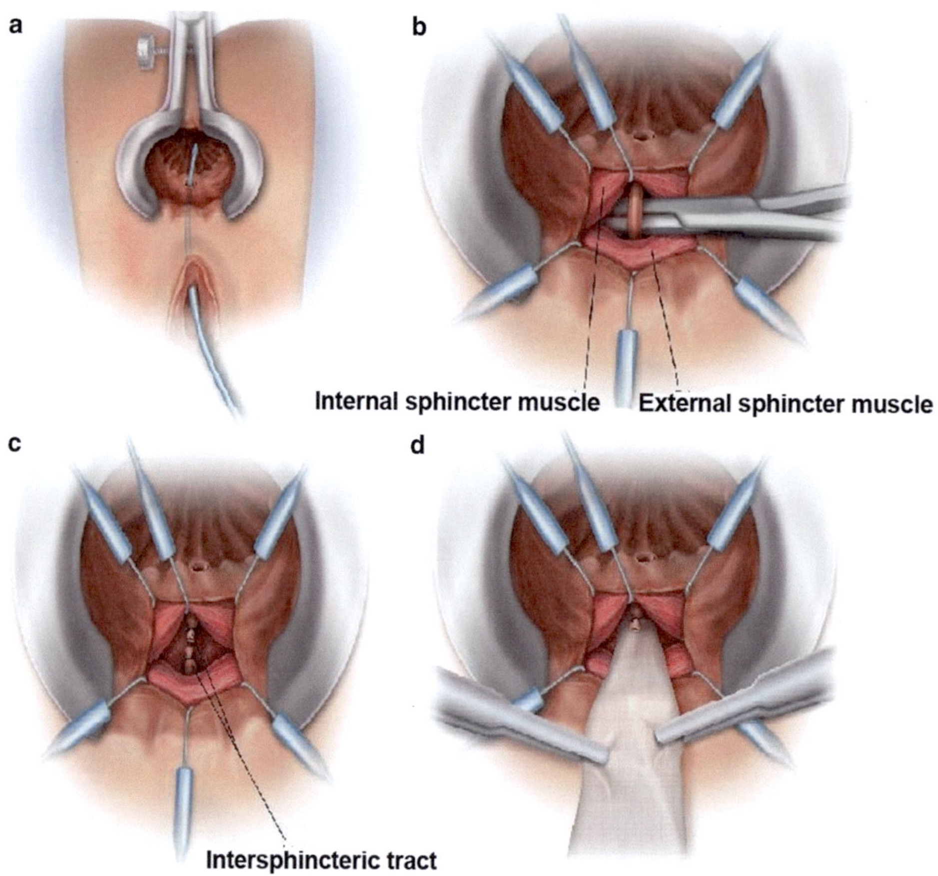

Fig. 19.11 (**a**) Incision for LIFT procedure; (**b**) identification of fistula tract in intersphincteric space; (**c**) ligation and division of fistula tract; (**d**) insertion of bioprosthetic material to separate ends of divided tract. (Adapted from Wexner SD, Fleshman JW. Colon and Rectal Surgery. Anoretal Operations 2012; 102–103, with permission)

performed by making a longitudinal incision in the labia majora and dissecting out the bulbocavernosus muscle and the labial fat pad. The muscle and fat pad are transected at the ventral extent of the pedicle and tunneled underneath the labia minora to the fistula site and sutured into place. Many of the earlier reports described the Martius flap for the treatment of radiation-induced rectal vaginal fistulas. More recently, McNevin et al. retrospectively reviewed 16 patients with complex, low RVFs with multiple etiologies who were treated with combination bulbocavernosus and labial fat pad grafts, and reported only one fistula recurrence. However, dyspareunia was observed in 31 % [63]. Songne et al. described their experience using a labial fat pad graft in the treatment of RVFs including seven Crohn's patients. All fistulas healed within 3 months, though two of the seven patients with Crohn's ultimately underwent proctectomy for worsening anal disease [64]. Given the close proximity of the graft to the operative field, the Martius flap is an attractive option for patients with low RVFs (Fig. 19.12).

An omental flap may be placed laparoscopically for high intersphincteric or transsphincteric RVFs. The fistula is divided as the cul de sac is exposed to the level of the fistula, and a piece of omentum interposed into the rectovaginal septum between the rectum and vagina. This technique may also be modified for low to mid RVFs using a combination laparoscopic and transperineal approach. The omentum is mobilized 2/3 of the way from the hepatic flexure to the splenic flexure, taking care to ligate the branches of the right gastroepiploic artery but to preserve the arcade. The anterior rectum is then mobilized, exposing the rectovaginal space. The fistula is excised, and the wound edges are approximated. The rectovaginal space is then opened up transperineally, and the omentum is pulled through this space and sutured to the subcutaneous tissue with a single suture (Fig. 19.13). Schloericke et al. reported no recurrences in nine patients treated with this approach, with a median follow-up of 22 months. Eight of these patients were diverted [65]. Though initial results appear promising, this technique is relatively new, and further studies are needed before conclusions are made regarding the efficacy of the procedure.

There are many surgical treatment options for patients with Crohn's RVFs. Unfortunately, recurrence rates are high with virtually all of these procedures. El-Gazzaz et al. looked at predictors for success and failure in women with Crohn's RVFs undergoing repair. They found that the use of immunomodulators was significantly associated with better

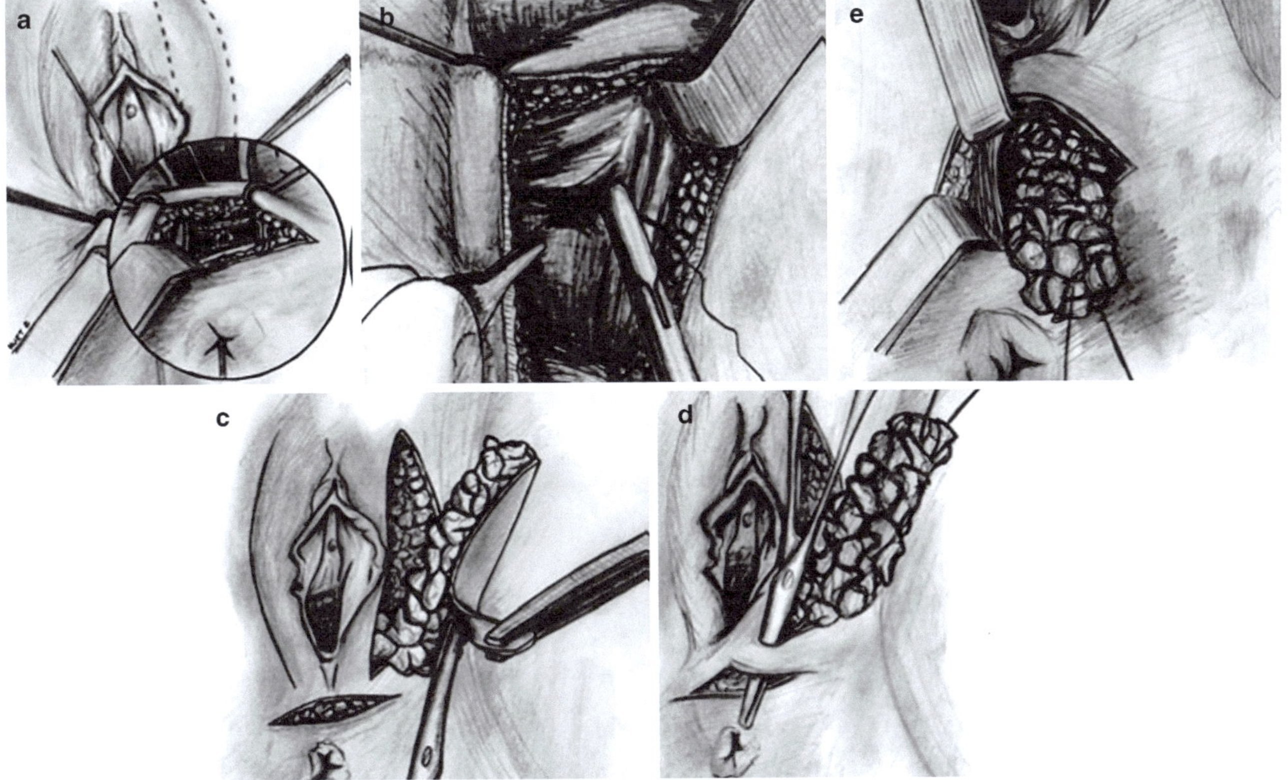

Fig. 19.12 Modified Martius graft procedure. (**a**) Identification of vaginal and rectal defects; (**b**) vaginal and rectal closure; (**c**) graft construction; (**d**) tunneling graft; and (**e**) interposition between the vaginal and rectal closures. (Adapted from Songne K et al. Treatment of anovaginal or rectovaginal fistulas with modified Martius graft. Colorectal Dis 2007;9(7):653–6. Reprinted with permission)

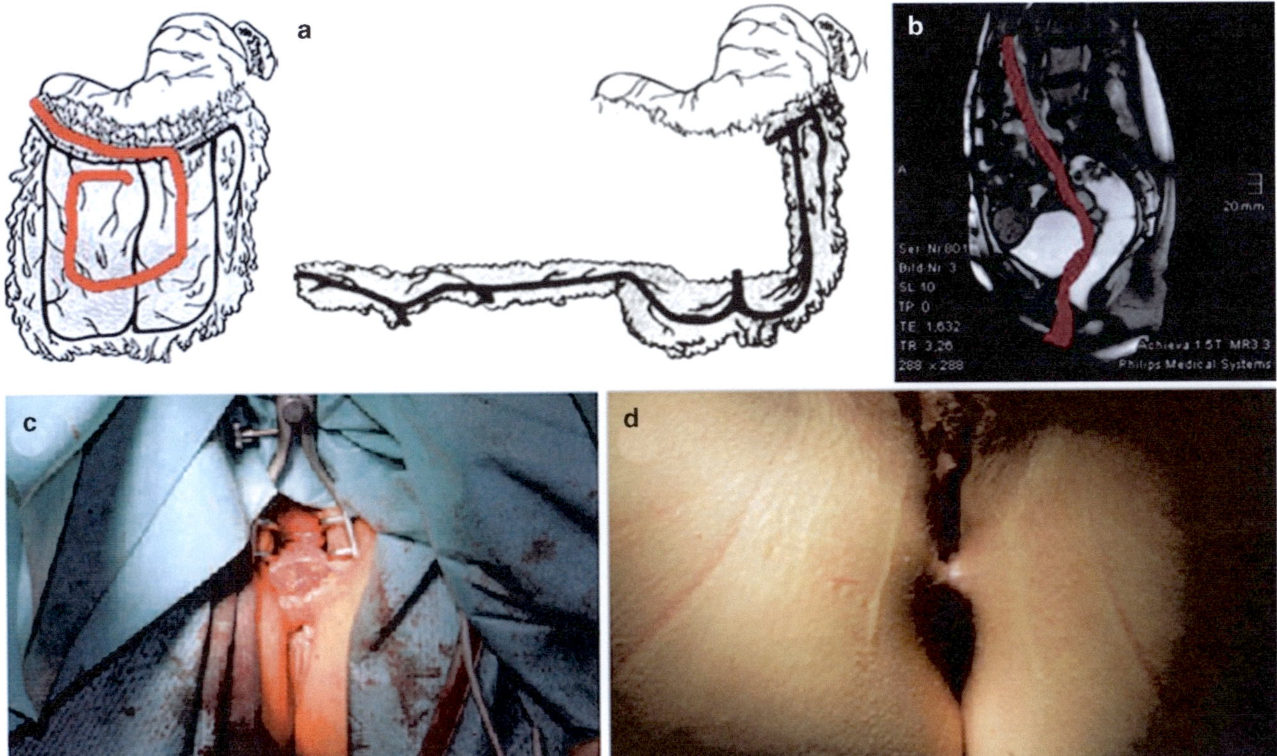

Fig. 19.13 (**a**) Mobilization of the greater omentum; (**b**) transperineal pull-through of the omental flap; (**c**) perineum immediately after fixation of the omental flap; (**d**) perineum 3 months after fixation of the omental flap. (Adapted from Schloericke E et al. Transperineal omentum flap for the anatomic reconstruction of the rectovaginal space in the therapy of rectovaginal fistulas. Colorectal Dis 2012;14(5):604–10. Reprinted with permission)

outcomes, and that smoking and steroid use were associated with higher failure rates [66]. Further studies are needed comparing long-term patient outcomes with each procedure.

Crohn's perianal fistulas and RVFs remain challenging medical and surgical problems. Healing is difficult to achieve and recurrence rates are high. Many advances have been made, particularly with regard to biologic agents, and with newer surgical techniques such as the LIFT procedure. More information is needed with regard to long-term outcome with various treatment modalities so the best option may be chosen for each patient.

References

1. Zawadzki A, Starck M, Bohe M, Thorlacius H. A unique 3D endo-anal ultrasound feature of perianal Crohn's fistula: the 'Crohn ultrasound fistula sign'. Colorectal Dis. 2012;9:e608–11.
2. Yousem DM, Fishman EK, Jones B. Crohn disease: perirectal and perianal findings at CT. Radiology. 1988;167:331–4.
3. Guillaumin E, Jeffrey Jr RB, Shea WJ, Asling CW, Goldberg HI. Perirectal inflammatory disease: CT findings. Radiology. 1986; 161:153–7.
4. Leyendecker J, Bloomfield R, DiSantis D, Waters G, Mott R, Bechtold R. MR enterography in the management of patients with Crohn disease. Radiographics. 2009;6:1827–46.
5. Buchanan G, Halligan S, Williams A, Cohen CR, Tarroni D, Phillips RK, et al. Effect of MRI on clinical outcome of recurrent fistula-in-ano. Lancet. 2002;360:1661–2.
6. Law PJ, Talbot RW, Bartram CI, Northover JM. Anal endosonography in the evaluation of perianal sepsis and fistula in ano. Br J Surg. 1989;76(7):752–5.
7. Hildebrandt U, Feifel G, Schwarz HP, Scherr O. Endorectal ultrasound: instrumentation and clinical aspects. Int J Colorectal Dis. 1986;1(4):203–7.
8. Navarro-Luna A, García-Comingo MI, Rius-Macías J, Marco-Molina C. Ultrasound study of anal fistulas with hydrogen peroxide enhancement. Dis Colon Rectum. 2004;47(1):108–14.
9. Lengyel AJ, Hurst NG, Williams JG. Pre-operative assessment of anal fistulas using endoanal ultrasound. Colorectal Dis. 2002;4(6): 436–40.
10. Halligan S, Stoker J. Imaging of fistula in ano. Radiology. 2006; 239(1):18–33.
11. Schwartz DA, Wiersema MI, Dudiak KM, et al. A comparison of endoscopic ultrasound, magnetic resonance imaging, and exam under anesthesia for evaluation of Crohn's perianal fistulas. Gastroenterology. 2001;121:1064–72.
12. Sahni VA, Ahmad R, Burling D. Which method is best for imaging of perianal fistula? Abdom Imaging. 2008;33:26–30.
13. West RL, van der Woude CJ, Hansen BE, Felt-Bersma RJ, van Tilburg AJ, Drapers JA, Kuipers EJ. Clinical and endosonographic effect of ciprofloxacin on the treatment of perianal fistulae in Crohn's disease with infliximab: a double-blind placebo-controlled study. Aliment Pharmacol Ther. 2004;20(11–12):1329–36.
14. Bernstein LH, Frank MS, Brandt LJ, Boley SJ. Healing of perineal Crohn's disease with metronidazole. Gastroenterology. 1987;79: 357–65.
15. Thia KT, Mahadevan U, Feagan BG, Wong C, Cockeram A, Bitton A, Bernstein CN, Sandborn WJ. Ciprofloxacin or metronidazole for the treatment of perianal fistulas in patients with Crohn's disease: a randomized, double-blind, placebo-controlled pilot study. Inflamm Bowel Dis. 2009;15(1):17–24.
16. Lecomte T, Contou JF, Beaugerie L, Carbonnel F, Cattan S, Gendre JP, Cosnes J. Predictive factors of response of perianal Crohn's disease to azathioprine or 6-mercaptopurine. Dis Colon Rectum. 2003;46(11):1469–75.
17. Korelitz BI, Present DH. Favorable effect of 6-mercaptopurine on fistulae of Crohn's disease. Dig Dis Sci. 1985;30(1):58–64.
18. Present DH, Korelitz BI, Wisch N, Glass JL, Sachar DB, Pasternack BS. Treatment of Crohn's disease with 6-mercaptopurine. A long-term, randomized, double-blind study. N Engl J Med. 1980; 302(18):981–7.
19. Jeshion WC, Larsen KL, Jawad AF, Piccoli DA, Verma R, Maller ES, Baldassano RN. Azathioprine and 6-mercaptopurine for the treatment of perianal Crohn's disease in children. J Clin Gastroenterol. 2000;30(3):294–8.
20. Ochsenkühn T, Göke B, Sackmann M. Combining infliximab with 6 mercaptopurine/azathioprine for fistula therapy in Crohn's disease. Am J Gastroenterol. 2002;97(8):2022–5.
21. Kornbluth A. Infliximab approved for use in Crohn's disease: a report on the FDA GI advisory committee conference. Inflamm Bowel Dis. 1998;4(4):328–9.
22. Present DH, Rutgeerts P, Targan S, Hanauer S, Mayer L, van Hogezand RA, Podolsky D, Sands B, Braakman T, DeWoody KL, Schaible TF, van Deventer SJH. Infliximab for the treatment of fistulas in patients with Crohn's disease. N Engl J Med. 1999; 340:1398–405.
23. Lichtiger S, Binion DG, Wolf DC, Present DH, Bensimon AG, Wu E, Yu AP, Cardoso AT, Chao J, Mulani PM, Lomax KG, Kent JD. The CHOICE trial: adalimumab demonstrates safety, fistula healing, improved quality of life and increased work productivity in patients with Crohn's disease who failed prior infliximab therapy. Aliment Pharmacol Ther. 2010;32(10):1228–39.
24. Schreiber S, Lawrance IC, Thomsen OØ, Hanauer SB, Bloomfield R, Sandborn WJ. Randomised clinical trial: certolizumab pegol for fistulas in Crohn's disease—subgroup results from a placebo-controlled study. Aliment Pharmacol Ther. 2011;33(2):185–93.
25. D'Haens GR, Panaccione R, Higgins PD, Vermeire S, Gassull M, Chowers Y, Hanauer SB, Herfarth H, Hommes DW, Kamm M, Löfberg R, Quary A, Sands B, Sood A, Watermeyer G, Lashner B, Lémann M, Plevy S, Reinisch W, Schreiber S, Siegel C, Targan S, Watanabe M, Feagan B, Sandborn WJ, Colombel JF, Travis S. The London position statement of the world congress of gastroenterology on biological therapy for IBD with the European Crohn's and colitis organization: when to start, when to stop, which drug to choose, and how to predict response? Am J Gastroenterol. 2011;106(2):199–212.
26. Takesue Y, Ohge H, Yokoyama T, Murakami Y, Imamura Y, Sueda T. Long-term results of seton drainage on complex anal fistulae in patients with Crohn's disease. J Gastroenterol. 2002;37(11):912–5.
27. Soltani A, Kaiser AM. Endorectal advancement flap for cryptoglandular or Crohn's fistula-in-ano. Dis Colon Rectum. 2010;53(4): 486–95.
28. Kodner IJ, Mazor A, Shemesh EI, Fry RD, Fleshman JW, Birnbaum EH. Endorectal advancement flap repair of rectovaginal and other complicated anorectal fistulas. Surgery. 1993;114(4):682–9.
29. Grimaud JC, Munoz-Bongrand N, Siproudhis L, Abramowitz L, Sénéjoux A, Vitton V, Gambiez L, Flourié B, Hébuterne X, Louis E, Coffin B, De Parades V, Savoye G, Soulé JC, Bouhnik Y, Colombel JF, Contou JF, François Y, Mary JY, Lémann M. Fibrin glue is effective healing perianal fistulas in patients with Crohn's disease. Gastroenterology. 2010;138(7):2275–81.
30. O'Riordan JM, Datta I, Johnston C, Baxter NN. A systematic review of the anal fistula plug for patients with Crohn's and non-Crohn's related fistula-in-ano. Dis Colon Rectum. 2012;55(3):351–8.
31. Taxonera C, Schwartz D, García-Olmo D. Emerging treatments for complex perianal fistula in Crohn's disease. World J Gastroenterol. 2009;15(34):4263–72.

32. Guadalajara H, Herreros D, De-La-Quintana P, Trebol J, Garcia-Arranz M, Garcia-Olmo D. Long-term follow-up of patients undergoing adipose-derived adult stem cell administration to treat complex perianal fistulas. Int J Colorectal Dis. 2012;27(5):595–600.

33. Rojanasakul A, Pattanaarun J, Sahakitrungruang C, Tantiphlachiva K. Total anal sphincter saving technique for fistula-in-ano; the ligation of intersphincteric fistula tract. J Med Assoc Thai. 2007; 90(3):581–6.

34. Sileri P, Franceschilli L, Angelucci GP, D'Ugo S, Milito G, Cadeddu F, Selvaggio I, Lazzaro S, Gaspari AL. Ligation of the intersphincteric fistula tract (LIFT) to treat anal fistula: early results from a prospective observational study. Tech Coloproctol. 2011; 15(4):413–6.

35. Tan KK, Alsuwaigh R, Tan AM, Tan IJ, Liu X, Koh DC, Tsang CB. To LIFT or to flap? Which surgery to perform following seton insertion for high anal fistula? Dis Colon Rectum. 2012;55(12): 1273–7.

36. Han JG, Yi BQ, Wang ZJ, Zheng Y, Cui JJ, Yu XQ, Zhao BC, Yang XQ. Ligation of the intersphincteric fistula tract plus bioprosthetic anal fistula plug (LIFT-Plug): a new technique for fistula-in-ano. Colorectal Dis. 2013;15(5):582–6.

37. Rehg KL, Sanchez JE, Krieger BR, Marcet JE. Fecal diversion in perirectal fistulizing Crohn's disease is an underutilized and potentially temporary means of successful treatment. Am Surg. 2009;75(8):715–8.

38. Galandiuk S, Kimberling J, Al-Mishlab TG, Stromberg AJ. Perianal Crohn disease: predictors of need for permanent diversion. Ann Surg. 2005;241(5):796–801.

39. Genua JC, Vivas DA. Management of nonhealing perineal wounds. Clin Colon Rectal Surg. 2007;20(4):322–8.

40. Ky A, Sohn N, Weinstein MA, Korelitz BI. Carcinoma arising in anorectal fistulas of Crohn's disease. Dis Colon Rectum. 1998;41(8):992–6. Review.

41. Korelitz BI. Carcinoma of the intestinal tract in Crohn's disease: results of a survey conducted by the National Foundation for ileitis and colitis. Am J Gastroenterol. 1983;78(1):44–6.

42. Schwartz DA, Loftus Jr EV, Tremaine WJ, Panaccione R, Harmsen WS, Zinsmeister AR, Sandborn WJ. The natural history of fistulizing Crohn's disease in Olmsted County, Minnesota. Gastroenterology. 2002;122(4):875–80.

43. Sands BE, Blank MA, Patel K, van Deventer SJ. Longterm treatment of rectovaginal fistulas in Crohn's disease: response to infliximab in the ACCENT II study. Clin Gastroenterol Hepatol. 2004;2(10):912–20.

44. Shobeiri SA, Quiroz L, Nihira M. Rectovaginal fistulography: a technique for the identification of recurrent elusive fistulas. Int Urogynecol J Pelvic Floor Dysfunct. 2009;20(5):571–3.

45. Stoker J, Rociu E, Schouten WR, Laméris JS. Anovaginal and rectovaginal fistulas: endoluminal sonography versus endoluminal MR imaging. AJR Am J Roentgenol. 2002;178(3):737–41.

46. Maconi G, Ardizzone S, Greco S, Radice E, Bezzio C, Bianchi Porro G. Transperineal ultrasound in the detection of perianal and rectovaginal fistulae in Crohn's disease. Am J Gastroenterol. 2007;102(10):2214–9. Epub 2006 Aug 4.

47. Coller JA. Clinical application of anorectal manometry. Gastroenterol Clin North Am. 1987;16(1):17–33.

48. Tsang CB, Madoff RD, Wong WD, Rothenberger DA, Finne CO, Singer D, Lowry AC. Anal sphincter integrity and function influences outcome in rectovaginal fistula repair. Dis Colon Rectum. 1998;41(9):1141–6.

49. Buchanan GN, Bartram CI, Phillips RK, Gould SW, Halligan S, Rockall TA, Sibbons P, Cohen RG. Efficacy of fibrin sealant in the management of complex anal fistula: a prospective trial. Dis Colon Rectum. 2003;46(9):1167–74.

50. Abel ME, Chiu YS, Russell TR, Volpe PA. Autologous fibrin glue in the treatment of rectovaginal and complex fistulas. Dis Colon Rectum. 1993;36(5):447–9.

51. Gajsek U, McArthur DR, Sagar PM. Long-term efficacy of the button fistula plug in the treatment of ileal pouch-vaginal and Crohn's-related rectovaginal fistulas. Dis Colon Rectum. 2011; 54(8):999–1002.

52. MacRae HM, McLeod RS, Cohen Z, Stern H, Reznick R. Treatment of rectovaginal fistulas that has failed previous repair attempts. Dis Colon Rectum. 1995;38(9):921–5.

53. Khanduja KS, Padmanabhan A, Kerner BA, Wise WE, Aguilar PS. Reconstruction of rectovaginal fistula with sphincter disruption by combining rectal mucosal advancement flap and anal sphincteroplasty. Dis Colon Rectum. 1999;42(11):1432–7.

54. Wise Jr WE, Aguilar PS, Padmanabhan A, Meesig DM, Arnold MW, Stewart WR. Surgical treatment of low rectovaginal fistulas. Dis Colon Rectum. 1991;34(3):271–4.

55. Bravo Gutierrez A, Madoff RD, Lowry AC, Parker SC, Buie WD, Baxter NN. Long-term results of anterior sphincteroplasty. Dis Colon Rectum. 2004;47(5):727–31.

56. Malouf AJ, Norton CS, Engel AF, Nicholls RJ, Kamm MA. Long-term results of overlapping anterior anal-sphincter repair for obstetric trauma. Lancet. 2000;355(9200):260–5.

57. Ellis CN. Outcomes after repair of rectovaginal fistulas using bioprosthetics. Dis Colon Rectum. 2008;51(7):1084–8.

58. Haray PN, Stiff G, Foster ME. New option for recurrent rectovaginal fistulas. Dis Colon Rectum. 1996;39:463–4.

59. Ruffolo C, Scarpa M, Bassi N, Angriman I. A systematic review on advancement flaps for rectovaginal fistula in Crohn's disease: transrectal vs transvaginal approach. Colorectal Dis. 2010;12(12): 1183–91.

60. Marchesa P, Hull TL, Fazio VW. Advancement sleeve flaps for treatment of severe perianal Crohn's disease. Br J Surg. 1998;85: 1695–8.

61. Hull TL, Fazio VW. Surgical approaches to low anovaginal fistula in Crohn's disease. Am J Surg. 1997;173(2):95–8.

62. Fürst A, Schmidbauer C, Swol-Ben J, Iesalnieks I, Schwandner O, Agha A. Gracilis transposition for repair of recurrent anovaginal and rectovaginal fistulas in Crohn's disease. Int J Colorectal Dis. 2008;23(4):349–53.

63. McNevin MS, Lee PYH, Bax TW. Martius flap: an adjunct for repair of complex, low rectovaginal fistula. Am J Surg. 2007; 193(5):597–9.

64. Songne K, Scotté M, Lubrano J, Huet E, Lefébure B, Surlemont Y, Leroy S, Michot F, Ténière P. Treatment of anovaginal or rectovaginal fistulas with modified Martius graft. Colorectal Dis. 2007; 9(7):653–6.

65. Schloericke E, Hoffman M, Zimmermann M, Kraus M, Bouchard R, Roblick UJ, Hildebrand P, Nolde J, Bruch HP, Limmer S. Transperineal omentum flap for the anatomic reconstruction of the rectovaginal space in the therapy of rectovaginal fistulas. Colorectal Dis. 2012;14(5):604–10.

66. El-Gazzaz G, Hull T, Mignanelli E, Hammel J, Gurland B, Zutshi M. Analysis of function and predictors of failure in women undergoing repair of Crohn's related rectovaginal fistula. J Gastrointest Surg. 2010;14(5):824–9.

Tuberculosis Fistulas

Pravin Jaiprakash Gupta

Introduction

Anal fistula is a very common condition found in 34–66 % of all anorectal abscesses, and while most of the anal fistulas are thought to arise because of cryptoglandular infection, they are found in patients with inflammatory bowel disease, particularly Crohn's disease. Resurgence in tuberculosis during the HIV era has produced a new spectrum of presentations for the surgeon and, therefore, invasion by tubercle bacilli is often seen at unusual sites of the gut and ano-perianal region [1]. Anal fistulas can also be associated with actinomycosis, chlamydia, syphilis, lymphogranuloma venereum, radiation exposure, diverticulitis, foreign-body reactions, and fungal infections [2]. Approximately 30 % of patients with HIV disease develop anorectal abscesses and fistulas.

Tuberculosis (TB) is an infectious granulomatous disease caused mainly by *Mycobacterium tuberculosis*, an acid-fast bacillus that is primarily transmitted via the respiratory system [3]. In 1882, Robert Koch isolated the bacillus, grew it in pure culture, and demonstrated its pathogenic capacity. Thus, tubercular disease is also called as Koch's disease. Tuberculosis around the anus is a rare extrapulmonary form of the disease. Although it is described as one of the cause of granulomatous diseases within the anorectal region, yet perianal tuberculosis, without the presence of any previous or active pulmonary infection, is extremely rare.

Gastrointestinal tuberculosis represents 1 % of extrapulmonary tuberculosis and only sporadic cases of anal tuberculosis have been reported in the literature [4]. Tuberculosis is a neglected cause of anal sepsis. Often it is not recognized and, therefore, is not treated properly. Although the symptoms are often misleading and thus go unrecognized, they ought to be recognized, because they require specific treatment. Else, this results in recurrence of fistulas after routine surgical treatment. Extrapulmonary tuberculosis can attack any organ; ano-perineal disease (1 % of digestive tract incidence) is much more rare [5].

TB, known also as the white plague, has been around for millennia and is responsible for more human deaths than any other single pathogen today. The combination with HIV coinfection, which dramatically compromises host resistance to TB, leads to high disease prevalence in affected endemic populations. Currently, each year more than 1.5 million people die of TB, and more than nine million newly develop TB [6]. This dire situation is further compromised by the increasing prevalence of multidrug-resistant (MDR) and extensively drug-resistant (XDR) strains, and the more recent occurrence of TDR (totally drug-resistant) strains, which are virtually untreatable.

Tuberculosis of gastrointestinal tract may be primary or secondary to a primary focus elsewhere. Primary intestinal tuberculosis is attributable to bovine tubercle bacilli entering the system through milk intake. The incidence of primary tuberculosis is on a decline due to public preference for pasteurized milk [7].

Infection by Koch's bacillus is still a public health problem both in underdeveloped and in developed countries where the epidemic of human immunodeficiency virus (HIV), the appearance of multiresistant bacilli, large immigrant populations, and poverty all play their part in the increased incidence of the disease. Although anal tuberculosis is relatively rare, it is not as uncommon as one may think. The disease will not be found unless it is thought of and looked for. There is no ground for complacency; tuberculosis remains a menacing disease. According to the World Health Organization (2007), tuberculosis is spreading and currently a third of the world's population is infected with *M. tuberculosis* [8].

Growing immigrant populations in the developed countries has reversed the decline in the incidence of tuberculosis in these countries in comparison to the previous decades. A recent resurgence in the incidence of anal tuberculosis

P.J. Gupta, M.S., F.I.C.A., F.A.I.S., F.I.C.S., F.A.C.S. (✉)
Fine Morning Hospital and Research Center, Gupta Nursing
Home, D/9, Laxaminagar, Nagpur 440 022, India
e-mail: drpjg@yahoo.co.in; piles@drpravingupta.com

H. Abcarian (ed.), *Anal Fistula: Principles and Management*, DOI 10.1007/978-1-4614-9014-2_20,
© Springer Science+Business Media New York 2014

has been reported at two areas, shelters for the homeless and nursing homes, which are fast becoming fertile places for the transmission of tubercular infection [9].

Tuberculosis is not always a stigma of the poor; even well-to-do are not immune to it. Louis XIII, the king of France died of abdominal tuberculosis. Byron, Keats, and Chopin were affected by tuberculosis. Dr. Anton Chekhov, Maxim Gorki, and D.H. Lawrence had it [10]. Throughout history, there runs a suggestion that the intellectually gifted are the most likely to contract the disease, but there is no evidence that tuberculosis breeds genius. The probability is rather the eagerness for achievements leads to a way of life that renders the body less resistant to infections.

The most frequently encountered anorectal tuberculous lesions are suppurations and fistulae [11]. Anal tubercular sepsis seems to have characteristic clinical features. It should be considered in cases of known pulmonary or extrapulmonary tuberculosis or if anal sepsis is persistent, recurrent, or complex in nature.

Anal fistula occurring due to tuberculosis is rare in western countries; it has clearly regressed in the developing countries due to early detection of pulmonary tuberculosis, availability of specific antibiotics, and widespread immunization.

Extrapulmonary TB can be found in any organ, with or without the lungs being affected, and can be diffuse. Anal contamination is usually caused by the swallowing of respiratory secretions that contain a large quantity of Koch's bacillus; more rarely, it may be caused through the blood or the lymphatic system. A pre-existing anal lesion (fissure, erosion, fistula, pilonidal sinus, or scar) is often found which makes way for the bacillus to invade [12].

Etiology

Perianal tuberculosis comprises less than 10 % of all perianal diseases and 0.7 % of all tuberculosis cases. In a report from India, 19 (15.6 %) of 122 cases of anal fistula were diagnosed as having tubercular etiology [13]. Only three cases presented with a clinical picture of concomitant pulmonary tuberculosis; none was HIV-positive. Another study showed 14 % of 64 patients with extrapulmonary tuberculosis had tubercular anal fistula [14]. It is speculated that perianal tuberculosis may be the result of hematogenous or lymphatic dissemination from a distant pulmonary focus in a few patients, and it is estimated that tuberculous fistulae to be 13 times more common in tuberculous subjects than in nontuberculous types. In others, it is usually associated with gastrointestinal tract tuberculosis.

Two hypotheses can explain anal involvement by tuberculosis: swallowing of respiratory secretions containing large quantity of Koch's bacillus or following reactivation of a latent focus.

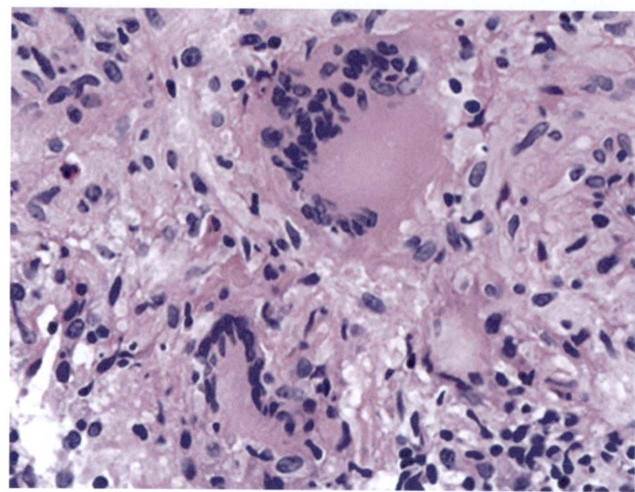

Fig. 20.1 Histology of a tubercular lesion with caseation, multinucleated giant cells, macrophages, and lymphocytes

For many years in the past, the common belief held was that majority of anal fistulae are tuberculous. However, exhaustive work by various authors has shown that only a small percentage of fistulae are tuberculous in nature. Opinions have varied widely as to the percentage of anal fistulae that are tuberculous in nature and as to the part tuberculosis plays in anal fistula. Buie et al. [15] have described two reasons for this difference of opinion. The first is that the criteria on which the diagnosis is made differs; at one extreme are those who make demonstration of tubercle bacilli in fistula a requisite for positive diagnosis. At the other are those who feel that the clinical picture or even the demonstration of tuberculosis elsewhere in the body, is enough to establish the diagnosis of a tuberculous fistula. The second reason for the variance of opinion is the difference in the source of material investigated. All now agree it that the laboratory methods are the only exact means of determining the tuberculous nature of fistula. These methods consist of demonstration of tuberculous granulation tissue (fibroblasts, lymphocytes, capillaries, and fibrin) with typical Langhans type of giant cell, characteristic tubercle formation with caseation and monocytic and lymphocytic infiltration on histopathological examination (Fig. 20.1), a positive guinea pig inoculation or a positive culture of tubercle bacilli. However, most of the researchers are now of the opinion that only histopathological examination can confirm the diagnosis of tuberculous fistula.

Pathogenesis

An active extrarectal tuberculous lesion or a history of previous infection can usually be elicited in these patients. Perianal tuberculosis appears in several forms. The commonest are the perirectal abscess, usually with secondary infection, fistula in ano, and a soft, indolent perianal ulcer. If an abscess is formed, it may appear as the typical perianal or ischiorectal variety with secondary infection, or it may remain for a time as a non-tender swelling with induration of the subcutaneous tissues near the mucous margin. Eventually this becomes secondarily infected to soften and break and then to persist as an indolent swelling with profuse thin purulent or watery discharge and the edges of the opening heaped up with pale unhealthy granulations. When a fistula is present, the external opening is large with purplish, overhanging edges and there is a copious, thin, creamy discharge. As in the non-tuberculous fistulae, there may be multiple external openings with extensive spread of the infection to the surrounding tissues of the ischiorectal fosse and perineum and eventually even to the buttocks. There is usually only one internal opening and this is generally superficial or between the sphincters. A fistula may complicate or can be complicated by a perirectal abscess; in the former instance, it may be of the blind external variety due to inadequate drainage of the original abscess.

Infection leading to fistula is generally supposed to originate from an infected anal gland. The infection usually occurs from the bowel lumen, the patient swallowing the sputum laden with tubercle bacilli. This is the commonest route of infection in patients suffering from pulmonary tuberculosis. The anal glands are at the base of the anal crypts and are located at the level of the dentate line. Most people have between six and eight such glands, which extend down into the internal sphincter up to or including the intersphincteric groove. Obstruction of these glands leads to stasis, bacterial overgrowth, and ultimately abscesses that are located in the intersphincteric groove. These abscesses have several routes of egress, the most common of which are downward extension to the anoderm (perianal abscess) or across the external sphincter into the ischiorectal fossa (ischiorectal abscess) [16]. Less common routes of spread are superiorly up the intersphincteric groove to the supralevator space or in the submucosal plane. When the abscess is drained either surgically or spontaneously, persistence of the septic foci and epithelization of the draining tract may occur and lead to a fistula-in-ano.

The tubercle bacillus has a predilection for lymphoid tissue and so the infection usually spreads from the rectum through lymph channels and forms an abscess in the perianal tissues, though sometimes it may travel from the rectum to the perianal tissues by blood vessels or by direct extension [17]. The tubercle bacilli may also gain entrance into the blood stream from some extrarectal focus and may lodge in the fat of ischiorectal fossa to start there as an abscess. Fissures and abrasions round the anus may be infected by direct external inoculation or autoinoculation. These patients are commonly subjected to increased anal trauma, as both

diarrhea and constipation are common in their disease. There is a diminution in the subcutaneous adipose tissue because of the patient's poor general condition and thus the anal and perianal tissues can be traumatized easily. Lesions, such as abrasions or tears of the mucosa or skin at the mucocutaneous junction may be secondarily infected with local infective organism leading to an abscess.

This perianal abscess on rupture leaves a draining fistula. It rarely may be the result of a spread of the infection from the neighboring organs, which are the seat of tuberculosis, e.g., prostate, seminal vesicles, spine or sacroiliac joints [18].

In patients with a fistula, the abscesses are more likely to contain multiple different organisms. Fistula formation allows for increased bacterial invasion in the abscess. Most aerobic and anaerobic organisms isolated from such abscesses are of gastrointestinal tract and skin flora origin [19]. The incidence of gut-derived microorganisms including *E. coli*, *B. fragilis*, and *Enterococci* cultured from perirectal abscesses has been reported as between 70 and 80 %.

Clinical Presentations

Since these fistulae are commonly a complication of pulmonary tuberculosis, the majority of the patients are found to be in the third and fourth decades of life. Constitutional symptoms as anorexia, fever, weight loss, or malaise usually are not present. A previous history of perirectal abscess either drained spontaneously or surgically can usually be elicited. Patients often report a cyclical pattern of pain, swelling, and drainage. Moisture can cause skin irritation, excoriation, and pruritus (Fig. 20.2). Prior TB infection as a child, immunocompromised states such as human immunodeficiency virus/acquired immunodeficiency syndrome, immunosuppression with organ transplantation, travel to endemic areas, and immigration are important considerations while obtaining a

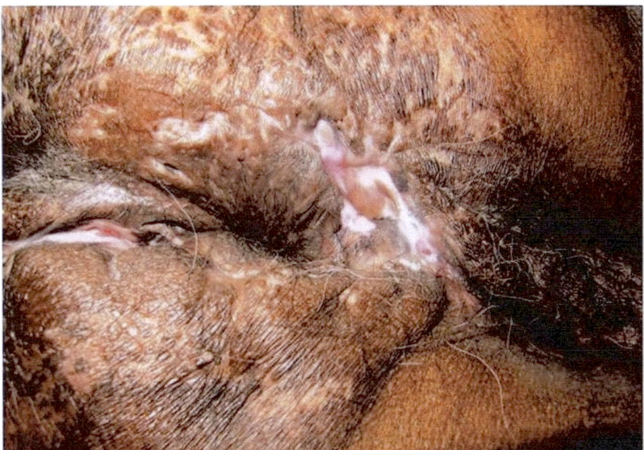

Fig. 20.2 Tubercular anal fistulae with scarring

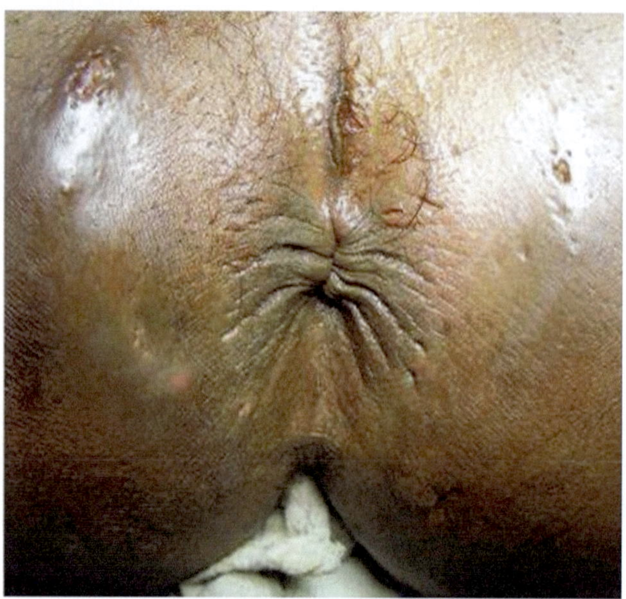

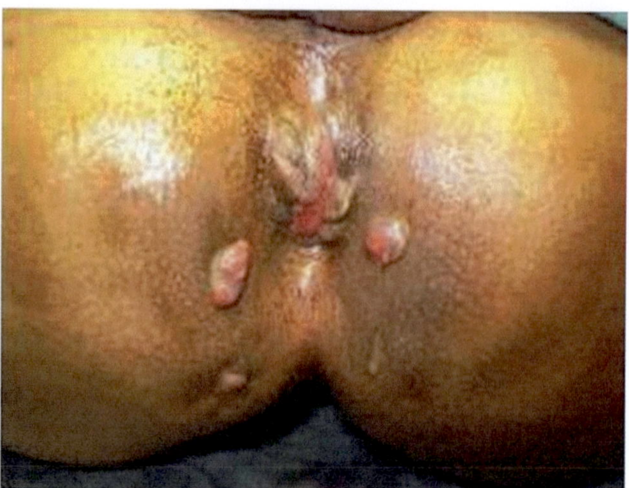

Fig. 20.4 A horseshoe tubercular fistula

Fig. 20.3 Multiple pin-like openings of a tubercular fistula

medical history [20]. There is a general agreement that tuberculosis is rarely if ever primary in fistula; in more than 98 % of the cases the original focus is elsewhere. It may, however, be the initial sign of the disease, which should always be suspected with the appearance of a fistula in a susceptible individual from the situations mentioned above.

A good digital examination is usually sufficient for the diagnosis and the treatment planning of anal fistula. There is no functional sign or preferred site that allows a tuberculous fistula to be distinguished from a cryptoglandular fistula. The external opening may be a pinhole or appear as an irregular ulcer of varying size (Fig. 20.3). The fistulous tract is patulous due to the absence of induration. The granulations are pale and flabby. A gaping external fistulous orifice with detached margins and highly vascular in nature is suggestive [21]. The discharge is frequently continuous and is thin and milky. These form the majority of the tuberculous fistulae and are labeled as the superficial or low variety. The deep or high tuberculous fistula forms a tract with little induration and often leads to a palpable submucous thickening high up (Fig. 20.4). Most authors report a higher frequency of complex tuberculous fistula forms (62–100 %) which sometimes puts the sphincter and continence at risk [22]. A long period of development and the recurrence of the fistula despite well-managed surgical treatment have been found in a majority of patients. The tract of the fistula and its relationship to the sphincter muscle can be investigated by probing and/or dyeing intraoperatively with the patient under anesthesia.

It is not necessary that all reported cases of anorectal tuberculosis are patients with old tuberculotic lesions or with active pulmonary tuberculosis in the lung. Diagnosis can be delayed, because physicians may neglect to perform a general physical examination in patients with a positive sputum smear and the typical chest X-ray. It is emphasize that all patients with pulmonary tuberculosis must undergo a complete physical examination. Chest physicians must remember that patients may not mention anal complaints if not asked. The possibility of tuberculosis must never be forgotten in the etiology of anal nodular and ulcerated lesions, regardless of the presence or absence of pulmonary tuberculosis [23]. The patient's continence is another important facet that needs to be included, as well as any history of anorectal surgery.

Investigations

As tuberculosis of anal region is a rare entity and there is no characteristic clinical picture, it is very difficult to diagnose it preoperatively. The diagnosis of anal TB is difficult and may be missed for months or even years. Nevertheless, overlooking the diagnosis of perianal tuberculosis can result in chronic morbidity and often mortality, especially among immunocompromised patients. The physician must take a thorough history, look for acid-fast bacilli in the discharge from the lesion, carefully examine excised tissue, and culture for *M. tuberculosis* to make the correct diagnosis of this potentially curable disease [24]. Positive Siebert purified protein derivative (PPD) or of tuberculin test supports TB infection, but a negative test does not rule it out.

The tuberculin skin test is one of the few investigations dating from the nineteenth century that is still widely used as an important test for diagnosing tuberculosis. It was developed by Koch in 1890, but it was Charles Mantoux, who described the intradermal technique currently in use in 1912. Short of demonstrating viable organisms in body tissues and fluids, the tuberculin skin test (TST) is the only method of detecting *M. tuberculosis* infection in an individual and is used in the diagnosis of TB in individual patients. The tuberculin most widely used is purified protein derivative (PPD), which is derived from cultures of M. tuberculosis. The reaction to intracutaneously injected tuberculin is the classic example of a delayed (cellular) hypersensitivity reaction [25].

A standard dose of five tuberculin units (TU) (0.1 mL) is injected intradermally and read 48–72 h later. A person who has been exposed to the bacteria is expected to mount an immune response in the skin containing the bacterial proteins. TST indurations >10 mm are considered positive, 5–10 mm intermediate; and <5 mm as negative [26].

The Mantoux test does not measure immunity to TB but the degree of hypersensitivity to tuberculin. There is no correlation between the size of induration and likelihood of current active TB disease but the reaction size is correlated with the future risk of developing TB disease. The test has a poor positive predictive value for current active disease. The formation of vesicles, bullae, or necrosis at the test site indicates high degree of tuberculin sensitivity and thus presence of infection with tubercle bacilli [27].

Negative tests can be interpreted to mean that the person has not been infected with the TB bacteria or that the person has been infected recently and not enough time has elapsed for the body to react to the skin test. There is disagreement about the role of Mantoux testing in people who have been vaccinated. The US recommendation is that TST is not contraindicated for BCG-vaccinated persons and that prior BCG vaccination should not influence the interpretation of the test [28].

Positive diagnosis of anal TB depends on histological or bacteriologic analysis. The typical histological lesion is the epithelioid and giant cell tubercle around a zone of caseous necrosis, but the pathognomonic presence of caseation is not constant and presents diagnostic problems, especially in the case of Crohn's disease with anoperineal localization. And though this histological picture of granulomatous inflammation is characteristic of *Mycobacterium* infection, it can also be found in other disease entities such as sarcoidosis, leprosy, and systemic lupus erythematosus [29]. Tuberculosis, even when present, is frequently missed; in that too few sections are studied. Tissue for microscopical examination should be carefully selected and even then, there may be presence of such a large number of acute and chronic inflammatory cells, that the underlying tuberculosis may be missed. Diagnosis can also be done by looking for Koch's bacillus in the anal lesions by direct examination (Ziehl–Nielsen stain) and culture. To overcome the slowness of the culture (3–4 weeks), new diagnostic techniques for TB have been proposed, in particular genomic amplification by polymerase chain reaction (PCR), which can detect the presence of the bacterial DNA in 48 h with high sensitivity and specificity when several samples are tested [30]. TB-nested

PCR using pus or tissue specimens is a good alternative method with exquisite sensitivity and specificity for rapid and early detection of the disease. However, one of the disadvantages of PCR is its inability to detect whether the TB infection is biologically active or in its latent phase. New enzyme-linked immunosorbent assays for the diagnosis of digestive tract TB that appear to be highly specific and sensitive are currently undergoing evaluation [31]. Histological examination is mandatory if the patient has had or still has tuberculosis elsewhere in the body. Stool cultures are rarely useful and they are not routinely performed.

Transanal and endorectal sonography and other sonographic techniques may evaluate the nature and course of fistula [32]. This procedure is simple, fast, can be done in the same office visit, and provides information about the fistula track, the type, and complexity and whether the anal sphincter muscle is normal, scarred, or disrupted, as well as the presence of an abscess cavity. With the use of high-frequency linear or curved array probes on the perineum in both transverse and longitudinal planes, fistulous and sinus tracts, collections in the perineum, buttocks, scrotum, and labia can be assessed and followed in a retrograde direction to their connection with the anal canal. A high sensitivity of 96 % is reported for the detection of tracts, with a negative predictive value of close to 100 % on perianal sonography [33]. The advantage of endosonography is that it is easy and cheap to use, but it does depend to a high degree on the examiner's experience.

Identified tracts appear on a sonographic scan as hypoechoic linear areas or fluid-containing tubular areas, depending on their size and activity, with contained particulate fluid or hyperechoic moving reflections created by air bubbles and pus. Highly complex trans-sphincteric tracts, which may extend to involve the deep tissues of the buttocks, the perineum, the scrotum in men, and the labia and vagina in women, can also be documented, along with horseshoe fistulas. Perianal fluid collections and abscesses present as oval hypo to anechoic masses, most often with a direct association with a fistulous tract [34]. This documentation of fluid collections formed by fistulas and of the relationship of inflammatory tracts to the sphincter mechanism is important for surgical treatment.

Sonography can identify the internal opening in the upper anal canal with a high accuracy in more than 90 % of patients. Further, 3D imaging may better map the course of a fistula than 2D imaging. However, for some authors, hydrogen peroxide or SH U 508A (Levovist, Schering) injection of the external opening and a 3D reconstruction during transrectal sonography may better demarcate small fistulous tracts, internal openings, and secondary extensions and may facilitate differentiation between an active fistulous tract and fibrotic tissue, thereby providing a dynamic depiction of perianal fistulas, although with some limits and possible pitfalls [35]. Anal ultrasound is operator dependent; scars and defects may confuse sonographic interpretation and might render delineation of the fistulous track difficult.

Cross-sectional imaging techniques can accurately identify deep abscesses and characterize complex fistulae. MRI is well suited for this examination, with almost no motion artifact, excellent contrast between muscles and fatty spaces, and multiplanar acquisition. The cryptoglandular anal fistulae are nonspecific in origin and are usually simple, whereas specific fistulae-like tuberculosis are at time complex. MRI appears useful in the cases with recurrent fistulae, when the secondary orifice is atypically placed, during a multistep treatment for complex fistulae, or when an anal stenosis forbids a clinical or ultrasound examination [36].

A good knowledge of the perineum anatomy is required for analyzing the fistula tracts. The muscle planes separate fatty spaces which have an important role in the spread of the disease: sub-mucosal space, marginal space, intersphincteric space, postanal space of Courtney, supralevator space, and the two ischioanal spaces on both sides of the anal canal, all have their role to play in the formation and spread of infection.

MRI examination is performed with an external phased array coil, where a canula is placed to identify the anal canal. The T2W sequences give the more interesting information, but the sequences with fat-suppression and gadolinium chelate injection are also very useful. Digital subtraction MR-fistulography is a new, noninvasive imaging technique for the detection of perianal fistulas and abscesses [37].

However, MRI is cost intensive, not always available, and its diagnostic value depends on technical conditions; nonetheless, it is to be preferred to endosonography for lesions distant from the anus. Other advantages of MRI are that it allows pain-free acquisition of images that can be evaluated independently of the examiner.

Because of the radiation burden, visualization of fistulas using contrast media like fistulogram and computed tomography (CT) is regarded as obsolete.

Although anal manometry may provide information about sphincter pressures, obtaining a fecal incontinence score will also yield clinically relevant information. Collectively, this information will help select the best choice for treatment and allows the surgeon to counsel the patient about expectations and probabilities of success.

The other investigative tools proposed for the diagnosis of tuberculosis includes the ELISA, Rapid Immunochromatographic assay (ICT Tuberculosis), Fluid adenosine deaminase estimation, Interferon gamma and the radiometric BACTEC system studies, The Xpert MTB/RIF assay, and QuantiFERON®-TB Gold test [38]. Fine needle aspiration cytology (FNAC) of the perianal lesions can also be performed as a supportive investigation.

The serodiagnosis of tuberculosis has long been the subject of controversy, as we still lack a test with widespread clinical utility. The poor sensitivity and specificity of commercial assays preclude their use as the sole means of diagnosis. All these assays use mycobacterial antigens adsorbed onto a surface. There is a high possibility of false positive and false negative reactions. The overall sensitivity of these tests for extrapulmonary tuberculosis is as low as 16 % [39].

The relatively low sensitivities and specificities of these serologic tests make them poor tools for the diagnosis of tuberculosis. For the EIA-IgA, the sensitivity reported was 74 % and the specificity was 68 % when a cutoff determined by a receiver operator characteristic curve was used. For the EIA-IgG, the sensitivity was 69 % and the specificity was 64 % [40].

Experience shows that a triad of fine needle aspiration cytology, AFB smear, and culture are cheaper, foolproof, and confirmatory when compared to costlier tests like TB IgG, IgM, or ICT tests.

Similarly, an elevated erythrocyte sedimentation rate (ESR) may be expected in patients with tuberculosis, but it has been found that one-third of patients with TB had a normal ESR at the time of diagnosis, and consequently there would seem to be little value in using ESR as a diagnostic test for tuberculosis.

Sometimes, a cluster of epidemiologic, clinical, histological, radiologic, and evolutive arguments can contribute to the diagnosis of tubercular anal fistula. These may include the origin and social class of the patient, previous history of TB, recurrent anal suppuration, weight loss, fever, night sweats, chronic dry cough, positive reaction to the tuberculin skin test, epithelioid granulomas without caseous necrosis on a sample from the lesion, associated evaluative pulmonary or digestive TB, and favorable and rapid response to antituberculosis treatment [41].

Differential Diagnosis

Differential diagnosis of anal TB must be done specially with Crohn's disease, due to similar clinical, radiological, and endoscopic features [42]. While Crohn's disease occurs in a relatively younger age group, TB is seen mostly in the elderly. Tubercular disease is predominantly a disease of the males; however, no gender is immune to Crohn's. Tuberculosis presentations are nonspecific in general (recurring fistula, superficial ulceration); Crohn's features are either typical (deep ulceration) or nonspecific (fissure, abscess, or recurring fistula). X-ray of the lungs would be usually normal in Crohn's, while it would depict active lesions in the lungs or may show the sequel of the disease. Tuberculin test would obviously be positive in TB patients but would be negative in Crohn's. The digestive tract in Crohn's is frequently seen affected in the form of an ileocecal lesion, while it is rare to find such involvement in TB [43].

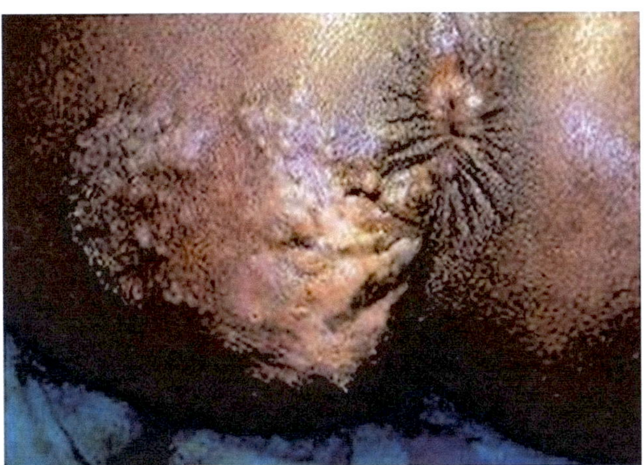

Fig. 20.5 Perianal actinomycosis with multiple pus discharging openings

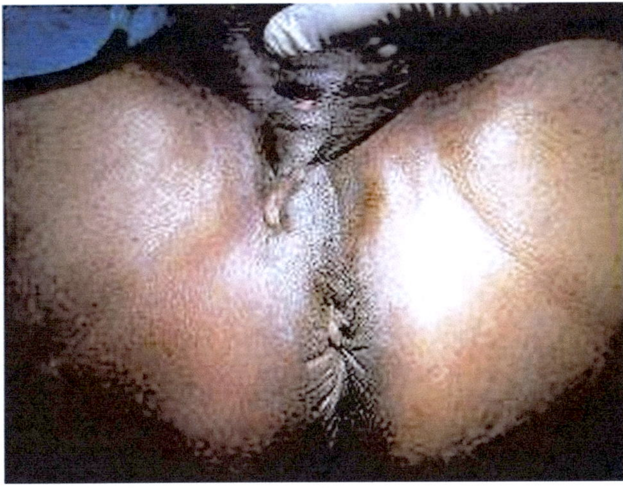

Fig. 20.6 Anal syphilis with pus discharging opening in the perineum

The histological features of Crohn's disease is a granuloma without caseation or a nonspecific granuloma, while tubercular granulomas are more numerous, larger, often merging together and rich in multinucleated giant cells with or without caseation.

Culture of Koch's bacillus is negative in Crohn's while it may be positive or negative when observed in the excised tissue, urine, or gastric secretion. Relapses are common in Crohn's disease even after a full course of therapy, while the tubercular infection is fully cured after the prescribed antitubercular therapy (ATT).

Other possible granulomatous diseases of the anus can mimic anal fistula, such as amoebiasis, actinomycosis (Fig. 20.5), reaction to a foreign body, sarcoidosis, syphilis (Fig. 20.6), and venereal lymphogranuloma with *Chlamydia trachomatis*. In rare cases, anoperineal TB can simulate cancer, particularly colloid cancer; here, histology is vital to make the correct diagnosis [44].

HIV and Tuberculosis

Because of the absence of diagnostic symptoms and signs, the diagnosis of perianal tuberculosis can be much more complicated among HIV-positive patients, although it is considered an important marker of HIV infection. The development of active TB is dramatically accelerated by coinfection with HIV, which increases *M. tuberculosis* reactivation rates from 3–10 % per lifetime to 5–10 % per life-year [45].

AIDS patients seem to be particularly susceptible to tuberculosis, which is of extrapulmonary type in almost three-fourth of the cases. HIV has been a major factor contributing to the resurgence of tuberculosis in developed and developing countries alike. The virus has altered the balance between human beings and Koch's bacillus, as well as having a noticeable impact on the epidemiology, natural history, and clinical evolution of tuberculosis. Coinfection with tuberculosis/HIV results in higher mortality rates than does HIV infection alone.

Antituberculosis drug resistance and an increased risk of transmission have also emerged as problems due to noncompliance with the tuberculosis treatment [46]. Because of impaired immune response, HIV-infected patients are at increased risk of reactivation of latent tuberculosis infection, and AIDS is a strong risk factor for death in patients with tuberculosis. In coinfected patients, mortality is commonly related to delayed diagnosis, because some HIV-infected individuals postpone seeking health care in order to avoid receiving an AIDS diagnosis, which may result in their social ostracism [47].

Tuberculosis as a frequent complicating infection of HIV-positive patients, often diagnosed some time before the AIDS infection. There is a high prevalence of anal lesions because of acquired immunodeficiency syndrome that is estimated as being between 16 and 34 %. Although the incidence of TB is increasing in these patients, especially in extrapulmonary forms, occurrence of fistula is relatively uncommon [48]. When it does exist, it is often believed to be of secondary importance, whereas TB of other sites is given more attention. There appears to be a reciprocal Koch's bacillus/HIV potentiation; in fact, Koch's bacillus stimulates the propagation of HIV through released growth factors. The immunosuppression caused by HIV brings about a deterioration in the functions of different types of cells (B and T lymphocytes), natural killer cells, and macrophages that leads to reactivation of latent seats of mycobacteria, which are generally localized in pulmonary adenopathies or in the digestive tract [49]. AIDS seems to render the tubercle bacillus more virulent, the tuberculosis is severe and has unusual presentations with much higher morbidity and mortality.

Sexual transmission of Koch's bacillus during anal intercourse has already been postulated but never proved.

Tuberculosis and AIDS are diseases of such magnitude that they are not confined by biological barriers, constituting a serious social problem. Individuals become vulnerable when they assume that they are not at risk and therefore neglect self-care; in addition, limited access to health care increases patient vulnerability. The epidemiological aspects of the association between tuberculosis and AIDS represent a major challenge, given the difficulties in coordinating tuberculosis and AIDS control measures [50]. These measures are performed under separate programs, which do not coordinate efforts and which adopt control policies at different levels of health care.

Treatment

As in most of the cases, the diagnosis of tubercular infection in anal fistula is made only after receiving the histopathological reports, the approach is similar as to the fistula of cryptoglandular origin, i.e., surgical.

Surgical Treatment

A diagnosis of anal fistula is usually an indication for surgery in order to prevent a recurring septic process. The choice of operative technique is governed by the fistula tract and its relation to the anal sphincter. The most common operative technique in use is fistulotomy, that is, division of the tissue between the fistula tract and the anal canal. Healing rates are between 74 and 100 %. Rates of impaired continence vary between 0 and 45 %. For low fistulas, a healing rate of almost 100 % can be achieved [51]. Postoperative incontinence rates described in the literature as relatively low, but this is still a sequel to be taken seriously. In all cases, the incontinence rate rises with the amount of sphincter that is divided. Extensive division should always be avoided.

Placement of a seton drain is another frequently employed technique in anal fistula surgery. The material used is either a strong braided non-resorbable suture or a plastic (vessel-loop, etc.) suture thread. Three different techniques which are in use include the cutting seton, the fibrosing seton, and the draining or loose seton [52].

Other techniques of fistula treatment include the flaps, use of biomaterials, fulguration of the tract, stapling, etc. [53].

In all high anal fistulas, a sphincter-sparing procedure should be carried out. The results of the various techniques for surgical reconstruction are largely identical. In general, occlusion using biomaterials leads to not only lower healing rates but also lower incontinence rates [54].

Postoperative care after tubercular fistula surgery does not need any special care and can be managed exactly as like any cryptoglandular fistula. The external wound heals by secondary intention and should be regularly cleaned by sitz bath two times a day plus a good local hygiene.

Medical Treatment

ATT is highly effective, and in most cases curative. The remits obtained in tubercular anal fistula in which surgery is performed and is immediately followed by appropriate antitubercular treatment are most gratifying [55]. This supplementation shortens postoperative period required for the healing of the wound, reduces postoperative wound discharge, ensures against recurrence, and protect against spread or flaring up of the associated pulmonary tuberculosis during healing of the wound [56]. It is seen that combining with medical therapy, the wound usually heals within 4–6 weeks as like any other anal fistula wound.

Since 1982, the American Thoracic Society and the Centers for Disease Control have recommended a 9-month course of isoniazid and rifampicin for the routine treatment of TB in the USA [57]. However, a shorter course of 4 or 6 months of chemotherapy is sufficient for the treatment of anal tuberculosis. The treatment of choice is chemotherapy using three to four anti-TB drugs. Isoniazid, rifampicin, and pyrazinamide, with or without ethambutol, are normally used initially for 6–12 weeks [58]. After this 6–12-week course, isoniazid and rifampin should be continued for an additional 3–6 months. However, resistance is reportedly developing, particularly to rifampicin, isoniazid, and streptomycin wherever it is being used [59].

Nevertheless, patient compliance and follow-up are important factors that affect and can complicate the success of anti-TB chemotherapy. The role of the DOTS (Directly Observed Therapy Shortcourse) program that has been successfully tried in pulmonary TB is being evaluated in extrapulmonary TB to improve patient compliance [60]. It has also been found that micronutrient supplementation in patients with TB decrease the risk of adverse TB treatment outcomes, mortality, and morbidity and improve nutritional and immunological parameters. Daily supplements of micronutrients vitamins A, B-complex, C, E, and selenium may reduce the recurrence of tuberculosis during standard treatment.

However, the standard 6- or 9-month course of chemotherapy may not be suitable for patients infected with HIV, because relapses have been reported. Infection with HIV increases the risk of TB and is thought to decrease the effectiveness of antituberculosis treatment [61]. Moreover, the outbreaks of multidrug-resistant tuberculosis (MDR-TB) in persons with or without HIV infection are associated with higher mortality. Thus, a different strategy should be applied in patients with MDR-TB or HIV or other severely immunocompromised status [62]. Newer drugs like Rifapentine,

Rifabutin, Linezolid, Capreomycin, Ethionamide, and Diarylquinoline R207910 are under evaluation for patients who show resistance or toxicity to the first-line antitubercular drugs [63].

Vaccination

BCG vaccine was isolated by and named after Calmette and Gue'rin in Lille, France. It is routinely administered to infants in many countries worldwide and provides significant protection against severe forms of TB, mostly disseminating and meningeal forms [64]. BCG is the one of the most widely administered vaccines, having been given over four billion times. BCG has been part of the expanded program on immunization (EPI) since the early 1970s and features relatively few serious adverse events. BCG's protective efficacy is found to last for over 50 years [65]. However, the protective efficacy of BCG against pulmonary TB in adults is inconsistent and incomplete, and BCG vaccination campaigns have had little impact on the occurrence of pulmonary TB, which represents the transmissible form of this disease. It is still unclear why the protective effect of neonatal or early-age BCG vaccination often begins to wane in early adolescence, at least in TB-endemic areas. And only fairly recently has it become apparent that individuals with genetic defects in key immune genes or infants with clinically active HIV infection are highly susceptible to developing disseminating BCG disease [66]. So now, the WHO Global Advisory Committee on Vaccine Safety has recommended that BCG should not be used in HIV positive children.

This implies that BCG is clearly insufficient for worldwide TB control, and there is a strong need to develop vaccines that can either boost BCG's initial priming and protective effects, or replace BCG by superior vaccines [67]. There is a need that TB vaccines need to be developed that not only have a superior ability to induce protective immunity against TB but also have a better safety profile compared to BCG. As of now, more than 12 novel TB vaccines have been or are being evaluated in clinical trials in humans [68]. Moreover, many new approaches and strategies are under evaluation for further improvement of these and other vaccines [69]. This raises hope that vaccines can be developed which are better than BCG.

Conclusions

Extrapulmonary TB can be found in any organ, with or without the lungs being affected, and can be diffuse; it is more frequent in immigrants and subjects with immunosuppression, especially those infected with HIV. Anal fistula is the most frequent symptom of anorectal tuberculosis. Although the symptoms are often misleading and thus go unrecognized, they ought to be recognized, because they require specific treatment.

A tubercular fistula-in-ano is seldom diagnosed preoperatively on the basis of clinical picture. There is no functional sign or preferred site that allows a tuberculous fistula to be distinguished from a cryptoglandular fistula. A long period of development and the recurrence of the fistula despite well-managed surgical treatment may give a hint of possibility of tubercular affliction of the fistula. Positive diagnosis of anal TB depends on histological or bacteriologic analysis. Chest X-rays and tuberculin skin tests should also be performed. New diagnostic techniques for TB have been proposed, in particular genomic amplification by polymerase chain reaction, which can detect the presence of the bacterial DNA in 48 h with high sensitivity and specificity. Sometimes a cluster of epidemiologic, clinical, histological, radiologic, and evolutive arguments can contribute to the diagnosis of anal TB. The differential diagnosis for anoperineal TB is primarily Crohn's disease, which has remarkable clinical similarities with mycobacterial infections.

Therefore, in all cases of recurrent fistula-in-ano, histopathological examination of the excised fistula is mandatory. The treatment is twofold: surgical for the suppuration as like any other cryptoglandular fistula with various surgical approaches along with pharmacological treatment for the TB. Once tuberculosis is confirmed, antituberculous treatment should be immediately started to ensure early healing and cure of the disease. As with all other forms, anal TB necessitates specific antibiotic therapy under rigorous supervision. Despite the increase in the incidence of TB in patients infected with HIV, ano-perineal TB does not seem to have risen in parallel.

Summary

- Anorectal mycobacterial infection is very rare with the decline in the general incidence of tuberculosis, but should be taken into consideration as a cause of anal fistula.
- The clinical features, which include symptoms and signs of anal pain or discharge, multiple or recurrent fistula-in-ano, are not characteristically distinct from other anal lesions.
- Although the incidence of TB is increasing in HIV patients, especially in extrapulmonary forms, anoperineal region is rarely affected.
- It is very difficult to diagnose tubercular anal fistula prior to surgery unless patients has systemic tubercular disease.
- Histological examination of specimens taken from suspicious anal lesions is mandatory for a correct diagnosis of *M. tuberculosis* infection, which is curable by antituberculosis drug regimen.

References

1. Candela F, Serrano P, Arriero JM, Teruel A, Reyes D, Calpena R. Perianal disease of tuberculous origin: report of a case and review of the literature. Dis Colon Rectum. 1999;42:110–2.

2. Harland RW, Varkey B. Anal tuberculosis: report of two cases and literature review. Am J Gastroenterol. 1992;87:1488–91.

3. Marshall JB. Tuberculosis of the gastrointestinal tract and peritoneum. Am J Gastroenterol. 1993;88:989–99.

4. Archimandritis A, Kolitsopoulos A, Tzivras M, Fertakis A, Papalambrou E, Kittas C. Tuberculosis of the anal canal. J Clin Gastroenterol. 1993;16:89–90.

5. Shukla HS, Gupta SC, Singh G, Singh PA. Tubercular fistula in ano. Br J Surg. 1988;75:38–9.

6. International Union Against Tuberculosis and Lung Disease. Tuberculosis: a guide to the essentials of good clinical practice. Paris: International Union Against Tuberculosis and Lung Disease; 2010.

7. Gupta PJ. Ano-perianal tuberculosis—solving a clinical dilemma. Afr Health Sci. 2005;5:345–7.

8. Aït-Khaled N, Alarcon E, Armengol R, Bissell K, Boillot F, Caminero JA. Management of tuberculosis: a guide to the essentials of good clinical practice. Paris: International Union Against Tuberculosis and Lung Disease; 2010.

9. Ottenhoff TH. Overcoming the global crisis: "yes, we can", but also for TB … ? Eur J Immunol. 2009;39:2014–20.

10. Ducati RG, Rufinno-Netto A, Basso LA, Santos DS. The resumption of consumption: a review on tuberculosis. Mem Inst Oswaldo Cruz. 2006;01:697–714.

11. Romelaer C, Abramowitz L. Anal abscess with a tuberculous origin: report of two cases and review of the literature. Gastroenterol Clin Biol. 2007;31:94–6.

12. Myers SR. Tuberculous fissure-in ano. J R Soc Med. 1994;87:46.

13. Seghal VN, Jain MK, Srivastava G. Changing pattern of cutaneous tuberculosis: a prospective study. Int J Dermatol. 1989;28:231–6.

14. Ilgazli A, Boyaci H, Basyigit I, Yildiz F. Extrapulmonary tuberculosis: clinical and epidemiologic spectrum of 636 cases. Arch Med Res. 2004;35:435–41.

15. Buie LA, Smith ND, Jackman RJ. The role of tuberculosis in anal fistula. Surg Gynecol Obstet. 1939;68:191–5.

16. Abcarian H. Anorectal infection: abscess-fistula. Clin Colon Rectal Surg. 2011;24:14–21.

17. Chung CC, Choi CL, Kwok SP, Leung KL, Lau WY, Li AK. Anal and perianal tuberculosis: a report of three cases in 10 years. J R Coll Surg Edinb. 1997;42:189–90.

18. Abdelwahab IF, Kenan S, Hermann G, Klein MJ. Tuberculous gluteal abscess without bone involvement. Skeletal Radiol. 1998;27:36–9.

19. Seow-Choen F, Hay AJ, Heard S, Philips RK. Bacteriology of anal fistula. Br J Surg. 1992;79:27–8.

20. Korman TM, Mijch AM, Bassily R, Grayson ML. Fistula in-ano: don't forget tuberculosis. Med J Aust. 1996;166:387–8.

21. Rocha M, Carrasco C, Naquira N, Venegas J, Kauer G, Coñoman H. Anal tuberculosis: report of a case. Rev Med Chil. 1997;125: 1199–203.

22. Gupta PJ. A case of multiple (eight external openings) tubercular anal fistulae: a case report. Eur Rev Med Pharmacol Sci. 2007;11:359–61.

23. Alvarez Conde JL, Gutierrez Alonso VM, Del Riego TJ, Garcia Martinez I, Arizcun Sanchez-Morate A, Vaquero PC. Perianal ulcers of tubercular origin. A report of 3 new cases. Rev Esp Enferm Dig. 1992;81:46–8.

24. Miteva L, Bardarov E. Perianal tuberculosis: a rare case of skin ulceration? Acta Derm Venereol. 2002;82:481–2.

25. Aris EA, Bakari M, Chonde TM, Kitinya J, Swai AB. Diagnosis of tuberculosis in sputum-negative patients in Dar es Salaam. East Afr Med J. 1999;76:630–4.

26. Rose DN, Schechter CB, Adler JJ. Interpretation of the tuberculin skin test. J Gen Intern Med. 1995;10:635–42.

27. Nayak S, Acharjya B. Mantoux test and its interpretation. Indian Dermatol Online J. 2012;3:2–6.

28. Consensus Expert Committee API. API TB Consensus Guidelines 2006: management of pulmonary tuberculosis, extra-pulmonary tuberculosis and tuberculosis in special situations. Assoc Phys India. 2006;54:219–34.

29. Pai M, Minion J, Steingart K, Ramsay A. New and improved tuberculosis diagnostics: evidence, policy, practice, and impact. Curr Opin Pulm Med. 2012;16:271–84.

30. Faizal M, Jimenez G, Burgos C, Portillo PD, Romero RE, Patarroya ME. Diagnosis of cutaneous tuberculosis by polymerase chain reaction using a species specific gene. Int J Dermatol. 1996;35: 185–8.

31. Mori T, Sakatani M, Yamagishi F, Takashima T, Kawabe Y, Nagao K, et al. Specific detection of tuberculosis infection: an interferon-gamma-based assay using new antigen. Am J Respir Crit Care Med. 2004;170:59–64.

32. Halligan S, Stoker J. Imaging of fistula in ano. Radiology. 2006;239:18–33.

33. Gustafsson UM, Kahvecioglu B, Astrom G, Ahlstrom H, Graf W. Endoanal ultrasound or magnetic resonance imaging for preoperative assessment of anal fistula: a comparative study. Colorectal Dis. 2001;3:189–97.

34. Lunniss PJ, Barker PG, Sultan AH, Armstrong P, Reznek RH, Bartram CI, et al. Magnetic resonance imaging of fistula-in-ano. Dis Colon Rectum. 1994;37:708–18.

35. Gravante G, Giordano P. The role of three-dimensional endoluminal ultrasound imaging in the evaluation of anorectal diseases: a review. Surg Endosc. 2008;22:1570–8.

36. Maier AG, Funovics MA, Kreuzer SH, Herbst F, Wunderlich M, Teleky BK, et al. Evaluation of perianal sepsis: comparison of anal endosonography and magnetic resonance imaging. J Magn Reson Imaging. 2001;14:254–60.

37. Schaefer O, Lohrmann C, Langer M. Assessment of anal fistulas with high resolution subtraction MR-fistulography: comparison with surgical findings. J Magn Reson Imaging. 2004;19:91–8.

38. Gan H, Ouyang Q, Bu H, et al. Value of polymerase chain reaction assay in diagnosis of intestinal tuberculosis and differentiation from Crohn's disease. Chin Med J (Engl). 1994;107:215–20.

39. Portillo-Gomez L, Morris SL, Panduro A. Rapid and efficient detection of extra-pulmonary Mycobacterium tuberculosis by PCR analysis. Int J Tuberc Lung Dis. 2000;4:361–70.

40. Haldar S, Bose M, Chakrabarti P, Daginawala HF, Harinath BC, Kashyap RS, et al. Improved laboratory diagnosis of tuberculosis—the Indian experience. Tuberculosis. 2011;91:414–26.

41. Parida SK, Kaufmann SH. The quest for biomarkers in tuberculosis. Drug Discov Today. 2010;15:148–57.

42. Epstein D, Watermeyer G, Kirsch R. Review article: the diagnosis and management of Crohn's disease in populations with high- risk rates for tuberculosis. Aliment Pharmacol Ther. 2007;25:1373–88.

43. Al-Ghamdi AS, Al-Mofleh IA, Al-Rashed RS, et al. Epidemiology and outcome of Crohns disease in a teaching hospital in Riyadh. World J Gastroenterol. 2004;10:1341–4.

44. Gupta PJ. Tubercular infection in the sacrococcygeal pilonidal sinus disease—a case report. Int Wound J. 2008;5:648–50.

45. Schluger NW, Burzynski J. Tuberculosis and HIV infection: epidemiology, immunology, and treatment. HIV Clin Trials. 2001;2: 356–65.

46. Ghiya R, Sharma A, Marfatia YS. Perianal ulcer as a marker of tuberculosis in the HIV infected. Indian J Dermatol Venereol Leprol. 2008;74:386–8.

47. Corbett EL, Watt CJ, Walker N, Maher D, Williams BG, et al. The growing burden of tuberculosis: global trends and interactions with the HIV epidemic. Arch Intern Med. 2003;163: 1009–21.
48. Lax JD, Haroutiounian G, Attia A, Rodriguez R, Thayaparan R, Bashist B. Tuberculosis of the rectum in a patient with acquired immune deficiency syndrome: report of a case. Dis Colon Rectum. 1988;31:394–7.
49. Barone B, Kreuzig PL, Gusmão PM, Chamié D, Bezerra S, Pinheiro P, et al. Case report of lymph nodal, hepatic and splenic tuberculosis in an HIV-positive patient. Braz J Infect Dis. 2006;10:149–53.
50. Mehta JB, Dutt A, Harvill L, Mathews KM. Epidemiology of extrapulmonary tuberculosis. A comparative analysis with pre-AIDS era. Chest. 1991;99:1134–8.
51. Garcia-Aguilar J, Belmonte C, Wong WD, Goldberg SM, Madoff RD. Anal fistula surgery. Factors associated with recurrence and incontinence. Dis Colon Rectum. 1996;39:723–9.
52. Malik AI, Nelson RL. Surgical management of anal fistulae: a systematic review. Colorectal Dis. 2008;10:420–30.
53. Dudukgian H, Abcarian H. Why do we have so much trouble treating anal fistula? World J Gastroenterol. 2011;17:3292–6.
54. Blumetti J, Abcarian A, Quinteros F, Chaudhry V, Prasad L, Abcarian H. Evolution of treatment of fistula in ano. World J Surg. 2012;36:1162–7.
55. World Health Organization: Treatment of tuberculosis: guidelines for national programmes. 3rd ed. Geneva, WHO; 2003. http://www.who.int/mediacentre/factsheets/fs104/en.
56. Peloquin CA. Pharmacological issues in the treatment of tuberculosis. Ann N Y Acad Sci. 2001;953:157–64.
57. Heifets LB. Antimycobacterial drugs. Sem Respir Infect. 1994; 9:84–103.
58. Israili ZH, Rogers CM, el-Attar H. Pharmacokinetics of antituberculosis drugs in patients. J Clin Pharmacol. 1987;27:78–83.
59. Somoskovi A, Parsons LM, Salfinger M. The molecular basis of resistance to isoniazid, rifampin, and pyrazinamide in Mycobacterium tuberculosis. Resp Res. 2001;2:164–8.
60. World Health Organization. An expanded DOTS framework for effective tuberculosis control. WHO/CDS/TB/2002.297. Geneva: WHO; 2002.
61. Burman WJ, Gallicano K, Peloquin C. Therapeutic implications of drug interactions in the treatment of human immunodeficiency virus-related tuberculosis. Clin Infect Dis. 1999;28:419–29.
62. WHO. Treatment of tuberculosis: guidelines for national programmes. WHO/CDS/TB 2003.313. Geneva: WHO; 2003.
63. Mitnick CD, McGee B, Peloquin CA. Tuberculosis pharmacotherapy: strategies to optimize patient care. Expert Opin Pharmacother. 2009;10:381–401.
64. Ottenhoff THM, Kaufmann SHE. Vaccines against tuberculosis: where are we and where do we need to go? PLoS Pathog. 2012;8:e1002607.
65. Hoft DF, Blazevic A, Abate G, Hanekom WA, Kaplan G, et al. A new recombinant bacille Calmette-Guerin vaccine safely induces significantly enhanced tuberculosis-specific immunity in human volunteers. J Infect Dis. 2008;198:1491–501.
66. Hesseling AC, Marais BJ, Gie RP, Schaaf HS, Fine PE, et al. The risk of disseminated Bacille Calmette-Guerin (BCG) disease in HIV-infected children. Vaccine. 2007;25:14–8.
67. Kaufmann SH. Future vaccination strategies against tuberculosis: thinking outside the box. Immunity. 2010;33:567–77.
68. Aagaard C, Hoang T, Dietrich J, Cardona PJ, Izzo A, et al. A multistage tuberculosis vaccine that confers efficient protection before and after exposure. Nat Med. 2011;17:189–94.
69. Lin PL, Dietrich J, Tan E, Abalos RM, Burgos J, et al. The multistage vaccine H56 boosts the effects of BCG to protect cynomolgus macaques against active tuberculosis and reactivation of latent Mycobacterium tuberculosis infection. J Clin Invest. 2012;122: 303–14.

Fistula Surgery in the Era of Evidence-Based Medicine

21

Richard L. Nelson and Herand Abcarian

We live in an era when at least in the academic and scientific circles, evidence-based medicine has definitely replaced its eminence based counterpart. Readers of medical literature now often evaluate the quality of reported data (e.g., randomized control trials, etc.) and grade the level of evidence presented in the paper searching from level I evidence in support of the published conclusions. The Cochrane database, celebrating its twentieth anniversary this year is replete with such data.

It is however clearly obvious that despite the frustrating difficulty we have in treating anal fistulas [1], a disease regularly treated with results regularly reported since the mid-nineteenth century, there is very little in the Cochrane data base to rely on. The efficacy of nonrandomized case series vary tremendously in published articles on fistula-in-ano. The problem is that contrary to numerous randomized controlled trials in anal fissure comparing new techniques or chemicals to the gold standard, i.e., partial lateral internal sphincterotomy [2], there are no such trials comparing sphincter sparing techniques to anal fistulotomy (a true and tested procedure), due to concern regarding operation-related fecal incontinence. Therefore many new procedures have appeared in the literature without solid evidence as to their efficacy. In addition where "biologics" have been added to the surgical procedure, randomized studies comparing these biologics to a gold standards, which is essential to evaluate both the "biologic" product as well as the surgical technique are sorely missing, again due to concerns about risk of incontinence in trans-sphincteric fistulas [3]. Is the reported risk of fecal incontinence exceptionally high? This clearly varies from fistula to fistula and from surgeon to surgeon [4]. On the other hand, the expectation of patients as to the treatment outcomes and their acceptance of various degrees of fecal incontinence differ greatly from country to country as well [5]. The risk and benefits of fistulotomy is extensively detailed in Chap. 9.

So how are we to proceed in the absence of credible RCTs? Lewis et al. suggested that "the alternative is an adequately powered single-arm observational study in clearly defined populations" [6]. They also recommend documenting fistula healing by postoperative MRI in order to distinguish real healing from mere closure of the external opening, and the duration of follow-ups should be sufficiently long to validate claims of successful healing. Finally, they conclude that, "In the interim, appropriately constructed registries allowing consistent data capture of the long term would be desirable" [6]. What the authors do not address is the real question. How long is a longer or adequate follow-up? One does not hesitate to follow cancer patients for at least 5 years to accurately collect data on 5-year survival, but there are no established end points for assessing fistula healing. Frequently reported successes in short term follow-ups (e.g., 5 months) are downgraded in longer term follow-up of 12–18 months let alone longer periods. This has been recently documented for the LIFT procedure with the authors concluding that "LIFT has a significant risk of failure (40 %) but good functional outcome in patients with no recurrence" [7].

A review of clinical trials.gov shows a large number of currently registered randomized trials listed by Nelson [3] in his commentary on the paper by Lewis and colleagues [6]. These are reproduced in Table 21.1. As one can easily conclude, new operations are being compared to another group of procedures which also have uncertain outcomes. In reality if fecal incontinence was not a concern, the comparator would be fistulotomy.

So what do we know about published trials, however imperfect. A paradigm shift occurred in the mid-1990s in treatment of trans-sphincteric fistulas from fistulotomy to sphincter sparing operations. This is well documented in a 25-year time trends of fistula operations which documents a definite decline in fistulotomies commensurate with a steep rise in sphincter-sparing procedures [8]. Also because most

R.L. Nelson, M.D., F.A.C.S.
Northern General Hospital, Herr Road Sheffield, South Yorkshire, S5 7AU, UK
e-mail: kerber@uni-bayreuth.de

H. Abcarian, M.D., F.A.C.S. (✉)
The University of Illinois at Chicago, Division of Colon and Rectal Surgery, John Stroger Hospital of Cook Country, IL 60612, USA
e-mail: abcarian@uic.edu

H. Abcarian (ed.), *Anal Fistula: Principles and Management*, DOI 10.1007/978-1-4614-9014-2_21,
© Springer Science+Business Media New York 2014

Table 21.1 Clinical trials.gov registered randomized trials [3]

Experimental therapy	Control group
Stem cell + glue	Glue
Plug	Cutting seton
Stem cell	Stem cell + glue
Plug	Rectal flap
Plug	LIFT
Glue	Seton
Plug	Flap
LIFT + plug	LIFT
Stem cell (Crohn's)	Placebo (Crohn's)
Flap + platelet injection	Flap

of these procedures include closure of the primary opening, it seems that insertion of seton to drain the fistula tract and prior elimination of acute sepsis and preparation of the fistula for definitive procedure is mandatory. This has resulted in far greater use of setons than before [8]. Also if these procedures fail, the patient will have continued drainage or a new abscess which has to be treated with drainage and insertion of a new seton. In essence we have traded a single operation, i.e., fistulotomy for multiple procedures in an attempt to preserve continence. This fact must be stressed to the patient in the process of preoperative informed consent. And of course in addition to the risk of incontinence, anal fistulotomy does not afford 100 % cure rates. Recurrence rates of 2–13 % (median 11 %) have been reported in selected series and when the study was limited to trans-sphincteric fistulas, recurrence rates climbs to 13–37 % [9–11].

There are two published Cochrane reviews for anal fistulas. Malik and Nelson looked at the results of incision and drainage of anorectal abscess alone vs. combined with primary fistulotomy [12]. They found six studies with a total of 474 patients. The recurrence risk was 0.13 (0.07–0.24) and the incontinence risk was 3.06 (0.7–13.45). There are two problems with this study. One is the incidence of fistula found during incision and drainage of abscess which was seen in 88–100 % of the patients. This is a clearcut case of "overkill," because the reports from multiple case series place the incidence of fistula in post-I&D patients around 30–37 %. The second problem is the very poor quality of the studies. The review concluded that primary fistulotomy significantly reduced the odds of persistent fistula and need for reoperation and a small number of patients may have transient minor incontinence. One has to be careful not to apply these conclusions to patient at high risk of incontinence such as women with anterior fistulas and patients with IBD or HIV or previous anorectal surgery [12].

The second Cochrane review attempted to look at surgical operations for anal fistula. However of the ten studies collected for review many addressed the trivial issue of radiofrequency vs. diathermy or fistulotomy plus/minus marsupialization. Other studies looking at flap procedures with or without glue reported very small number of patients and some no data or risk of recurrence and incontinence [13].

The following are chronologic listing of additional randomized trials not included in the two Cochrane reviews:

Shukla compared Ayurvedic seton with fistulotomy or fistulotomy in a multicenter RCT of 502 patients. Forty percent of the patients were lost to follow-up and the study shows higher healing and lower recurrence in surgical vs. Ayurvedic seton [14].

Belmonte Montes and colleagues compared fistulotomy with fistulectomy in 40 patients. This is a question of high importance of fistula surgery but regretfully no outcome data was provided, only ultrasonographic evaluation of the sphincters [15].

Zimmerman and associates studied the impact of two different types of anal retractors in fistula surgery, demonstrating that even an innocuous retraction during surgery may have delectations effects on resting pressure and continence. In this study of 30 patients Scott retractors (same as LoneStar®) was compared with Parks' retractors. Use of Scott retractors resulted in better resting pressure ($p=0.035$) and better continence preservation ($p=0.038$) [16]. Singer, Cintron, and colleagues studying fibrin sealant, randomized 75 patients with trans-sphincteric fistulas to three groups attempting to address causes of treatment failure: infection vs. glue extrusion due to large internal openings. Fibrin sealant is covered in Chap. 11. One group received fibrin sealant with antibiotics, the second fibrin sealant and closure of the internal opening, and the third had fibrin sealant plus both antibiotics and closure of the internal opening [17]. The results were worse than their previously published data on fibrin sealant alone (healing of 25–55 %) [18].

Perez and associates studied the clinical and manometric results of advancement flaps vs. fistulotomy with sphincter reconstruction in complex fistulas in 60 patients [19]. There were two recurrences (2/30) in each arm and the postoperative incontinence rate was similar [19]. Gustafson and Graf postulated that failure of advancement flap in fistula-in-ano was a result of infection. They randomized 83 patients to flap and implantation of gentamicin collagen beneath the flaps vs. flap alone. There was no added benefit from this modification ($p=0.45$) [20]. Garcia-Olmo et al. have published the use of autologous adipose-derived stem cell in the treatment of complex fistulas. Injecting the stem cells suspended in fibrin sealant into the wall of the anal fistulas in Crohn's disease, they reported a significantly higher incidence of healing in 49 patients randomized in the group with fibrin sealant and autologous stem cells, 17/24 healed while in the fibrin glue alone arm 4/25 healed (OR = 4.43, CI 1.7–11.3) [21]. This topic is discussed in Chap. 18.

Hammond et al. reported on the use of cross-linked collagen suspended in fibrin sealant and compared them with fibrin sealant alone in 29 patients [22]. In the glue plus collagen arm 12/15 healed, while in the sealant alone group 7/13 healed, but the differences were not statistically significant (p=NS). Grimand Grimaud and colleagues compared fibrin sealant to no therapy in 71 patients with Crohn's fistulae. This is a rare and possibly the only controlled trail comparing treatment with observation (placebo). There was some benefit reported as "remission" in 13/34 patients in the glue arm vs. 6/37 patients in observation group [23]. Khafagy et al. randomized flap treatments for closure of the internal opening between full thickness flap and mucosal flap in 40 patients. The full thickness flap comprised of mucosa and smooth muscle (internal sphincter or lower rectal wall) had a statically significantly higher rate of healing (18/20) compared with mucosal flap (12/20) p=0.068. There were two cases of incontinence to flatus (10 %) in the former group [24].

A recent paper by Lewis et al. on novel biologic strategies in the management of anal fistulas is a compilation of 23 studies reviewing the use of biologics in fistula surgery warrants mentioning, even though none have results comparing to anal fistulotomy to the long-term eradication rate [6].

The following is a summary of the "biologics" and relevant studies in the above paper.

Cyanoacrylate Glue

There are three papers reporting the effectiveness of Glubran® (*N*-butyl 2 cyanoacrylate glue), a synthetic tissue adhesive for treatment of anal fistulas [25–27]. The reported success rate after one or more application was 67–95 % with follow-up ranging from 6 to 34 months. It is important to note the very small number of cohorts in all three papers (21, 20, and 24, respectively) [24–27]. Meinero and Mori have used cyanoacrylate to reinforce stapled closure of internal opening during video-assisted anal fistula repair (VAAFT) [28]. This technique is covered in a separate section (Chap. 17).

Gore Bio-A® Plug

The plug is made of bioabsorbable monofilament polyglycolic acid which has been shown historically to be absorbed completely in 7 months [29]. There is currently a multicenter prospective trail in accrual phase to study the 1 year healing rate of fistulas using Gore Bio-A® plug in 100 patients in the USA. There are three prospective case series in print to date. Bachman et al. compared healing rates of fistulas with Gore BioA® plug. Cook Surgisis plug® and reported a better outcome with Gore Bio-A® plug (54 of healing rate in 61.5 day follow-up period in 10 case) [30]. The other two case series also included small number of patients and reported variable success rate of 16–73 %

depending on the follow-up period (2–12 months) [31, 32]. Again these three case series can be considered level III evidence at best. The subject of plug use in the treatment of fistulas is covered in Chaps. 12, 13).

Bioglue®

Bioglue® is made of purified bovine serum albumin and glutaraldehyde approved for use as hemostastic adjunct in cardiovascular surgery. Three small case series comprised of 6, 8, and 14 patients have been reported using Bioglue® in anal fistulas with disappointing cure rates of 0–21 % at 60 months follow-up [33–35]. Serious side effects and glutaraldehyde toxicity have also been reported.

Tissue Grafts

Allogenic Tissue Grafts

Two different allogenic grafts: Alloderm® made in the US and ADM® (acellular dermal matrix) from China has been tried in anal fistula repairs. Fistula healing of 54 % with a median follow-up of 19 months with 1–2 % incontinence has been reported with the use of ADM® (acellular dermal matrix) in 114 patients [36].

Xenogeneic Tissue Grafts

Surgisis® is acellular noncrosslinked extracellular matrix sheet derived from porcine intestinal mucosa. This material in sheet form has been used with variable success rate in treatment of retrovaginal fistulas as an interposition technique. The Surgisis® anal fistula plug, Surgisis AFP® has been used in the treatment of anal fistulas of diverse etiology with variable success rate. The most recent publication reports 73 patients (11 % Crohn's fistulas) treated with Surgisis AFP®. The overall patient success rate was 38 % and plug success rate of 39.5 %. There were no intraoperative complications and four (5 %) postoperative abscess [37].

Permacol® is porcine acellular dermal sheet which has been used as graft strips placed into fistulas tracts or Permacol® suspension in fibrin sealant injected into the tract [38].

Cytokine Therapy

Basic fibroblast growth factor (bFGF) from Japan has been used in treatment of nine infants with fistulas been the ages of 1–9 months. Fistulas were sprayed with bFGF twice daily for 2 weeks. After one or two courses of treatment all fistulas healed with no side effects [39]. Spontaneous fistula healing in infants and children occur not infrequently and the effect of bFGF in adults with anal fistulas is awaited.

Stem Cell Therapy

Injection of stem cells for treatment of anal fistulas has been reported recently [21, 40, 41]. Garcia-Olma and colleagues first reported adipose-derived stem cells in treatment of Crohn's fistula with 71 % healing vs. 16 % in control group (level 1B evidence) [21]. Unfortunately the success rate decreased to 53 % at 3 years (evidence level 1B) [40]. Stem cell therapy of anal fistulas is covered extensively in Chap. 18).

Conclusion

In the last few years, there has been an increased or concentrated activity of the use of "biologics" in the treatment of anal fistulas. Regretfully most studies included small cohorts, short follow-up, and no further publication from many of the authors, making the evidence at best a level III. The true effectiveness of these methods requires multicenter randomized controlled trials and long follow-up periods to warrant reliable conclusions, this despite anal fistulas being one of the most common ailments afflicting man. Until then large case series, longer follow-up, and validation of healing with postoperative MRI are needed to address the success rate of newer sphincter-sparing procedures and biologic materials.

References

1. Dudukjian H, Abcarian H. Why do we have so much trouble treating anal fistulas? World J Gastoenterol. 2011;17:3292–6.
2. Nelson RL, Thomas K, Morgan J, Jones A. Non surgical therapy for anal fissure. Cochrane Database Syst Rev. 2012;4, CD003431.
3. Nelson RL. Commentary on Lewis R et al. Colorectal Dis. 2012;14:1445–56.
4. Nicholls RJ. Anal fistulae. Colorectal Dis. 2012;14:535.
5. Ellis CN. Sphincter sparing fistula management: what patients want? Dis Colon Rectum. 2010;53:1652–5.
6. Lewis R, Lunniss PJ, Hammond TM. Novel biological strategies in the management of anal fistula. Colorectal Dis. 2012;14:1445–56.
7. Willem UG, Mellgren AF, Madoff RD, Goldberg SM. Does ligation of intersphincteric fistula tract raise the bar in fistula surgery? Dis Colon Rectum. 2012;55(11):1173–8.
8. Blumetti J, Abcarian A, Quinteros F, Chaudhry V, Prasad L, Abcarian H. Evolution of treatment of fistula in ano. World J Surg. 2012;26(5):1162–7.
9. Garcia-Augulas J, Belmonte C, Wang D, Goldberg SM, Maddoff RD. Anal fistula surgery. Factors associated with recurrence and incontinence. Dis Colon Rectum. 1996;39:723–9.
10. Vasilevsky CA, Gordon PH. Results of treatment of fistula-in-ano. Dis Colon Rectum. 1985;28:225–31.
11. Joy H, Williams JD. The outcome of surgery for high anal fistulas. Colorect Dis. 2000;2:17–21.
12. Malik AI, Nelson RL, Tou S. Incision and drainage of perianal abscess with or without treatment of fistula in ano. Cochrane Database Syst Rev. 2010;7, CD006827.
13. Jacob TJ, Perakath B, Keighley MR. Surgical intervention for anorectal fistula. Cochrane Database Syst Rev. 2010;12(5), CD006319.
14. Shurkla N. Multicentric randomized controlled clinical trial of Kshaarasootra (Ayurvedic medicated thread) in the management of fistula-in-ano. Indian Council of Medical Research. Indian J Med Res. 1991;94:177–85.
15. Belmonte Montes C, Ruiz Galindo GH, et al. Fistulotomy vs. fistulectomy. Ultrasonographic evaluation lesions of the anal sphincter fistula. Rev Gastroentrol. 1999;64:167–70.
16. Zimmerman DD, Gosselink MP, et al. Impact of two different types of anal retractors on fecal incontinence after fistula repair. A prospective randomized clinical trial. Dis Colon Rectum. 2003;46: 1674–9.
17. Singer M, Cintron J, Nelson R, et al. Treatment of fistulae in ano with fibrin sealant in combination with intra-adhesive antibiotics and or surgical closure of the internal fistula opening. Dis Colon Rectum. 2005;48:799–808.
18. Cintron JR, Park JJ, et al. Repair of anorectal fistulae with fibrin sealant—long-term follow-up. Dis Colon Rectum. 2000;43: 949–50.
19. Perez F, Arroyo A, et al. Randomized clinical and manometric study of advancement flap versus fistulotomy wit sphincter reconstruction in the management of complex fistula-in-ano. Am J Surg. 2006;192:34–40.
20. Gustafsson UM, Graf W. Randomized clinical trial of local gentamicin–collagen treatment in advancement flap repair of anal fistula. Br J Surg. 2006;93:1202–7.
21. Garcia-Olmo D, Herreros D, Pascual I, et al. Expanded adipose-derived stem cells for the treatment of complex perianal fistulas: a phase II clinical trial. Dis Colon Rectum. 2009;52:79–86.
22. Hammond TM, Porrett TR, Scott SM, et al. Management of idiopathic anal fistula using cross-linked collagen: a prospective phase I study. Colorectal Dis. 2010;13:94–104.
23. Grimand JC, Munoz-Bouguard N, et al. Fibrin glue effective in healing perianal fistulas in patients with Crohn's disease. Gastroenterology. 2010;138:2257–81.
24. Khafagy W, Omar W, et al. Treatment of anal fistulas by partial rectal wall advancement flap or mucosal advancement flaps: a prospective randomized study. Int J Surg. 2010;8:321–35.
25. Basillari P, Basso L, et al. Cyanoacrylate glue in the treatment of anorectal fistulas. Int J Colorectal Dis. 2006;21:791–4.
26. Jain SK, Kaza RL, et al. Role of cyanocrylate in the management of fistula in ano—a prospective study. Int J Colorectal Dis. 2008; 23:355–8.
27. Queralto M, Portier G, Bonnaud G, et al. Efficacy of synthetic glue treatment of high cryptoglandular fistula-in-ano. Gastroenterol Clin Biol. 2010;34(8–9):477–82.
28. Merinero P, Mori L. Video-assisted anal fistula treatment (VAAFT): a novel sphincter saving procedure for treating complex anal fistulas. Tech Coloproctol. 2011;15:417–22.
29. Katz AR, Mukherjee DP, et al. A new synthetic microfilament absorbable suture made from polytrimethylene carbonate. Surg Gynecol Obstet. 1985;161:213–27.
30. Buchberg B, Masommi H, et al. A tale of two (anal fistula) plugs: if there a difference in short term outcome. Am Surg. 2010;76:1150–3.
31. De la Portillo F, Rada R, et al. Evaluation of a new synthetic plug in the treatment of anal fistulas. Results of a pilot study. Dis Colon Rectum. 2011;54:1419–22.
32. Ratto C, Lilla F, et al. Gore Bio A® fistula plug. A new sphincter-sparing procedure for complex anal fistula. Colorectal Dis. 2012; 41:264–9.
33. Abbas M, Tejirian T. Bioglue for treatment of anal fistula is associated with acute anal sepsis. Dis Colon Rectum. 2008;51:115–1158.

34. Alexander SM, Mitalas LE, et al. Obliteration of the fistulous tract with Bioglue adversely affects the outcomes of transanal advancement flap repairs. Tech Coloproctol. 2008;12:225–8.

35. De la Portillo F, Rada R, et al. Long-term results change conclusions in Bioglue in the treatment of high transsphincteric anal fistula. Dis Colon Rectum. 2010;53:1220–1.

36. Han JG, Wang ZS, Zhao BL, et al. Long term outcomes of human acellular dermal matrix plug in closure of complex and fistulas with a single tract. Dis Colon Rectum. 2011;54:1412–8.

37. Cintron JR, Abcarian H, Chaudhry V, Singer M, et al. Treatment of fistula-in-ano using a porcine small intestinal submucosa anal fistula plug. Tech Coloproctol. 2013;17(2):187–91.

38. Sileri P, Franceschilli L, et al. Porcine dermal collagen matrix injection may enhance flap repair surgery for complex anal fistula. Int J Colorectal Dis. 2011;26:345–9.

39. Kubota M, Hirayama Y, Okuyama N. Usefulness of bFGF spray in the treatment of perianal abscess and fistula in ano. Pediatr Surg Int. 2010;26:1037–40.

40. Guadalajara H, Herreros D, et al. Long term follow-up of patients undergoing adipose derived adult stem cell administration to tract complex perianal fistulas. Int J Colorectal Dis. 2012;27:595–600.

41. Ciccociopp R, Bernardo ME, et al. Autologous bone marrow-derived mesenchymal stromal cells in the treatment of fistulising Crohn's disease. Gut. 2011;60:788–98.

Mohammad Ali Abbass and Maher Aref Abbas

Introduction

Anal fistula is one of the commonest benign anorectal conditions treated by colorectal and general surgeons. Patients with this condition can initially present with an acute or recurrent abscess or a chronically draining fistula [1]. Patients with an established fistula are often symptomatic. Symptoms include pain, drainage, bleeding, itching, and swelling. The severity of symptoms can vary. The majority of patients with anal fistula require operative treatment for resolution of the symptoms and healing of the fistula. The goal of surgical intervention is to eradicate the disease, preserve continence, minimize postoperative complications, and prevent recurrence. Three factors determine the outcome of patients with anal fistula: fistula-related characteristics, patient-related features, and surgical factors (Fig. 22.1) [2, 3]. While the first two factors are not modifiable, the surgeon can have a significant impact on outcome. The decision to treat medically in some patients such as those with inflammatory bowel disease or atypical infections as well as the choice of the right operation for an individual patient are critical in order to optimize the result and avoid failure and complications. But equally as important is the actual technical conduct of an operation by the surgeon. While anal fistulas heal in most patients following one or two surgical interventions, some fistulas persist. Failure of surgical intervention can be costly to the patient and often leads to additional interventions to treat potential postoperative septic complications and/or to resolve the persistent fistula. In addition to pain, suffering, and prolong recovery, all of which negatively impact quality of life, multiple operations can lead to permanent continence disturbance. Thus a thorough understanding of the factors that impact success or failure and complications of anal fistula surgery is of paramount importance to surgeons treating this condition.

The aim of this chapter is to discuss the causes of operative failure and risk factors for complications. A detailed description of the predictors of outcome for anal fistula surgery is reviewed in order to provide the surgeon with an appreciation of the fistula characteristics and patient-related factors that determine operative outcome. Furthermore the results of the various operative options available today are examined in order to provide a framework for operative decision-making.

The Impact of Fistula-Related Characteristics

Etiology of the Fistula

Anal fistulas are classified based on etiology and anatomy of the fistulous tract. Table 22.1 summarizes the various conditions that contribute to the development of anal fistula. The most common etiology of anal fistula is cryptoglandular disease caused by an infected anal gland. Crohn's disease, an inflammatory bowel disease, can lead to the development of gastrointestinal fistulas including anal fistula. Other etiologies include radiation, malignancy, obstetrical trauma, prior anal operations, and atypical infections such as actinomycosis and tuberculosis (Fig. 22.2a, b). Fistulas caused by such atypical infections are best treated medically and can often resolve once the infection is eradicated with surgical intervention reserved for the treatment of acute sepsis or recurrent or persistent fistulas [4–7].

Fistulas related to cryptoglandular disease are often single, while Crohn's fistulas can be multiple (Fig. 22.3). The anal mucosa is normal in the setting of cryptoglandular disease. In Crohn's disease the anal mucosa is often inflamed and/or scarred and can be associated with anal stricture, tags, and perianal skin ulceration (Fig. 22.4). Because of these findings, the surgical outcome of patients with anal fistula from

M.A. Abbass, M.D. • M.A. Abbas, M.D., F.A.C.S., F.A.S.C.R.S. (✉)
Department of Surgery, Kaiser Permanente, Los Angeles Medical Center, 4760 Sunset Blvd, 3rd floor, Los Angeles, CA 90027, USA
e-mail: maher.a.abbas@kp.org

H. Abcarian (ed.), *Anal Fistula: Principles and Management*, DOI 10.1007/978-1-4614-9014-2_22,
© Springer Science+Business Media New York 2014

cryptoglandular disease is different than those with Crohn's disease. Mizrahi and colleagues from the Cleveland Clinic in Florida reported their results with the endorectal advancement flap in 94 patients with anal fistula [8]. The failure rate was significantly higher in patients with Crohn's disease compared to patients with cryptoglandular disease (57.1 % vs. 33.3 %, respectively). A similar finding was published by Sonoda and colleagues from the Cleveland Clinic in Ohio [9].

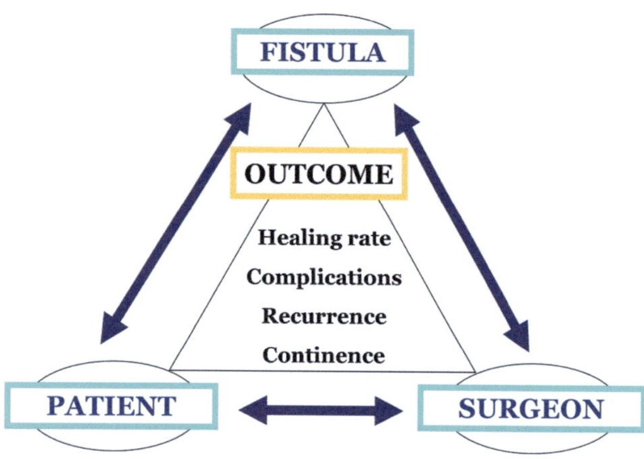

Fig. 22.1 The impact of various factors on outcome of anal fistula surgery

Table 22.1 Etiology of anal fistula

Cryptoglandular disease
Crohn's disease
Prior anal surgery
Obstetrical injury
Atypical infections (tuberculosis, actinomycosis)
Radiation therapy
Malignancy
Trauma

A review of 99 patients who underwent the endorectal advancement flap revealed a failure rate of 50 % in Crohn's patient compared to 23 % in non-Crohn's patients. Pinto and colleagues investigated the impact of Crohn's disease on rectovaginal fistula surgery results in 125 patients who were operated at the Cleveland Clinic Florida [10]. The patients underwent a variety of operative techniques. The recurrence rate of the fistula was highest in patients with Crohn's disease (55.8 %) compared to patients with obstetrical related fistula (33.3 %) and trauma (30 %). The increased failure rate noted in patients with Crohn's disease can be attributed to the complexity of the fistulous tract (course of the tracts and/or multiplicity), the presence of anal mucosa scarring and/or the presence of any associated stricture, and the level of disease activity.

In patients with active Crohn's inflammation in the anorectal region, the placement of a non-cutting seton for drainage followed by medical therapy is the most prudent course of action. Some patients require multiple setons placement due to multiple complex tracts (Fig. 22.5). Definitive fistula repair should be deferred to a later stage after the resolution of active inflammation in order to avoid operative failure. Some patients will heal with medical therapy alone and operative intervention can be undertaken in those with persistent fistula once the mucosal inflammation subsides. The University of Calgary from Canada reported their results with Infliximab 5 mg/kg (anti-TNFα) in 29 patients with fistulizing Crohn's disease [11]. Twenty-one patients had perianal fistulas, eight had rectovaginal fistulas, and four had combined fistulas. The selective use of seton combined with infliximab infusion and maintenance immunosuppression resulted in complete healing in 67 % of the patients with perianal fistula and a partial response with symptomatic improvement was noted in 19 % of the patients (mean follow-up of 9 months). Another study from the Cleveland Clinic Ohio reported the outcome of 218

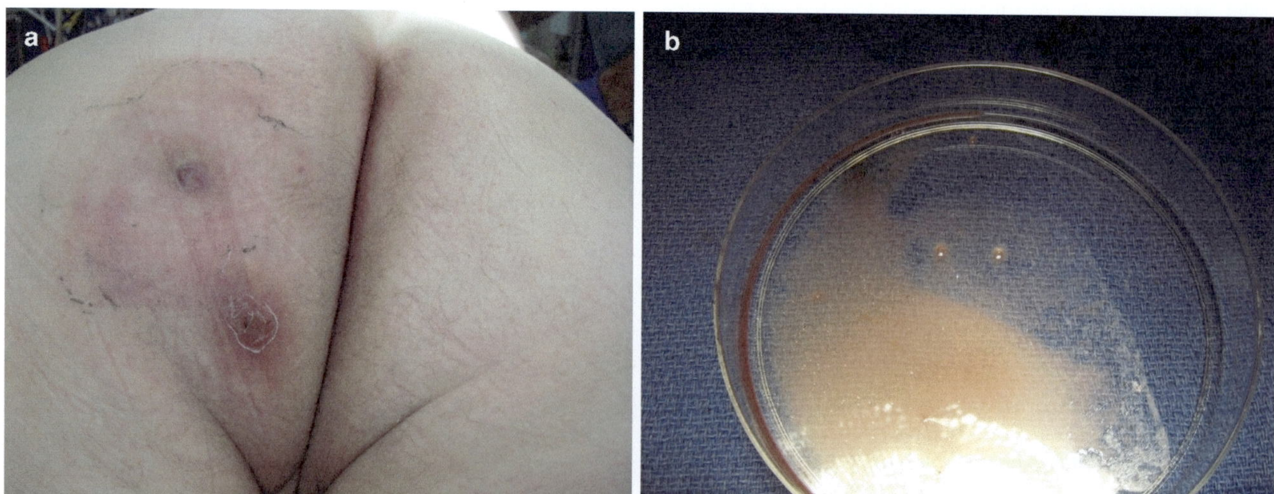

Fig. 22.2 (**a**) Patient with complex anal fistula from actinomycosis. (**b**) Silver granules noted in liquid content of fistula tract

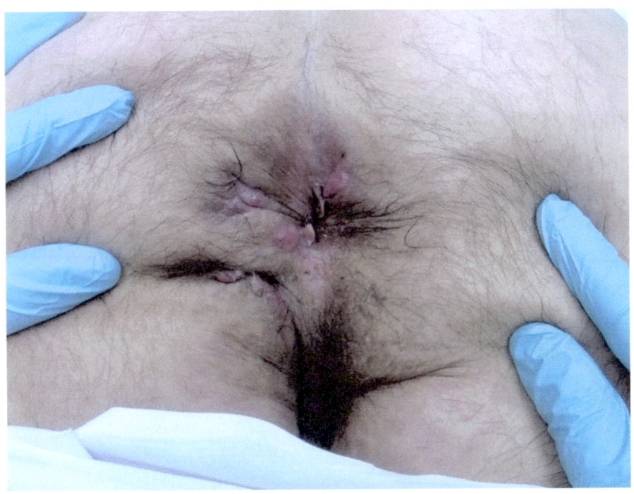

Fig. 22.3 Patient with Crohn's disease and multiple anal fistulas

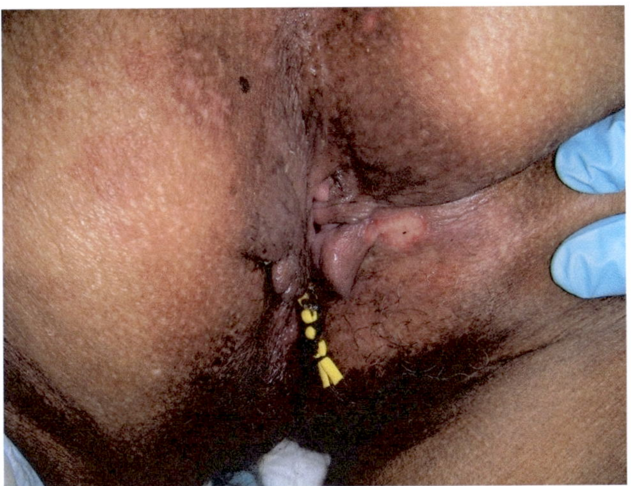

Fig. 22.4 Patient with Crohn's disease with anal fistula (seton in place), skin tags, and skin ulceration

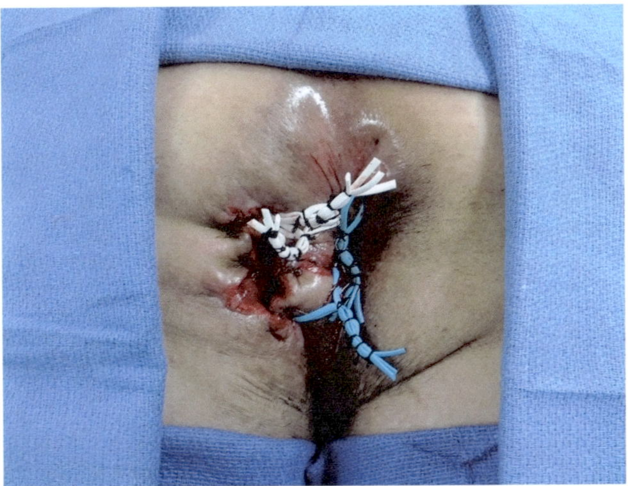

Fig. 22.5 Several non-cutting setons in a patient with multiple anal fistulas from Crohn's disease

patients with Crohn's disease and compared patients who underwent surgery alone for anal fistula to those who received biologic immunomodulator treatment in addition to surgery [12]. Overall improvement was higher in patients who received biologic therapy (71.3 % vs. 35.9 %, $p=0.001$). It is important to note that biologic treatment should be initiated only after drainage of any active perianal sepsis. A study from the University of Pittsburgh reported the outcome of 32 patients with perianal fistulizing Crohn's disease who received infliximab [13]. Patients who underwent an exam under anesthesia with placement of a draining seton had a lower recurrence rate compared to those who received the medical therapy alone (44 % vs. 79 %, $p=0.001$). Furthermore the time to recurrence was longer in patients with draining setons (13.5 vs. 3.6 months, $p=0.0001$). But it is essential to keep in mind that while medical therapy can be beneficial in some patients, it is ineffective in others. Iesalnieks and colleagues from Germany reported their experience with 66 Crohn's patients with perianal fistulas who underwent a total of 100 surgical interventions such as fistulotomy or non-cutting seton placement followed by azathioprine and/or infliximab therapy [14]. While 67 % of the patients benefited from the medical therapy, 33 % of patients failed. Predictors of poor outcome included presence of Crohn's colitis, age at the onset disease <20 years, and higher fistulas.

Anatomical Classification of the Fistula

The anatomy of an anal fistula has a direct impact on the outcome of operative intervention. Anal fistula is classified based on the course of the fistulous tract and its relationship to both the internal and external sphincter muscles. The most widely accepted fistula classification is the Parks' classification (Table 22.2). It was based on the analysis of 400 cases of anal fistulas treated over a 15-year period [15]. According to Parks and colleagues the majority of anal fistulas can be described as the following four types: (1) intersphincteric, (2) trans-sphincteric, (3) suprasphincteric, and (4) extrasphincteric. Each type has variations as reported in Table 22.2. Furthermore, some patients have combined types or horseshoe variation. Other types of fistulas that involve adjacent organs include anoperineal, anovaginal or rectovaginal, and rectourethral. Traditionally the fistula anatomy in an individual patient is determined by physical examination or delineated at time of operative intervention (Fig. 22.6). Routine imaging of anal fistula is not warranted but the selective use of radiologic studies can be helpful in patients with recurrent or complex fistulas and may decrease operative failure [16–19]. Preoperative three-dimensional ultrasound (Fig. 22.7a, b), computed tomography scan (Figs. 22.8 and 22.9), and magnetic resonance imaging (Fig. 22.10) can provide the surgeon with valuable information to guide the care of patients with prior failed surgery and/or complex anatomy such as multiple fistulous openings.

Garcia-Aguilar and colleagues from the University of Minnesota reported their results in 624 patients with anal fistula [2]. The overall fistula recurrence rate was 8 and 45 % of the patients complained of some degree of incontinence after surgery. Significant differences were noted in the recurrence rate between fistula types: intersphincteric 4 %, trans-sphincteric 7 %, suprasphincteric 33 %, extrasphincteric 33 %, and unclassified 16 %. Similarly a significant difference was noted in the incontinence rate amongst the various fistula types: extrasphincteric 83 %, suprasphincteric 80 %, trans-sphincteric 54 %, unclassified 49 %, and intersphincteric 37 %. In an analysis of 179 patients treated for anal fistula at Kaiser Permanente Los Angeles, a regional tertiary referral center for the 14 Kaiser Permanente hospitals in Southern California, Abbas and colleagues found similar associations between fistula type, operative failure rate, and incontinence rate [3]. The overall operative failure rate in their study was 15.6 % and de novo incontinence developed in 15.6 % of the patients. The fistula-specific operative failure rates were 0 % for subcutaneous, 9.5 % for intersphincteric, 10.7 % for low trans-sphincteric, 37.8 % for high trans-sphincteric, 27.3 % for suprasphincteric, and 44.4 % for horseshoe fistula.

Table 22.2 Parks anal fistula classification

Intersphincteric
Simple low track
High blind track
High track with opening into rectum
High fistula without a perineal opening
High fistula with extrarectal or pelvic extension
Trans-sphincteric
Uncomplicated
High blind tract
Suprasphincteric
Uncomplicated
High blind tract
Extrasphincteric
Secondary to trans-sphincteric fistula
Secondary to trauma
Secondary to anorectal disease
Secondary to pelvic inflammation
Combined/Horseshoe
Intersphincteric
Trans-sphincteric

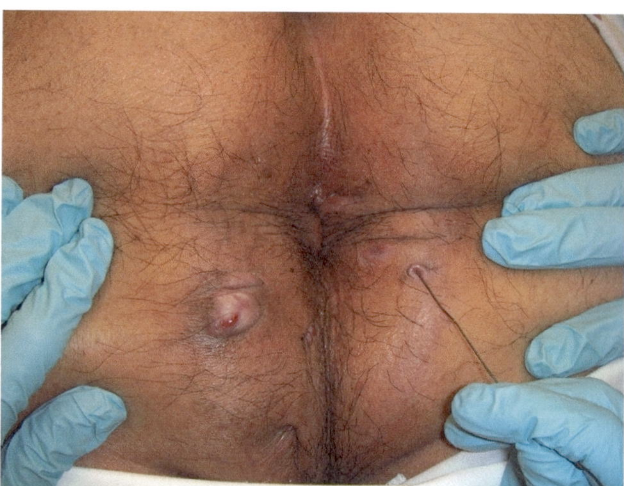

Fig. 22.6 Two external fistulous openings in a patient with an anterior-based horseshoe fistula

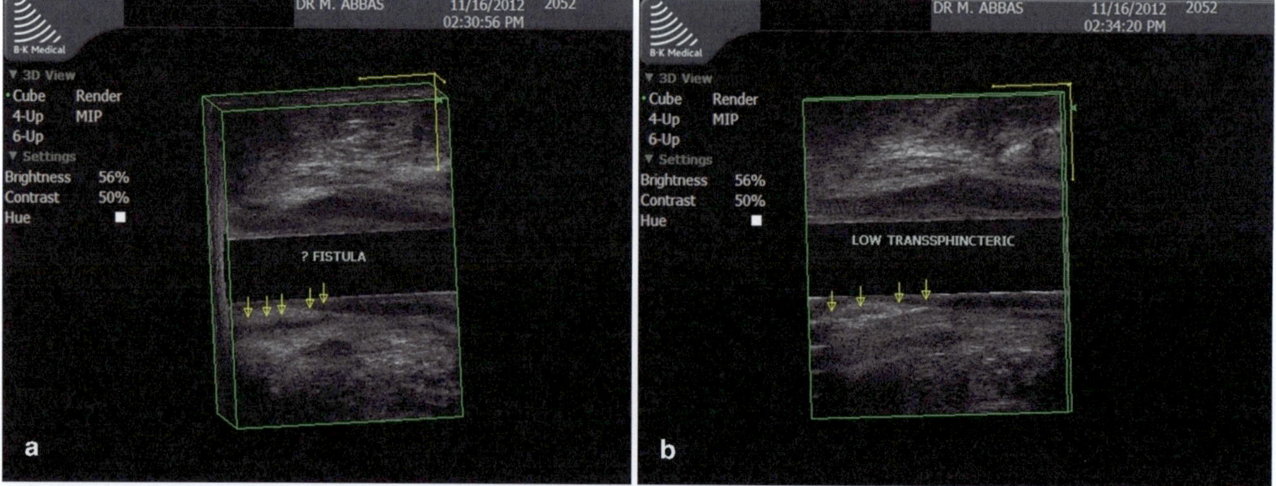

Fig. 22.7 (**a**) Three-dimensional ultrasound view of low trans-sphincteric fistula (*sagittal view*). (**b**) Post-hydrogen peroxide enhancement of low trans-sphincteric fistula (*sagittal view*)

Fecal incontinence rate was reported for the various fistula types: subcutaneous 4.2 %, intersphincteric 10.5 %, low trans-sphincteric 7.6 %, high trans-sphincteric 40 %, suprasphincteric 55.6 %, and horseshoe 44.4 %. High trans-sphincteric and suprasphincteric fistulas were predictors of incontinence (adjusted odds ratio, 22.9 [95% CI, 2.2–242.0; $p=0.009$] and 61.5 [4.5–844.0; $p=0.002$], respectively, compared to subcutaneous fistula). Another study from Spain reported by Jordan and colleagues analyzed the impact of fistula classification on postoperative outcome in 279 patients with anal fistula [20]. Persistence or recurrence of the fistula was noted in 7.2 % of the patients during a median follow-up of 4 months. Suprasphincteric and extrasphincteric fistulas were associated with the highest failure rates (28.1 % and 33.3 %, respectively). Similarly, the highest incontinence rates were noted in patients with suprasphincteric fistula and extrasphincteric fistula (42.3 % and 40 %, respectively). In general suprasphincteric fistula has been associated with some of the highest failure/recurrence rate and incontinence risk in numerous studies including a German study that reported the outcome of 224 patients [21]. Postoperative incontinence was noted in 43 % of patients with suprasphincteric fistula compared to 21 % of patients with trans-sphincteric fistula.

Anal fistulas that involve the vagina have been associated with a higher operative failure rate. The majority of anovaginal and rectovaginal fistulas are secondary to obstetrical trauma or Crohn's disease. In general such fistulas are more complex because of various factors including anal sphincter defects, multiple and/or higher tracts, and/or active mucosal inflammation. Several studies have compared the surgical outcome of patients with anal fistula to those with rectovaginal fistula. Abbas and colleagues from Kaiser Permanente Los

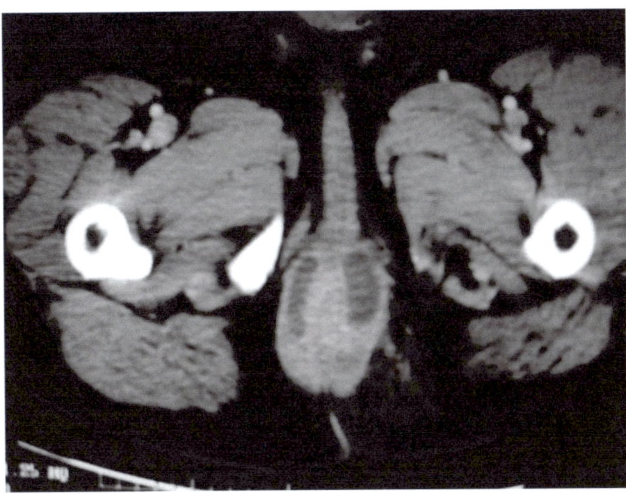

Fig. 22.8 Computed tomography scan view of patient with a posterior-based horseshoe fistula

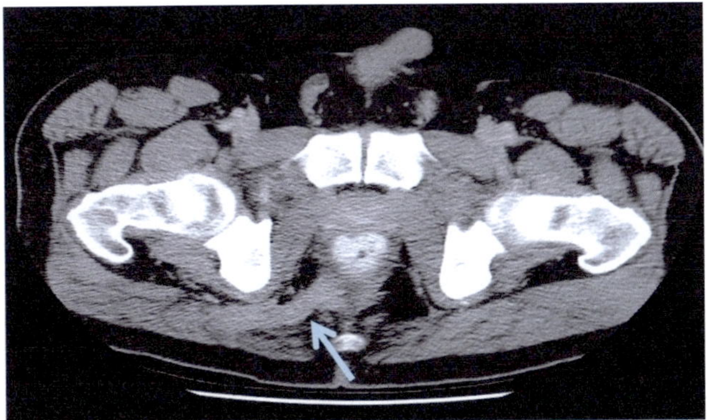

Fig. 22.9 Computed tomography scan view of patient with right suprasphincteric anal fistula

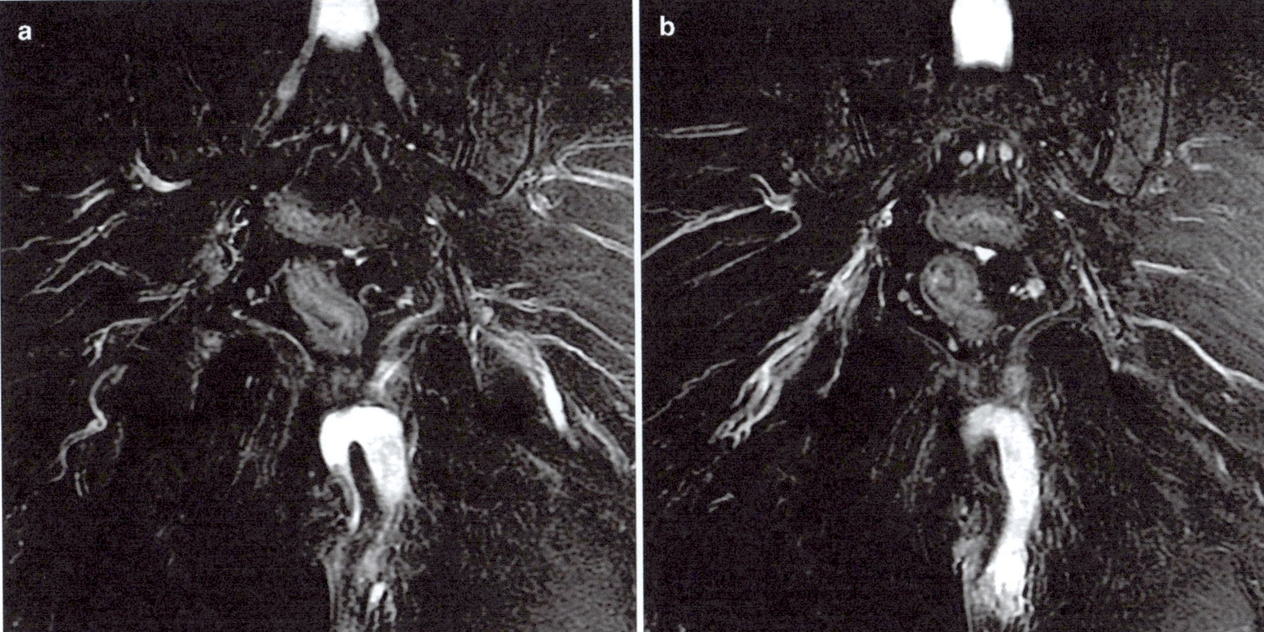

Fig. 22.10 (**a**, **b**) Magnetic resonance imaging of patient with left suprasphincteric anal fistula

Angeles reported their results with 36 patients who underwent 38 endorectal advancement flaps [22]. The overall success rate was 83 %. Patients with rectovaginal fistula had a higher failure rate compared to patients with anal fistula (67 % vs. 4 %, respectively). In a review of the Cleveland Clinic Ohio experience with 99 endorectal flaps, Sonada and colleagues noted a higher failure rate in patients rectovaginal fistula compared to those with anal fistula (57 % vs. 24 %, $p=0.002$) [9]. In the previously mentioned Canadian study looking at the impact of selective use of seton combined with infliximab infusion in Crohn's patients, complete healing was noted in 67 % of patients with anal fistula compared to 12.5 % of patients with rectovaginal fistula [11]. Löffler and colleagues from Germany reported similar findings in patients with Crohn's disease [23]. Over a 10-year period, 147 Crohn's patients underwent 292 operations for anorectal or rectovaginal fistula. The majority of patients had Crohn's colitis (98 %). A higher recurrence rate was noted in patients with complex fistulas such as rectovaginal (45.6 %) compared to patients with simple submucosal fistulas (18.8 %). Furthermore the need for major operations including proctectomy was higher in patients with rectovaginal fistula compared to patients with submucosal fistula (56 % vs. 14 %, respectively).

The length of an anal fistula may also impact the outcome of surgical intervention. McGee and colleagues from Case Western University reported their experience with the anal fistula plug in 41 patients with anal fistula secondary to cryptoglandular disease [24]. The failure rate of the plug was 57 % in their study. Failure rate was higher in patients with a fistulous tract <4 cm compared to those with a tract >4 cm (79 % vs. 39 %, $p=0.004$).

Prior Fistula Repair

Several studies have examined the impact of prior fistula repair on the subsequent outcome of additional operative intervention. In general, a higher failure rate has been observed in patients with prior repair. This finding is most likely due to a combination of factors: failure following the initial operative intervention may be related to the complexity of the fistula which predisposes the patient to subsequent failure and prior failure may lead to alteration of the anatomy of the fistula and the quality of tissue (i.e., more complex tracts and scarring of the anal sphincter and anal canal). Ellis and colleagues from the University of Alabama reported their experience with 95 endorectal and anodermal flaps performed between 2000 and 2003 [25]. Recurrence rate was higher in patients with a prior repair compared to those with no prior repair (43 % vs. 23 %, $p<0.03$). In his review of the Cleveland Clinic Florida experience with Crohn's-related rectovaginal fistula over a 10 year period, Pinto reported a

similar finding in 125 patients [10]. Patient with no prior repair had a recurrence rate of 30.4 % compared to 47.1 % in patients with one to two repairs and 50 % in patients with more than three repairs. Comparable findings have been previously reported by another study from the Netherlands [26]. Schouten and colleagues examined 44 endorectal advancement flaps performed over a 5-year period. Patients with 1 or no prior repair had a failure rate of 13 % compared to 50 % in patients with two or more prior repairs. Similarly Nelson and colleagues from Chicago reported their results in 65 patients undergoing the island-flap anoplasty for trans-sphincteric fistula-in-ano [27]. Recurrence rate was 37 % in patients with prior repair compared to 20 % in patients with no prior repair. These findings were duplicated by Zimmerman and colleagues from the Netherlands who reported a recurrence rate of 22 % in patients with one or no previous repair compared to 71 % in patients with two or more prior repairs [28]. It is also important to note that patients with prior failed repair are at increased risk for developing fecal incontinence. A study reported by Mizrahi and colleagues from the Cleveland Clinic Florida looked at the incontinence rate in patients undergoing endorectal advancement flap [8]. The fecal incontinence rate was 5.3 % in patients with no prior repair compared to 19 % in patients who had a prior repair. Toyonaga and colleagues from Japan also reported that multiple previous surgeries were an independent risk factor for postoperative incontinence [29].

The Impact of Patient-Related Characteristics

Age

Population-based studies have reported an annual incidence of anal fistula of 6.8–10/100,000 persons with an age-specific incidence [30, 31]. Infants and children can develop anal fistula but the majority of patients present in adulthood [32–36]. Most patients present between the third and fifth decade of life [1, 30, 32–38]. The initial presentation of anal fistula includes an acute abscess, a recurrent abscess, or a chronically draining fistula. A study from Kaiser Permanente Los Angeles examined the risk of developing recurrent perianal sepsis and/or chronic fistula following one episode of acute perianal sepsis [1]. Patients younger than 40 years had greater than twofold increase in incidence of recurrent perianal sepsis compared to those 40 years or older. Based on the results of that study, it appears that young age is a predisposing factor for recurrent perianal sepsis or developing a chronic anal fistula. In addition, young age seems to increase the risk of operative failure. In their review of the Cleveland Clinic Ohio experience with anorectal and rectovaginal fistulas, Sonada and colleagues reported an association between age and operative failure [9]. In their study, the operative failure rate was 54.3 % in patients younger than 40 years compared to 32.1 % in patients between 40 and 60 years and 0 % in patients older than 60 years. It is important to note however that no difference in recurrence has been noted in other studies that have looked at age as predictor of outcome [25]. In their review of the University of Alabama's experience with anal flap, Ellis and Clark found no difference in recurrence rate between patients younger than 40 years compared to those older than 40 years. Age can impact the functional outcome following anal fistula surgery. Abbas and colleagues analyzed the functional outcome of 179 patients operated at Kaiser Permanente Los Angeles over a 5-year period [3]. Patients older than 45 years had a higher postoperative incontinence rate compared with patients younger than 45 years (adjusted odds ratio, 2.8 [95 % CI, 1.0–7.7]; $p=0.04$). This finding is not surprising considering that aging can lead to weakness of the anal and pelvic floor musculature. Anal fistula surgery can further decrease baseline resting and squeeze pressure as previously demonstrated by anal manometry measurements in several studies [21, 39, 40].

Gender

Gender has been implicated as a risk factor for developing anal sepsis and chronic anal fistula. The incidence of anal fistula in males is two- to fourfold higher than females [37, 41–45]. Fistula-in-ano is uncommon in the pediatric population, but the majority of infants who present with anal fistula are males [32–36]. Interestingly a higher incidence of fistula-in-ano has been documented in male dogs compared to females [46]. It has also been observed that neutered dogs are less susceptible to develop anal fistula, raising the possibility of a hormonal influence on the pathogenesis of this condition [46]. Another proposed theory for the higher incidence of anal fistula in males is the higher sphincter tone compared to females which may contribute to duct obstruction and glandular inflammation [1].

Based on the above, it is clear that gender plays a role in the development of anal fistula but beyond the incidence of this condition, this finding has prompted many researchers to investigate the impact of gender on anal fistula surgery outcome. Hyman and colleagues reviewed the results of the prospective, multicenter outcomes registry of the New England Regional Society of the American Society of Colon and Rectal Surgeons [47]. A female gender was associated a higher failure rate ($p=0.04$). While some studies have reported an association between gender and operative outcome, Ellis and Clark found no difference in fistula recurrence rate between males and females who underwent anal flap [25]. A similar finding was reported by the Cleveland Clinic Florida group when analyzing the outcome of patients

who underwent advancement flap (recurrence rate 35.7 % in females and 47.3 % in males, $p=$NS) [8]. Van Koperen and colleagues from the Netherlands reported their results in 179 patients treated for anal fistula over an 8-year period [48]. In both groups that underwent fistulotomy or rectal advancement flap, no difference in recurrence rate was noted between genders. Garcia-Aguilar and colleagues from the University of Minnesota surveyed 375 patients who had undergone anal fistula surgery [2]. During a mean follow-up of 29 months, 45 % of the patients reported some degree of incontinence. A female gender was associated with a higher risk of incontinence.

Smoking

Smoking has been implicated as a risk factor for the development of anal fistula. A study reported from the Department of Veterans Affairs hospital in San Diego compared the risk of developing anal abscess and fistula in smokers vs. nonsmokers [49]. Smoking was associated with a significant increased risk (odds ratio 2.15, 95 % CI 1.34–3.48, $p=0.0025$). Smoking has been associated with a higher rate of postoperative complications following various anorectal operations including anal fistula surgery. Zimmerman and colleagues from the Netherlands compared the outcome of endorectal advancement flap in patients who smoked vs. those who did not [50]. One hundred and five patients were followed for a median time of 14 months. Healing rate was 60 % in smokers compared to 79 % in nonsmokers ($p=0.037$). In an effort to understand the effect of smoking on healing, a subsequent study by the same researchers measured blood flow during endorectal advancement flap procedures. Blood flow was significantly lower in smokers compared to nonsmokers [51]. The negative impact of smoking on healing following advancement flap repair was confirmed by Ellis and Clark from the University of Alabama [25]. The overall recurrence rate was 32.6 % in 94 patients who underwent mucosal or anodermal advancement flap. Smokers had a higher recurrence rate compared to nonsmokers (42 % vs. 19 %, $p<0.05$). Schwander and colleagues from Germany reported their results with the anal fistula plug in 60 patients [52]. Smokers had a higher failure rate compared to nonsmokers ($p=0.005$).

Obesity

Obesity and large body habitus present significant technical challenges to the surgeon operating on the anus. This is due to a variety of factors including deep buttock cleft, poor exposure, and difficulty with positioning the patient on the operating room table. There is a paucity of data on the impact of obesity on the outcome of anal fistula surgery. Schwandner from Germany reported his experience with 220 patients undergoing advancement flap repair of complex anal fistula [53]. Success rate was significantly different in obese [Body mass index (BMI) > 30 kg/m^2] compared to non-obese patients. In non-obese patients, recurrence rate of the fistula was 14 % compared to 28 % in obese patients ($p < 0.01$). In addition, the reoperation rate in the failed group was significantly higher in obese patients when compared to non-obese patients (73 % vs. 52 %, $p < 0.01$). Using multivariate analysis, obesity was identified as independent predictive factor of success or failure ($p < 0.02$).

The Impact of the Surgeon on Outcome

The surgeon has a significant impact on the outcome of anal fistula surgery. The choice of an operation and how it is technically performed by the surgeon are of paramount importance. Several operations are available to treat patients including fistulotomy, fistulectomy, anal flaps such anodermal and endorectal, ligating intersphincteric fistula tract (LIFT procedure), setons, and the anal fistula plug. The selection of an operation for an individual patient should take into consideration several factors including the anatomy of the fistula, its location, its etiology, prior intervention, baseline continence function, and body habitus. Several technical variations of the available operative interventions exist and yield different success rate. Technical details and intraoperative findings can determine outcome.

Intraoperative Findings and Technical Conduct

Described in simple terms, a fistula is a tunnel with two ends, an entrance and an exit. In order to successfully eradicate the fistula, the proper identification of both the internal opening (the entrance) and external opening (the exit) is necessary. This can be accomplished by probing of the fistulous tract or injecting the external opening with fluids such as hydrogen peroxide in order to identify the internal opening (Fig. 22.11a, b).

The inability to locate the internal opening is a predictor for a worse outcome. This finding has been confirmed by several studies. Sainio and Husa from Finland reported their results with 199 patients who underwent anal fistula surgery [54]. The overall recurrence rate was 11 % and the majority of the recurrences (91 %) were noted within 18 months of operation. The most common reason for recurrence was an undetected internal opening and incomplete laying open of the entire fistulous tract. Sangwan and colleagues from Pennsylvania evaluated the outcome of 523 patients with anal fistula [55]. Four hundred and sixty-three patients (89 %) were classified as simple fistula. The overall recurrence rate was 6.5 %. The recurrence was attributed to the inability to identify the internal opening in over half of the patients who recurred (53.3 %). Garcia-Aguilar and colleagues from the University of Minnesota examined the long-term outcome of 624 patients following anal fistula surgery [2]. In 4.3 % of the patients the internal opening couldn't be determined. The overall recurrence rate was 8 %. However the recurrence

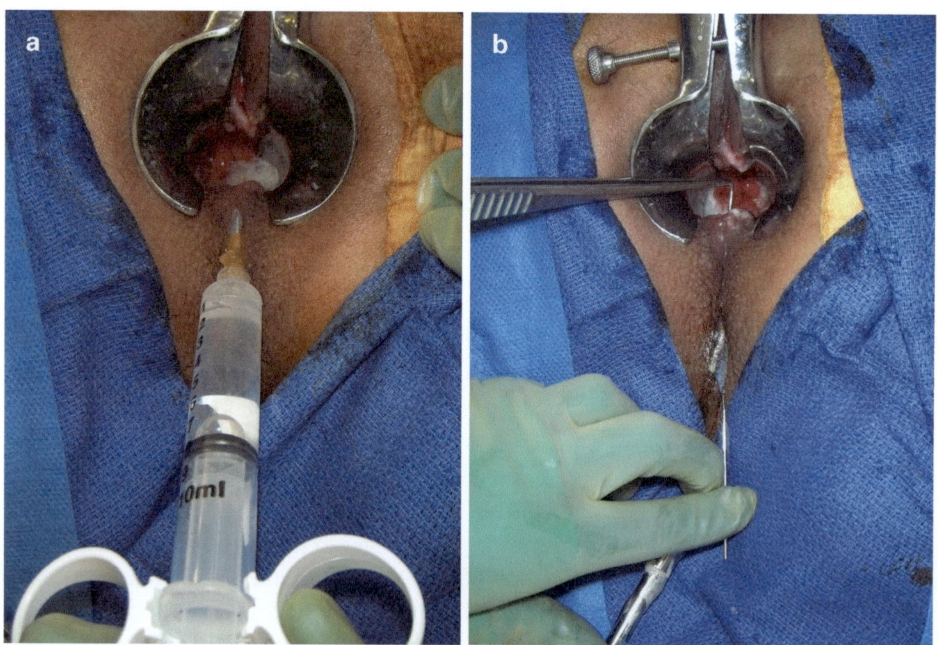

Fig. 22.11 (**a**) Hydrogen peroxide injection through external fistulous opening demonstrates the internal opening. (**b**) Probing of the tract is demonstrated

rate was much higher in the subgroup of patients whose internal opening could not be identified compared to those patients whose internal fistula opening was found (56 % vs. 7 %). Jordan and colleagues from Spain evaluated the impact of various factors on anal fistula recurrence [20]. The outcome of different techniques was compared in 279 patients. Recurrence rate was highest with the procedure of coring-out the fistula with internal opening closure compared to fistulotomy which yielded the lowest recurrence rate (42.9 % vs. 1.5 %). Multivariable analysis demonstrated a significant increased risk for recurrence in patients with complex fistula (odds ratio 10.5 (CI 95 %, 1.5–74.3) [$p<0.01$]) and in patients whose internal fistulous opening couldn't be determined at time of operative intervention (odds ratio 5.3 (CI 95 %, 1–27.9) [$p<0.01$]). Similarly Chi-Ming and colleagues looked at recurrence pattern in 135 Chinese patients treated for anal fistula over a 5-year period [56]. The overall recurrence rate was 13.3 % and median time to recurrence was 7.5 months. Univariate analysis identified six risk factors for recurrence including a prior history of perianal abscess and operation, complex fistula, perianal sinus, absence of internal opening, and the procedure of sinus tract excision. In logistic regression analysis, sinus tract excision was the only independent predictor of recurrence.

All the above studies highlight the importance of the identification of the internal opening. Selective preoperative imaging in some patients may be beneficial especially in those with prior failed surgery or complex fistulas. Furthermore if at time of operative intervention the internal opening is not identified by the surgeon or the anatomy of the fistula is ambiguous, the wisest course of action maybe to abort the operative procedure than risk failure, complication, and incontinence. Further investigation with imaging can be helpful prior to additional surgical intervention.

Choice of Operation

The armamentarium of anal fistula surgery includes a spectrum of procedures. In general, anal fistula operations can be divided into two groups: (1) partial sphincter-preserving procedures and (2) sphincter-conserving operations. The former group includes fistulotomy, fistulectomy, and cutting seton. The latter group consists of non-cutting seton, fibrin glue injection, anal fistula plug, the LIFT procedure, and flaps such as the anodermal and endorectal flaps.

A comprehensive overview of the literature as it pertains to the various anal fistula operations is beyond the scope of this chapter. The following section summarizes some of the outcome trends associated with commonly performed anal fistula operations. Heterogeneity of results exists in terms of success rate and impact on continence. Fistulotomy yields the highest success rate amongst all anal fistula procedures.

It involves laying open the fistulous tract. Toyonaga and colleagues from Japan reported a series of 35 patients who underwent fistulotomy [39]. During a mean follow-up of 12 months, the recurrence rate was very low (3 %). Most studies have reported a recurrence rate between 1 and 13 % following fistulotomy [3, 20, 40, 47, 57]. Most surgeons favor fistulotomy for the majority of patients with simple fistula because of its high success rate. However patient selection is critical as this procedure can lead to incontinence in some patients. Patients at risk for incontinence include those with high fistula, anterior fistula especially in females, multiple prior anal operations, and those with weak sphincter tone at baseline. Some degree of continence disturbance has been reported in 7–49 % of patients undergoing fistulotomy [3, 18, 29, 39, 40, 48, 58–60]. Preoperative three-dimensional ultrasound is helpful in determining the amount of muscle involvement by the fistula and may guide surgical therapy in order to minimize risk of incontinence [18].

Several sphincter-preserving operations have been advocated as an alternative to fistulotomy in order to minimize the risks of incontinence. The results of fibrin glue injection have been reported in several studies [61–69]. While the initial experience with fibrin glue was favorable with success rates ranging from 54 to 78 %, the results of more recent studies have not been encouraging [62, 65]. Buchanan and colleagues from St. Mark's Hospital in England reported a healing rate of 14 % in patients followed clinically and imaged with magnetic resonance imaging [63]. Similarly Loungnarath and colleagues from the University of Washington reported a healing rate of 31 % [66]. Fibrin glue alone carries no risk for incontinence and minimal recovery and thus it is reasonable to consider it in patients who are at risk for incontinence. Another surgical option that involves filling the fistulous tract without division of anal sphincter muscle is the anal fistula plug. Introduced into the surgical armamentarium of anal fistula surgery in the last decade, the anal plug has been extensively studied in patients with cryptoglandular disease as well as Crohn's disease [68–85]. A large variation in outcome has been reported by the various studies. Success rate has ranged from 14 to 83 % for patients with cryptoglandular disease and from 26.6 to 85.7 % for patients with Crohn's disease. It is unclear why success rate was high in some studies yet very low in others. Patient selection, technical variations, postoperative management, and length of follow-up may explain some of the differences. Failure of the plug is usually related to dislodgment or sepsis (Fig. 22.12). The original Surgisis® AFP™ plug by Cook Surgical (Bloomington, IN) was made of porcine submucosa. A second plug, the Gore Bio-A® is now available from Gore (Flagstaff, AZ) and is made of 100 % synthetic bioabsorbable scaffold. Early results with the Gore Bio-A® plug appeared promising [86, 87]. Several studies have compared the outcome of the anal fistula plug to anal flaps [88–91].

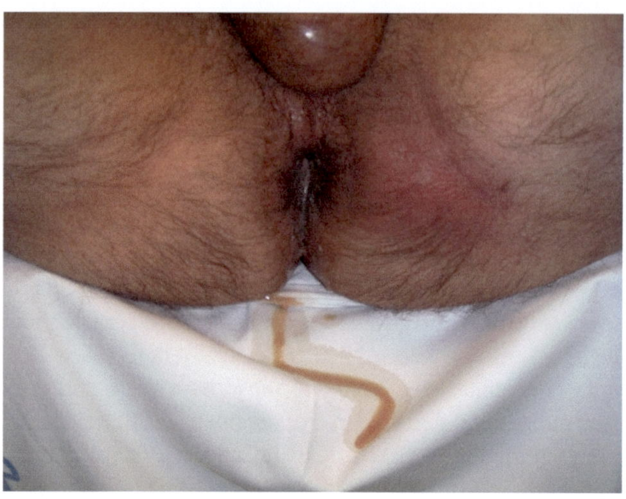

Fig. 22.12 Acute abscess after insertion of the anal fistula plug

Table 22.3 Published series: endorectal advancement flap

Authors	Year	N	Success (%)
Garcia-Aguilar et al. [2]	1984	151	99
Wedell et al. [105]	1987	31	100
Kodner et al. [106]	1993	107	84
Makowiec et al. [107]	1995	32	66
Kreis et al. [108]	1998	24	63
Shouten et al. [26]	1999	44	75
Ortiz and Marzo [109]	2000	103	93
Mizrahi et al. [8]	2002	94	60
Abbas et al. [3]	2008	38	83
Adamina et al. [110]	2010	12	33

In general the outcomes of anal flaps have been more favorable than the anal fistula plug. Wang and colleagues from the University of California in San Francisco reported 34 % closure rate with the plug compared to 62 % with Endorectal flap ($p=0.045$) [89]. Christoforidis and colleagues from the University of Minnesota found similar outcome with a healing rate of 63 % with the endorectal flap compared to 32 % with the anal fistula plug ($p=0.008$) [91]. Ortiz and colleagues from Spain conducted a randomized clinical trial comparing the anal fistula plug and the endorectal advancement flap [90]. The study was closed prematurely due a large difference in outcome in favor of the flap. Another multicenter randomized trial from the Netherlands found no significant difference in failure rate between the anal fistula plug and the mucosal advancement flap (71 % vs. 52 %, $p=0.126$) [88]. The outcome of the endorectal flap has been favorable in most reported series (Table 22.3) [2, 8, 22, 26, 105–110]. However the incontinence rate associated with the endorectal flap has ranged from 0 to 35 % (Table 22.4).

The LIFT procedure was recently introduced as a new sphincter-preserving option [92–94]. The procedure entails

Table 22.4 Published series: fecal incontinence rate following endorectal advancement flap

Authors	Year	N	Incontinence (%)
Garcia-Aguilar et al. [2]	1984	151	10
Wedell et al. [105]	1987	31	0
Kodner et al. [106]	1993	107	13
Makowiec et al. [107]	1995	32	3
Kreis et al. [108]	1998	24	13
Shouten et al. [26]	1999	44	35
Ortiz and Marzo [109]	2000	103	8
Mirzahi et al. [8]	2002	94	9
Uribe et al. [98]	2007	56	21
Abbas et al. [3]	2008	38	8

dissection in the intersphincteric plane with ligation and division of the fistulous tract in that location. Success rate has ranged from 60 to 95 %. More recently Ellis reported 31 patients with complex anal fistulas that were treated with a modification of the LIFT procedure called the BioLIFT [95]. A bioprosthetic graft was used to reinforce the LIFT procedure. Healing was achieved in 94% of the patients. More studies are needed to determine whether there are additional advantages to the use of biologic mesh.

Conclusions

Anal fistula is commonly treated by surgeons. Cryptoglandular disease contributes to the majority of fistula formation. Anal fistulas often require surgical intervention to drain the acute sepsis or to eradicate a chronic tract. Medical therapy can be helpful in subgroups of patients such as those with Crohn's disease in order to increase the success rate of operative intervention and minimize the risk of recurrence which is triggered by disease activity. The placement of a draining seton prior to instituting medical therapy can be helpful in such setting to control the fistula. While the majority of data available on the outcome of anal fistula surgery are derived from retrospective reviews of various institutions, several predictors of outcome have been identified. Factors such as Crohn's disease, complex fistulas such as suprasphincteric and extrasphincteric, rectovaginal fistula, prior failed operation, smoking, and obesity have been associated with a higher failure rate. More research is needed to further explore these associations and to identify treatment strategies that can mitigate the fistula-related characteristics and patient factors that lead to poor outcome. The surgeon can greatly impact the outcome of anal fistula surgery. The choice of operation and its technical conduct are of paramount importance. Various operations are available to treat this condition and can be generally categorized into sphincter-dividing or sphincter-preserving interventions. Success rate and long-term impact on continence defer greatly between the different surgical options available. Several technical modifications are available to enhance the outcome of these operations and some can yield better results while others are associated with higher failure rates. Surgeons treating anal fistula should be familiar with and be technically proficient in performing the various operations and should individualize the choice of operation based on the fistula and patient-related characteristics in order to optimize the outcome. Identification of the internal opening at time of operation remains critical to success. The selective use of imaging can be helpful in cases where the internal opening is not identified at time of operation, for complex fistulas such as those with multiple openings, high fistulas, and in those that failed prior surgical intervention.

Summary

- Goals of anal fistula surgery are to heal the fistula, minimize complications, preserve continence, and prevent recurrence
- Three things determine outcome of treatment: patient-related features, fistula characteristics, and surgeon's factor
- Choice and conduct of an operation is critical for treatment success.

References

1. Hamadani A, Haigh PI, Liu IA, Abbas MA. Who is at risk for developing chronic anal fistula or recurrent anal sepsis after initial perianal abscess? Dis Colon Rectum. 2009;52(2):217–21.
2. Garcia-Aguilar J, Belmonte C, Wong WD, Goldberg SM, Madoff RD. Anal fistula surgery. Factors associated with recurrence and incontinence. Dis Colon Rectum. 1996;39(7):723–9.
3. Abbas MA, Jackson CH, Haigh PI. Predictors of outcome for anal fistula surgery. Arch Surg. 2011;146(9):1011–6.
4. Adhami S, Duthie G, Greenstone M. A tuberculous anal fistula. J Roy Soc Med. 1999;92:467–8.
5. Alyoune M, Nadir S, Merzouk M, Mounadif A, Biadillah MC, Jamil D, Alaoui R, Cherkaoui A. Tuberculous anal fistulas. Ann Gastroenterol Hepatol. 1994;30(1):9–11.
6. Fry RD, Birnbaum EH, Lacey DL. Actinomyces as a cause of recurrent perianal fistula in the immunocompromised patient. Surgery. 1992;111(5):591–4.
7. Coremans G, Margaritis V, Van Poppel HP, Christiaens MR, Gruwez J, Geboes K, Wyndaele J, VAnbeckevoort D, Janssens J. Actinomycosis, a rare and unsuspected cause of anal fistulous abscess: report of three cases and review of the literature. Dis Colon Rectum. 2005;48(3):575–81.
8. Mizrahi N, Wexner SD, Zmora O, Da Silva G, Efron J, Weiss EG, Vernava 3rd AM, Nogueras JJ. Endorectal advancement flap: are there predictors of failure? Dis Colon Rectum. 2002;45(12):1616–21.
9. Sonada T, Hull T, Piedmonte MR, Fazio VW. Outcomes of primary repair of anorectal and rectovaginal fistulas using the endorectal advancement flap. Dis Colon Rectum. 2002;45:1622–8.
10. Pinto RA, Peterson TV, Shawki S, Davila GW, Wexner SD. Are there predictors of outcome following rectovaginal fistula? Dis Colon Rectum. 2010;53(9):1240–7.
11. Topstad DR, Panaccione R, Heine JA, Johnson DR, MacLean AR, Buie WD. Combined seton placement, infliximab infusion, and maintenance immunosuppressives improve healing rate in fistulizing anorectal Crohn's disease: a single center experience. Dis Colon Rectum. 2003;46(5):577–83.
12. El-Gazzaz G, Hull T, Church JM. Biologic immunomodulators improve the healing rate in surgically treated perianal Crohn's fistulas. Colorectal Dis. 2012;14(10):1217–23.
13. Regueiro M, Mardini H. Treatment of perianal fistulizing Crohn's disease with infliximab alone or as an adjunct to exam under anesthesia with seton placement. Inflamm Bowel Dis. 2003;9(2):98–103.
14. Iesalnieks I, Glass H, Kilger A, Ott C, Klebl F, Agha A, Schlitt HJ, Strauch U. Perianal fistulas in Crohn's disease: treatment results at an interdisciplinary unit. Chirurg. 2009;80(6):549–58.
15. Parks AG, Gordon PH, Hardcastle AG. A classification of fistula-in-ano. Br J Surg. 1976;63:1.
16. Ratto C, Grillo E, Parello A, Costamagna G, Doglietto GB. Endoanal ultrasound-guided surgery for anal fistula. Endoscopy. 2005;37:722–8.
17. Toyonaga T, Tanaka Y, Song JF, Katori R, Sogawa N, Kanyama H, Hatakeyama T, Matsushima M, Susuki S, Mibu R, Tanaka M. Comparison of accuracy of physical examination and endoanal ultrasonography for preoperative assessment in patients with acute and chronic fistula. Tech Coloproctol. 2008;12:217–23.
18. Murad-Regadas SM, Regadas FS, Rodrigues LV, Holanda EC, Barreto RG, Oliveira L. The role of 3-dimensional anorectal ultrasonography in the assessment of anterior transsphincteric fistula. Dis Colon Rectum. 2010;53(7):1035–40.
19. Joyce M, Venicro JC, Kiran RP. Magnetic resonance imaging in the management of anal fistula and anorectal sepsis. Clin Colon Rectal Surg. 2008;21(3):213–9.
20. Jordán J, Roig JV, García-Armengol J, García-Granero E, Solana A, Lledó S. Risk factors for recurrence and incontinence after anal fistula surgery. Colorectal Dis. 2010;12(3):254–60.
21. Athanasiadis S, Kohler A, Nafe M. Treatment of high anal fistulae by primary occlusion of the internal ostium, drainage of the intersphincteric space, and mucosal advancement flap. Int J Colorect Dis. 1994;9(3):153–7.
22. Abbas MA, Lemus-Rangel R, Hamadani A. Long-term outcome of endorectal advancement flap for complex anorectal fistulae. Am Surg. 2008;74(10):921–4.
23. Löffler T, Welsch T, Mühl S, Hinz U, Schmidt J, Kienle P. Long-term success rate after surgical treatment of anorectal and rectovaginal fistulas in Crohn's disease. Int J Colorectal Dis. 2009;24(5):521–6.
24. McGee MF, Champagne BJ, Stulberg JJ, Reynolds H, Marderstein E, Delaney CP. Tract length predicts successful closure with anal fistula plug in cryptoglandular fistulas. Dis Colon Rectum. 2010;53(8):1116–20.
25. Ellis CN, Clark S. Effect of tobacco smoking on advancement flap repair of complex anal fistulas. Dis Colon Rectum. 2007;50(4):459–63.
26. Schouten WR, Zimmerman DD, Briel JW. Transanal advancement flap repair of transsphincteric fistulas. Dis Colon Rectum. 1999;42(11):1419–22.
27. Nelson RL, Cintron J, Abcarian H. Dermal island-flap anoplasty for transsphincteric fistula-in-ano. Dis Colon Rectum. 2000;43(5):681–4.
28. Zimmerman DD, Briel JW, Gosselink MP, Schouten WR. Anocutaneous advancement flap repair of transsphincteric fistulas. Dis Colon Rectum. 2001;44(10):1474–80.
29. Toyonaga T, Matsushima M, Kiriu T, Sogawa N, Kanyama H, Matsumura N, Shimojima Y, Hatakeyama T, Tanaka Y, Suzuki K, Tanaka M. Factors affecting continence after fistulotomy for intersphincteric fistula-in-ano. Int J Colorect Dis. 2007;22(9):1071–5.

30. Sainio P. Fistula-in-ano in a defined population. Incidence and epidemiological aspects. Ann Chir Gynaecol. 1984;73:219–24.

31. Ewerth S, Ahlberg J, Collste G, Holmstrom B. Fistula-in-ano: a six year follow-up study of 143 operated patients. Acta Chir Scand. 1978;482:53–5.

32. Hill JR. Fistulas and fistulous abscesses in the anorectal region: personal experience in management. Dis Colon Rectum. 1967;10: 421–34.

33. Mazier WP. The treatment and care of anal fistulas: a study of 1000 patients. Dis Colon Rectum. 1971;14:134–44.

34. Matt JG. Anal fistula in infants and children. Dis Colon Rectum. 1960;3:258–61.

35. Venturo RC. Fistula-in-ano in infants. Am J Surg. 1953;86: 641–2.

36. Shafer AD, McGlone TP, Flanagan RA. Abnormal crypts of Morgagni: the cause of perirectal abscess and fistula-in-ano. J Pediatr Surg. 1987;22:203–4.

37. Read DR, Abcarian H. A prospective survey of 474 patients with anorectal abscess. Dis Colon Rectum. 1979;22:566–8.

38. Lai CK, Wong J, Ong GB. Anorectal suppuration: a review of 606 patients. Southeast Asian J Surg. 1983;6:22–6.

39. Toyonaga T, Matsushima M, Tanaka Y, Susuki K, Sogawa N, Kanyama H, Shimjima Y, Hatakeyama T, Tanaka M. Non-sphincter splitting fistulectomy vs conventional fistulotomy for high trans-sphincteric fistula-in-ano: a prospective functional and manometric study. Int J Colorectal Dis. 2007;22:1097–102.

40. Roig JV, Jordan J, Garcia-Armengol J, Esclapez P, Solana A. Changes in anorectal morphologic and functional parameters after fistula-in-ano. Dis Colon Rectum. 2009;52:1462–9.

41. Ramanujam PS, Prasad ML, Abcarian H, Tan AB. Perirectal abscesses and fistulas: a study of 1,023 patients. Dis Colon Rectum. 1984;27:593–7.

42. Winslett MC, Allan A, Ambrose NS. Anorectal sepsis as a presentation of occult rectal and systemic disease. Dis Colon Rectum. 1988;31:597–600.

43. Vasilevsky C, Gordon PH. The incidence of recurrent abscesses or fistula-in-ano following anorectal suppuration. Dis Colon Rectum. 1984;27:126–30.

44. Kronborg O, Olsen H. Incision and drainage vs. incision, curettage and suture under antibiotic cover in anorectal abscess: a randomized study with 3-year follow-up. Acta Chir Scand. 1984;150:689–92.

45. Marks CG, Ritchie JK. Anal fistulas at St. Mark's Hospital. Br J Surg. 1977;64:84–91.

46. Killingsworth CR, Walshaw R, Dunstan RW, Rosser Jr EJ. Bacterial population and histologic changes in dogs with perirectal fistula. Am J Vet Res. 1988;49:1736–41.

47. Hyman N, O'Brien S, Osler T. Outcomes after fistulotomy: results of a prospective, multicenter regional study. Dis Colon Rectum. 2009;52(12):2022–7.

48. Van Koperen PJ, Wind J, Bemelman WA, Bakx R, Reitsma JB, Slors JF. Long-term functional outcome and risk factors for recurrence after surgical treatment for low and high perianal fistulas of cryptoglandular origin. Dis Colon Rectum. 2008;51:1475–81.

49. Devaraj B, Khabassi S, Cosman B. Recent smoking is a risk factor for anal abscess and fistula. Dis Colon Rectum. 2011;54:681–5.

50. Zimmerman DD, Delemarre JB, Gosselink MP, Hop WC, Briel JW, Schouten WR. Smoking affects the outcome of transanal mucosal advancement flap repair of trans-sphincteric fistulas. Br J Surg. 2003;90:351–4.

51. Zimmerman DD, Gosselink MP, Mitalas LE, Mitalas LE, Delemarre JB, Hop WJ, Briel JW, Schouten WR. Smoking impairs rectal mucosal blood flow- a pilot study: possible implications for transanal advancement flap repair. Dis Colon Rectum. 2005;48: 1228–32.

52. Schwandner T, Roblick MH, Kierer W, Brom A, Padberg W, Hirschburger M. Surgical treatment of complex anal fistulas with the anal fistula plug: a prospective, multicenter study. D is Colon Rectum. 2009;52(9):1578–83.

53. Schwandner O. Obesity is a negative predictor of success after surgery for complex anal fistula. BMC Gastroenterol. 2011; 23(11):61.

54. Sainio P, Husa A. Fistula-in-ano. Clinical features and long-term results of surgery in 199 adults. Acta Chir Scand. 1985;151(2): 169–76.

55. Sangwan YP, Rosen L, Riether RD, Stasik JJ, Sheets JA, Khubchandani IT. Is simple fistula-in-ano simple? Dis Colon Rectum. 1994;37(9):885–9.

56. Poon CM, Ng DC, Ho-Yin MC, Li RS, Leong HT. Recurrence pattern of fistula-in-ano in a Chinese population. J Gastrointest Liver Dis. 2008;17(1):53–7.

57. Bokhari S, Lindsey I. Incontinence following sphincter division for treatment of anal fistula. Colorectal Dis. 2010;12((7 Online)): e135–9.

58. Cavanaugh M, Hyman N, Osler T. Fecal incontinence severity index after fistulotomy: a predictor of quality of life. Dis Colon Rectum. 2002;45(3):349–53.

59. Van Tets WF, Kuijpers HC. Continence disorders after anal fistulotomy. Dis Colon Rectum. 1994;37(12):1194–7.

60. Rosa G, Lolli P, Pccinelli D, Mazzola F, Bonomo S. Fistula in ano: anatomoclinical aspects, surgical therapy and results in 844 patients. Tech Coloproctol. 2006;10(3):215–21.

61. Lindsey I, Smilgin-Humphreys MM, Cunningham C, Mortensen NJ, George BD. A randomized, controlled trial of fibrin glue vs. conventional treatment for anal fistula. Dis Colon Rectum. 2002; 45:1608–15.

62. Sentovich SM. Fibrin glue for anal fistulas. Dis Colon Rectum. 2003;46:498–502.

63. Buchanan GN, Bartram CI, Phillips RK, Gould SW, Halligan S, Rockall TA, Sibbons P, Cohen RG. Efficacy of fibrin sealant in the management of complex anal fistula: a prospective trial. Dis Colon Rectum. 2003;46(9):1167–74.

64. Cirocchi R, Farinella E, La Mura F, Cattorini L, Rossetti B, Milani D, Ricci P, Covarelli P, Coccetta M, Noya G, Sciannameo F. Fibrin glue in the treatment of anal fistula: a systematic review. Ann Surg Innov Res. 2009;14(3):12.

65. Cintron JR, Park JJ, Orsay CP, Pearl RK, Nelson RL, Sone JH, Song R, Abcarian H. Repair of fistulas-in-ano using fibrin adhesive: long-term follow-up. Dis Colon Rectum. 2000;43(7):944–9.

66. Loungnarath R, Dietz DW, Mutch MG, Birnbaum EH, Kodner IJ, Fleshman JW. Fibrin glue treatment of complex anal fistulas has low success rate. Dis Colon Rectum. 2004;47(4):432–6.

67. de Oca J, Millán M, Jiménez A, Golda T, Biondo S. Long-term results of surgery plus fibrin sealant for anal fistula. Colorectal Dis. 2012;14(1):12–5.

68. Johnson EK, Gaw JU, Armstrong DN. Efficacy of anal fistula plug vs. fibrin glue in closure of anorectal fistulas. Dis Colon Rectum. 2006;49(3):371–6.

69. Tinay OE, El-Bakry AA. Treatment of chronic fistula-in-ano using commercial fibrin glue. Saudi Med J. 2004;25(8):1127–8.

70. Ellis CN, Clark S. Fibrin glue as an adjunct to flap repair of anal fistulas: a randomized, controlled study. Dis Colon Rectum. 2006;49(11):1736–40.

71. O'Connor L, Champagne BJ, Ferguson MA, Orangio GR, Schertzer ME, Armstrong DN. Efficacy of anal fistula plug in closure of Crohn's anorectal fistulas. Dis Colon Rectum. 2006; 49(10):1569–73.

72. Schwandner O, Stadler F, Dietl O, Wirsching RP, Fuerst A. Initial experience on efficacy in closure of cryptoglandular and Crohn's transsphincteric fistulas by the use of the anal fistula plug. Int J Colorectal Dis. 2008;23(3):319–24.

73. Champagne BJ, O'Connor LM, Ferguson M, Orangio GR, Schertzer ME, Armstrong DN. Efficacy of anal fistula plug in

closure of cryptoglandular fistulas: long-term follow-up. Dis Colon Rectum. 2006;49(12):1817–21.

74. van Koperen PJ, D'Hoore A, Wolthuis AM, Bemelman WA, Slors JF. Anal fistula plug for closure of difficult anorectal fistula: a prospective study. Dis Colon Rectum. 2007;50(12):2168–72.

75. Zubaidi A, Al-Obeed O. Anal fistula plug in high fistula-in-ano: an early Saudi experience. Dis Colon Rectum. 2009;52(9): 1584–8.

76. Schwandner T, Roblick MH, Kierer W, Brom A, Padberg W, Hirschburger M. Surgical treatment of complex anal fistulas with the anal fistula plug: a prospective, multicenter study. Dis Colon Rectum. 2009;52:1578–83.

77. Thekkinkattil DK, Botterill I, Ambrose NS, Lundby L, Sagar PM, Buntzen S, Finan PJ. Efficacy of the anal fistula plug in complex anorectal fistulae. Colorectal Dis. 2009;11(6):584–7.

78. Lenisa L, Espìn-Basany E, Rusconi A, Mascheroni L, Escoll-Rufino J, Lozoya-Trujillo R, Vallribera-Valls F, Mégevand J. Anal fistula plug is a valid alternative option for the treatment of complex anal fistula in the long term. Int J Colorectal Dis. 2010; 25(12):1487–93.

79. Han JG, Wang ZJ, Zhao BC, Zheng Y, Zhao B, Yi BQ, Yang XQ. Long-term outcomes of human acellular dermal matrix plug in closure of complex anal fistulas with a single tract. Dis Colon Rectum. 2011;54(11):1412–8.

80. Ky AJ, Sylla P, Steinhagen R, Steinhagen E, Khaitov S, Ly EK. Collagen fistula plug for the treatment of anal fistulas. Dis Colon Rectum. 2008;51(6):838–43.

81. Chung W, Kazemi P, Ko D, Sun C, Brown CJ, Raval M, Phang T. Anal fistula plug and fibrin glue versus conventional treatment in repair of complex anal fistulas. Am J Surg. 2009;197:604–8.

82. Lawes DA, Efron JE, Abbas M, Heppell J, Young-Fadok TM. Early experience with the bioabsorbable anal fistula plug. World J Surg. 2008;32(6):1157–9.

83. Christoforidis D, Etzioni DA, Goldberg SM, Madoff RD, Mellgren A. Treatment of complex anal fistulas with the collagen fistula plug. Dis Colon Rectum. 2008;51(10):1482–7.

84. Safar B, Jobanputra S, Sands D, Weiss EG, Nogueras JJ, Wexner SD. Anal fistula plug: initial experience and outcomes. Dis Colon Rectum. 2009;52(2):248–52.

85. O'Riordan JM, Datta I, Johnston C, Baxter NN. A systematic review of the anal fistula plug for patients with Crohn's and non-Crohn's related fistula-in-ano. Dis Colon Rectum. 2012;55:351–8.

86. Buchberg B, Masoomi H, Choi J, Bergman H, Mills S, Stamos MJ. A tale of two (anal fistula) plugs: is there a difference in short-term outcomes? Am Surg. 2010;76(10):1150–3.

87. Ratto C, Litta F, Parello A, Donisi L, Zaccone G, De Simone V. Gore Bio-A® Fistula Plug: a new sphincter-sparing procedure for complex anal fistula. Colorectal Dis. 2012;14(5):e264–9.

88. van Koperen PJ, Bemelman WA, Gerhards MF, Janssen LW, van Tets WF, van Dalsen AD, Slors JF. The anal fistula plug treatment compared with the mucosal advancement flap for cryptoglandular high transsphincteric perianal fistula: a double-blinded multicenter randomized trial. Dis Colon Rectum. 2011;54(4): 387–93.

89. Wang JY, Garcia-Aguilar J, Sternberg JA, Abel ME, Varma MG. Treatment of transsphincteric anal fistulas: are fistula plugs an acceptable alternative? Dis Colon Rectum. 2009;52(4):692–7.

90. Ortiz H, Marzo J, Ciga MA, Oteiza F, Armendáriz P, de Miguel M. Randomized clinical trial of anal fistula plug versus endorectal advancement flap for the treatment of high cryptoglandular fistula in ano. Br J Surg. 2009;6:608–12.

91. Christoforidis D, Pieh MC, Madoff RD, Mellgren AF. Treatment of transsphincteric anal fistulas by endorectal advancement flap or collagen fistula plug: a comparative study. Dis Colon Rectum. 2009;52(1):18–22.

92. Rojanasakul A, Pattanaarun J, Sahakitrungruang C, Tantiphlachiva K. Total anal sphincter saving technique for fistula-in-ano; the ligation of intersphincteric fistula tract. J Med Assoc Thai. 2007; 90(3):581–6.

93. Liu WY, Aboulian A, Kaji AH, Kumar RR. Long-term results of ligation of intersphincteric fistula tract (LIFT) for fistula-in-ano. Dis Colon Rectum. 2013;56(3):343–7.

94. Abcarian AM, Estrada JJ, Park J, Corning C, Chaudhry V, Cintron J, Prasad L, Abcarian H. Ligation of intersphincteric fistula tract: early results of a pilot study. Dis Colon Rectum. 2012;55(7): 778–82.

95. Ellis CN. Outcomes with the use of bioprosthetic grafts to reinforce the ligation of the intersphincteric fistula tract (BioLIFT procedure) for the management of complex anal fistulas. Dis Colon Rectum. 2010;53(10):1361–4.

96. Aguilar PS, Plasencia G, Hardy Jr TG, Hartmann RF, Stewart WR. Mucosal advancement in the treatment of anal fistula. Dis Colon Rectum. 1988;28(7):496–8.

97. Gustafsson UM, Graf W. Randomized clinical trial of local gentamicin-collagen treatment in advancement flap repair for anal fistula. Br J Surg. 2006;93(10):1202–7.

98. Uribe N, Millán M, Minguez M, Ballester C, Asencio F, Sanchiz V, Esclapez P, del Castillo JR. Clinical and manometric results of endorectal advancement flaps for complex anal fistula. Int J Colorectal Dis. 2007;22(3):259–64.

99. Dubsky PC, Stift A, Friedl J, Teleky B, Herbst F. Endorectal advancement flaps in the treatment of high anal fistula of cryptoglandular origin: full-thickness vs. mucosal-rectum flaps. Dis Colon Rectum. 2008;51:852–7.

100. Sileri P, Franceschilli L, Del Vecchio Blanco G, Stolfi VM, Angelucci GP, Gaspari AL. Porcine dermal collagen matrix injection may enhance flap repair surgery for complex anal fistula. Int J Colorectal Dis. 2011;26(3):345–9.

101. Jarrar A, Church J. Advancement flap repair: a good option for complex anorectal fistulas. Dis Colon Rectum. 2011;54(12):1537–41.

102. Hossack T, Solomon MJ, Young JM. Ano-cutaneous flap repair for complex and recurrent supra-sphincteric anal fistula. Colorectal Dis. 2005;7(2):187–92.

103. Tan KK, Tan IJ, Lim FS, Koh DC, Tsang CB. The anatomy of failures following the ligation of intersphincteric tract technique for anal fistula: a review of 93 patients over 4 years. Dis Colon Rectum. 2011;54(11):1368–72.

104. Sileri P, Franceschilli L, Angelucci GP, D'Ugo S, Milito G, Cadeddu F, Selvaggio I, Lazzaro S, Gaspari AL. Ligation of the intersphincteric fistula tract (LIFT) to treat anal fistula: early results from a prospective observational study. Tech Coloproctol. 2011;15(4):413–6.

105. Wedell J, Meier zu Eissen P, Banzhaf G, Kleine L. Sliding flap advancement for the treatment of high level fistulae. Br J Surg. 1987;74(5):390–1.

106. Kodner IJ, Mazor A, Shemesh EI, Fry RD, Fleshman JW, Birnbaum EH. Endorectal advancement flap repair of rectovaginal and other complicated anorectal fistulas. Surgery. 1993;114(4):682–9.

107. Makowiec F, Jehle EC, Becker HD, Starlinger M. Clinical course after transanal advancement flap repair of perianal fistula in patients with Crohn's disease. Br J Surg. 1995;82(5):603–6.

108. Kreis ME, Jehle EC, Ohlemann M, Becker HD, Starlinger MJ. Functional results after transanal rectal advancement flap repair of trans-sphincteric fistula. Br J Surg. 1998;85(2):240–2.

109. Ortíz H, Marzo J. Endorectal flap advancement repair and fistulectomy for high trans-sphincteric and suprasphincteric fistulas. Br J Surg. 2000;87(12):1680–3.

110. Adamina M, Hoch JS, Burnstein MJ. To plug or not to plug: a cost-effectiveness analysis for complex anal fistula. Surgery. 2010;147(1):72–8.

Recurrence/Persistence After Fistula Treatment: What Next?

Herand Abcarian

Anal fistula is amongst the most common affliction of man. The only therapeutic alternative to eradicate this disease is surgery. Despite the benign nature of the disease, recurrence or persistence after an operation is common and quite a disappointment for the patient and the surgeon. What prompts a fistula to heal after a single operation and another to recur after multiple procedures is not understood. The goal of an operation is primary healing, no recurrence, and preservation of continence. The conduct of the operation, especially the first one is critical. Why fistulas recur may be due to a factor related to the patient, the characteristic of the fistula itself and those related to the surgeon. There are discussed extensively in Chap. 22.

Evaluating the causes of recurrence especially when the patient is referred after one or two operations include the type of fistula, prior operation(s), presence or absence of inflammatory bowel disease, age of the patient, and persistence of sepsis associated with fistula. The adverse effects of obesity and smoking have also been discussed in Chap. 22. Dudukjian and Abcarian recently published a paper entitled "Why do we have so much trouble in treating fistulas?" [1]. However, the importance of the surgeon on the outcome of operative treatment is harder to pinpoint even though it is logical to conclude that specialists and experts with extensive experience in fistula surgery should have better results than surgeons who do one occasional fistula surgery intermingled with a variety of general surgical procedures.

Additionally the plethora of treatment alternatives in the surgical armamentum starting in mid-1990s has also contributed to an increase in the number of operative procedures per patient. A series of fistulas from a single institution reported the steady decline of anal fistulotomy from 98 % in 1975 to 50 % in 1999. Because many if not all sphincter sparing operations require placement of a marking seton as prerequisite, this factor contributes to the rise in the number of operations per patient, from 1.3 % during 1975–1979 timeline to 32.9 % during the 2005–2009 time period [2].

It is important that in the process of informed consent the patient be apprised of the realistic likelihood of complete healing and the probability of recurrence and disturbance of continence. The patient can thus make an informed decision as to the choice of surgical treatment and its potential consequences [3].

Even though tolerance of minor degrees of fecal incontinence is quite different in the USA vs. UK, the patient must be given all the information and be allowed to make a choice for fistulotomy vs. sphincter preserving procedure (Chap. 9). As discussed in Chap. 22, the fistula patient must be encouraged to lose weight and quite smoking to optimize their chance for postoperative healing especially if a flap procedure is being considered [4].

Considering that the intersphincteric fistulas can be managed safely with a low internal sphincterotomy and that the extrasphincteric fistulas are not amenable to ordinary fistula surgery, sphincter-sparing procedures are optimal in the treatment of trans-sphincteric and suprasphincteric fistulas (Chap. 7). The following alternatives can be used as strategies to deal with operative failures:

1. Fibrin sealant has been discussed in Chap. 11. In case of failure, a second attempt (salvage procedure) can be utilized. Sentovich reported an increase in success rate from 50 to 69 % [5]. Failure after a second attempt can be treated with either fistula plug or advancement flap.

2. The use of biologic plugs and synthetic plugs are covered in Chaps. 12 and 13. There is no good published evidence for superiority of one over the other. In case of failure, if an abscess develops, it should be drained with a draining seton. One can then redo the plug (although most patients are reluctant due to pain and repeat surgical procedure with potential for failure again) or go to advancement flap.

3. Advancement flaps are discussed in Chaps. 14 and 15. Advancement flaps are generally not suitable for fistulas

H. Abcarian, M.D., F.A.C.S. (✉)
The University of Illinois at Chicago, Division of Colon and Rectal Surgery, John Stroger Hospital of Cook Country, IL 60612, USA
e-mail: abcarian@uic.edu

H. Abcarian (ed.), *Anal Fistula: Principles and Management*, DOI 10.1007/978-1-4614-9014-2_23,
© Springer Science+Business Media New York 2014

secondary to Crohn's disease unless the rectal mucosa is normal. Also the endorectal advancement flap is very difficult if not impossible to perform for a posterior quadrant anal fistula. The flap cannot be readily mobilized due to posterior angulation of the anorectum. Usually if the primary opening is somewhat distally located in the anoderm, dermal advancement flap is preferable because endorectal advancement may lead to an ectropion and postoperative wet anus which is interpreted by most patients as fecal incontinence. Flap failures can be redone but salvage flaps have no better success rates. It is absolutely imperative for patients to quit smoking in order not to jeopardize the viability of the flaps [5].

4. The LIFT procedure is one operation that makes absolute sense. Ligation of the fistula tract in the intersphincteric grove, division of the tract, and suture closure of the proximal and distal ends should result in higher success rates. Also if the fistula recurs, it is often in the internal segment of the tract medializing, the fistula from trans-sphincteric to intersphincteric. A simple internal sphincterotomy can address this problem. Recurrence or persistence at the external end may mandate a repeat LIFT procedure.

5. The complex issue of Crohn's fistula has been addressed in Chaps. 19 and 22 and will not be discussed any further.

6. VAAFT procedure designed for complex and recurrent fistulas has yielded success rates of 77 %. This procedure is gradually expanding to more countries and continents and additional experience in larger patient population and longer follow-up will go a long way to popularize this technique. The learning curve of this procedure is fairly short.

7. The pioneering work of García–Olmo in the use of adipose derived stem cells in the treatment of complex anal Crohn's fistulas was ground breaking and is discussed in detail in Chap. 18. There is currently an explosion of studies using autologous and generic stem cells in the treatment of IBD related or complex anal fistulas. The interested individual should refer to the NIH Web site. Failure of the first treatment can be managed with a second round of stem cell therapy although cost may be a prohibiting factor.

What if all efforts fail to achieve complete healing? Most surgeons would resort to fecal diversion at this juncture. Before resorting to a stoma one should seriously consider a fistulotomy or fistulectomy with layered repair. As Phillips so aptly states, it is not how much muscle is divided, but how much muscle is left behind (Chap. 9). The patient needs to make this choice. Also repair of the divided sphincter after complete healing of fistula is not totally out of the question even though the results may be less than desirable. This can be accomplished with or without a covering stoma. Unquestionably the most difficult fistula to deal with is the

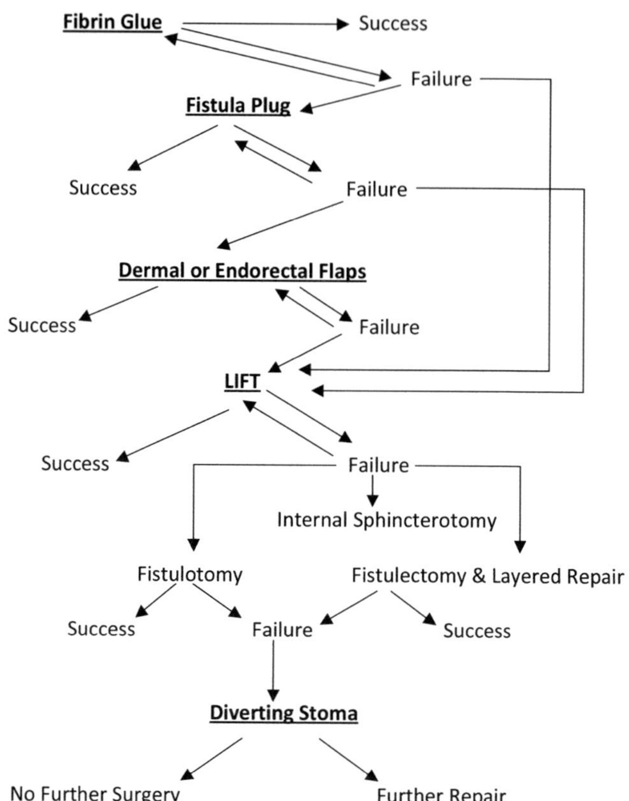

Fig. 23.1 Algorithm in treatment of trans-sphincteric fistulas

posterior high trans-sphincteric fistula in a male patient. If the amount of the sphincter mechanism involves is 50 % or less, the complete fistulectomy and layered repair by Herold is a likely alternative (Chap. 10). Also one has to consider that placing a stoma does not necessarily guarantee a successful outcome of the fistula treatment. However there are patients who have undergone multiple fistula operations with fecal incontinence and persistent fistula tracts. They suffer from constant leakage, wetness, and masceration of perianal and gluteal skin causing extreme itching and pain. For such patients fecal diversion changes their quality of life so much for the better that they elect to live with their stoma without any further operative intervention.

Figure 23.1 shows an algorithm for the treatment of trans-sphincteric fistulas.

Conclusion

This chapter follows the one on fistula surgery in the era of evidence-based medicine. The absence of a reliable level of evidence is discussed in Chap. 21. At the risk of committing blasphemy, the patients are less interested in the level of evidence than improving their quality of life. The moral compass of the surgeon dealing with fistula patients is to make every attempt to cure this disease. If he/she is capable and experienced, multiple alternatives may have to be resorted to. If the surgeon is not very experienced to deal with complex fistulas, it is better to refer the patient to an experienced surgeon or a center which deals with scores of fistulas every year. In short, the surgeon must tailor the procedure to specific patient and not vice versa. Colostomy should be considered as a last resort but it should not be withheld from the patient whose quality of life can be improved despite persistence of their fistulas.

References

1. Dudukjian H, Abcarian H. Why do we have so much trouble treating anal fistulas? World J Gastoenterol. 2011;17:3292–6.
2. Blumetti J, Abcarian A, Abcarian H, et al. Evolution of treatment of fistula in ano. World J Surg. 2012;26(5):1162–7.
3. Ellis CN. Sphincter preserving fistula management: what patients want? Dis Colon Rectum. 2010;53(12):1653–5.
4. Ellis CN, Clark S. Effect of tobacco smoking on advancement flap repair of complex anal fistula. Dis Colon Rectum. 2007;50(4): 459–63.
5. Sentovich SM. Fibrin glue for all anal fistulas. J Gastrointest Surg. 2001;5(2):158–61.

Index

H. Abcarian (ed.), *Anal Fistula: Principles and Management*, DOI 10.1007/978-1-4614-9014-2,
© Springer Science+Business Media New York 2014

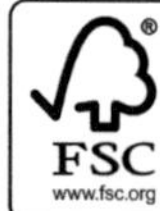